Signed by author BL $7.00 STORE

ASSOCIATED MEDICAL SERVICES

INCORPORATED

A HISTORY

To Jack Neilson:

Hope that you may find this book of some interest and I send it to you with the compliments of its co-author and your namesake

Jack Neilson M.D.

11 November 1987

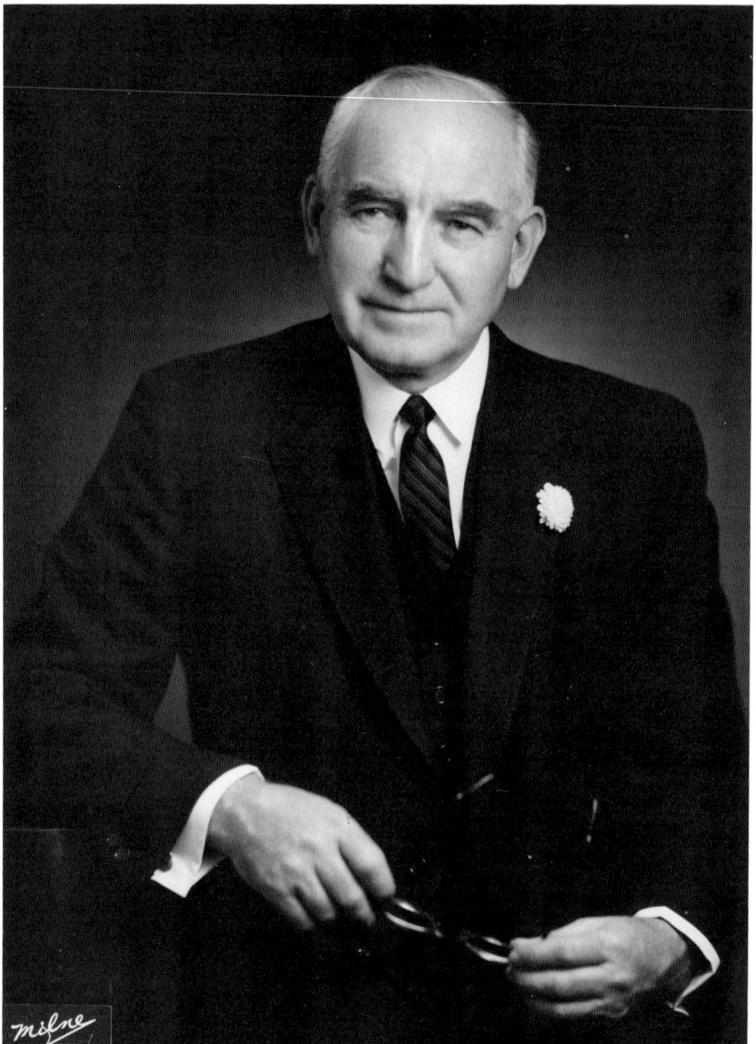

Jason A. Hannah, B.A., M.D., C.M., F.R.C.P.(C).
– Photograph by Milne, Toronto

Associated Medical Services

INCORPORATED

A History

by

John B. Neilson, M.D.
& G.R. Paterson, Ph.D.

Canadian Cataloguing in Publication Data

Neilson, John B., 1911–
Associated Medical Services, Incorporated: A History

Co-published by the Hannah Institute for the History of Medicine.
Bibliography: p.
Includes index.
ISBN 0-9691429-2-7

1. Associated Medical Services, Inc. – History. 2. Hannah Institute for the History of Medicine – History. 3. Hannah, Jason Albert, 1899-1977. 4. Insurance, Health – Ontario – History. I. Paterson, G.R., 1920- . II. Associated Medical Services, Inc. III. Hannah Institute for the History of Medicine. IV. Title.

RA413.3.A8N44 1987 368.3'82'0060713 C87-093439-2

– Front cover photo by Birgitte Nielsen

Produced by:

The Boston Mills Press
132 Main Street
Erin, Ontario
N0B 1T0

C • O • N • T • E • N • T • S

ACKNOWLEDGEMENTS

Associated Medical Services, Incorporated wishes to acknowledge the help and skills of the following in the preparation of this book:

Ms. Catherine Cragg, for her very able editing of the manuscript and for her understanding and good humour in the process; Mr. Christopher Blackburn, for compiling a comprehensive index; Ms. Donalda Taynen, for assistance in keyboarding the final copy; and Boston Mills Press for typesetting and printing the manuscript.

FOREWORD

On 9 April 1937, Associated Medical Services received its charter to provide medical care by prepayment. This activity flourished over the years. But when the provision of health care was eventually taken over by the provincial government, AMS had to reassess its activities. The result was the establishment of the Hannah Institute for the History of Medicine. Now, fifty years after AMS incorporation and after a decade of avowed interest in history, the Board has commissioned a work to cover the activities of AMS. It is a tribute to the founder of AMS, Dr. Jason A. Hannah, who served the corporation as its President and Managing Director for some thirty-eight years.

The Board was fortunate in obtaining two authors for this work, both of whom are very knowledgeable about the activities of AMS, having been associated with it in different capacities over many years. The decision was made to present the volume in two sections, one to outline the activities of the parent organization and the other the activities of the Hannah Institute.

John B. Neilson received his M.D. from the University of Toronto, but from his early days has always shown great interest in the administration of health care. He served the Hamilton Civic Hospitals for thirteen years, many of these as Superintendent. He was one of the first appointees to the Ontario Hospital Services Commission, eventually becoming its chairman. There followed eight years as Executive Director of the University Hospital, London, Ontario. During this period he held the position of director in several of the hospital associations. Dr. Neilson was a member of the Board of AMS from 1966 to 1984, serving as President for seven of those years. Who better to write this section of the book, in view of his long career and association with many aspects of health care and his direct involvement with an organization that was one of the first in providing a prepayment plan for health care?

Dr. G.R. Paterson received his Phm.B. from the University of Toronto, the B.S.P. and the M.Sc. from the University of Saskatchewan, and the Ph.D. from the University of Wisconsin. Dr. Paterson had a distinguished career in the Faculty of Pharmacy and the University of Toronto, and as an officer of the leading pharmaceutical associations both national and international. During this time, he also demonstrated a teaching and research interest and ability in the history of medicine. Accordingly, when Dr. Hannah was looking for a leader for his new Institute for the History of Medicine, Dr. Paterson was the appointee. In effect Dr. Paterson has been involved from day one and has been responsible for its growth and stature, which we are now reviewing at the end of its first decade. Who could have a better understanding and feel for this Institute? It is understandable that we are very pleased to have Dr. Paterson author the second section of the book.

With the publication of this book we hope to provide an insight into the activities and personalities of an organization that has had an impact on two entirely different aspects of Canadian life. The Board has been reviewing its alternatives for the future. It will continue its support of the History of Medicine and it is to be hoped that the future endeavours of AMS will be as productive as those of the past.

D.R. Wilson
President
Associated Medical Services, Inc.

PART ONE

Associated Medical Services and Medical Care by Prepayment

by

J.B. Neilson

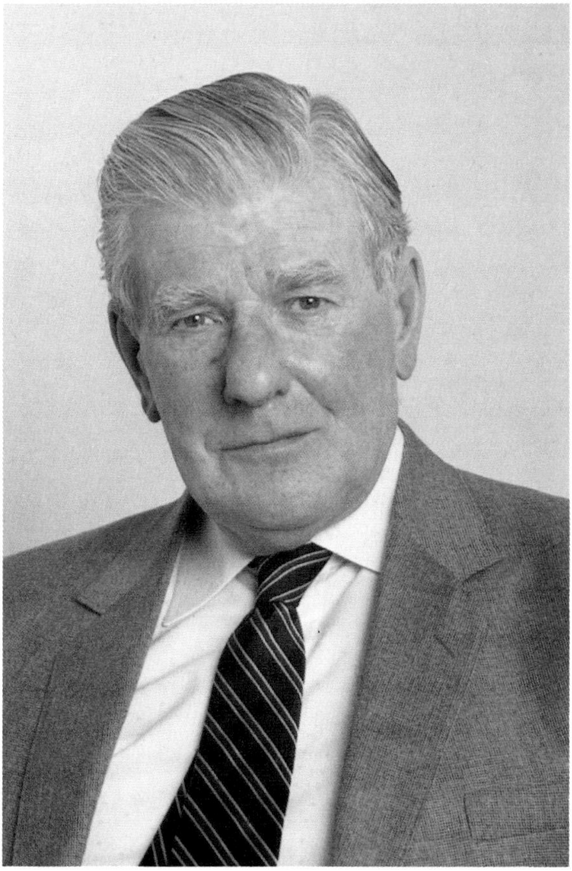

John B. Neilson, M.D. President of AMS, 1975-83. – Photograph by Birgitte Nielsen

ACKNOWLEDGEMENTS

I have tried to prepare, in an abbreviated form, a history of Associated Medical Services during the period 1937 to 1987. It is possible, and maybe historically desirable, that at some time in the future a much more competent historian than I am will write a definitive and detailed history of AMS with more particular reference to the involvement of AMS and its contemporary medical care prepayment plans in actuarial studies, rate setting, morbidity data analysis, and other subjects encompassed by "medical economics".

I would like to acknowledge and express my gratitude to several persons who have helped and encouraged me to the completion of this historical assignment.

—The preparation of the written words, the need to consult records, and the provision of space to do these things has made me a frequent, and often unexpected, visitor at the AMS offices. At all my appearances I have been made welcome with a large-sized cup of coffee and working space. For this and many other favours, I am grateful to Dr. D.R. Wilson, President of AMS, and to Mrs. Sheila Snelgrove, Administrative Assistant to Dr. G.R. Paterson.

—Miss Mary Wildridge, Secretary of AMS, was assigned the unenviable task of typing and revising my written material and putting it into some semblance of order, as well as compiling the appendix. She has been patient, understanding, and at all times encouraging to a historical neophyte and I express my thanks and gratitude to her.

—Along the way, as some problems in recollection have occurred, I have consulted with Dr. Boyd Upper, Dr. John Scott, and Dr. G.R. Paterson, all of whose association with AMS has equalled or exceeded mine. All of them have been helpful and encouraging and I thank them for being so readily available to me in time of need.

—Dr. John Norris, Dr. W.E. Noonan, and Dr. S.B. Upper have all read the manuscript and have contributed numerous helpful comments and criticisms. I am most grateful to them.

Sources

AMS was founded in April 1937 by Dr. Jason A. Hannah and functioned under his careful, and even autocratic, guidance, direction, and control, from 1937 until his retirement in April 1976. The opening chapter of the book is devoted appropriately to a biographical description of Dr. Hannah from his birth in 1899 to the founding of AMS in 1937. In large part the source for this biographical material is his own writings: four typewritten volumes of recollections and memoirs from his birth in November 1899 until April 1937, which he titled "The Hannah Saga".

The account of events leading up to the formation of AMS and its progress in the following years up to June 1972, when it ceased to operate as a provider of prepaid medical care, is based on the following reports, records, and writings:

—The corporate or "official records" of AMS contained in the reports of the meetings of the Board of Directors of AMS, usually held four times in each year, and the required annual meeting of members. These records are complete for the period 1937 to 1973 and include the minutes of meetings, reports of Dr. Hannah to the meetings, and financial reports. All of these records are in the custody of the Fisher Rare Book Library of the University of Toronto.

—A bound volume, prepared under the direction of Dr. Hannah and containing copies of forty-seven speeches, reports, presentations to committees, etc., prepared by Dr. Hannah chiefly during the period 1937 to 1947, all dealing with the development and progress of AMS in its early years. This volume is presently in the custody of the Toronto office of AMS.

—A 30-page pamphlet published by AMS in June 1947 with the title "The First Ten Years of Progress 1937-1947". This pamphlet contains historical information about AMS as well as several photographs of members of the Board of Directors and staff.

—A manuscript prepared by Mr. G. Howard Shillington with the title "Prepayment and the Medical Profession – the Evolution of an Idea". Mr. Shillington had held the position of Executive Director of Trans-Canada Medical Plans and was the author of *The Road to Medicare in Canada* (1972). In 1973 Dr. Hannah had engaged his services to write the above manuscript, which was described as history of the development of medical care prepayment plans under medical sponsorship across Canada. The text describes in considerable detail the events in Ontario in the 1937-1947 period and the involvement of the Ontario Medical Association in the problems of "medical care insurance"; there are numerous references to AMS. I have found the manuscript a most helpful and useful source; however, the exchanges of correspondence between them indicate that Dr. Hannah did not believe that Mr. Shillington had met his responsibilities in the agreement – for example, Mr. Shillington delivered the manuscript to Dr. Hannah three months beyond its due date, and several of the references to AMS in the manuscript failed to acknowledge the role of AMS as the principal proponent of prepayment principles in Canada. Dr. Hannah refused to submit the manuscript to a publisher and, as the correspondence reveals, refused to pay Mr. Shillington the third and last instalment of $5,000 of the $15,000 payment authorized by the Board. It was only after Mr. Shillington retained counsel that Dr. Hannah remitted the final payment. My first actual acquaintance with this matter came in mid-1977, some two to three months following the death of Dr. Hannah, when Mr. Shillington gave to me his copy of the manuscript and offered his help in the event that AMS might decide to publish it. My opinion at that time, which remains unchanged, was that the rather limited area of interest of the manuscript did not merit its publication; nonetheless, as a resource for the present endeavour, it has been valuable.

For the 1950-1960 period, the principal information source has again been the corporate or official records of AMS.

As well, some of the items in Dr. Hannah's diaries have pertinence to the coming in Ontario of a national plan of hospital insurance.

For the 1960-1973 period the principal source of historical information about AMS continues to be the corporate records in the Fisher Rare Book Library. In addition, in the custody of AMS are the "Hannah Diaries" covering the 1960-1970 period. These ten volumes include copies of correspondence to and from his daughter and members of his family, to staff members, to physicians who in his view did not subscribe to the rules and regulations of AMS, to Premiers of Ontario, to Ministers of Health, and to many others. The mostly irrelevant historical information, reports on holidays, and comments on inadequacies of staff members of AMS made necessary a lot of reading to find items with some direct relevance to the history of AMS. However, during this time Dr. Hannah was an active participant in the affairs of the College of Physicians and Surgeons of Ontario and a member of several committees at Queen's University, and his diary entries cover in detail meetings of the College and University.

During this same period Dr. Hannah found additional opportunity with little restriction to voice his opinions in most monthly issues of the *Ontario Medical Review* and the *Toronto Board of Trade Journal.* Several of these articles are of historical interest in that they express, often in pungent language, the strong objections of Dr. Hannah to the entry of government into the field of medical care insurance, while chiding the medical profession for its failure to recognize that in the near future the practice of medicine would be subservient to the control of government.

Access to the corporate records of AMS since 1973 was much easier, because they are retained in the offices of AMS. There are also available three published reports of AMS, covering the years 1972 to 1978, 1978 to 1980, and 1980 to 1982, and a further report covering the period 1982 to 1986, which will be published shortly.

As general background to these writings, I have read and re-read three books that I recommend to any student of health insurance as it has developed in Canada:

Health Insurance in Canada by Malcolm B. Taylor (Toronto: Oxford University Press, 1956).

The Road to Medicare in Canada by G. Howard Shillington (Toronto: DEL Graphics Publishing, 1972).

Health Insurance and Canadian Public Policy – The Seven Decisions That Created the Canadian Health Insurance System by Malcolm G. Taylor (Montreal: McGill-Queen's Press, 1978).

John B. Neilson

CHAPTER I

Jason Albert Hannah – Early Years

Jason Albert Hannah was born on 11 November 1899 in the farm home of his parents, near the village of Munster in Carleton County about twenty miles southwest of the city of Ottawa.

Jason's father, Samuel Hannah, born in 1854, was a son of Samuel Hannah, whose family had migrated to Canada from Northern Ireland about 1820 and had settled as homesteaders in the southwest area of Carleton County. In his memoirs, written during the period 1967 to 1972, Dr. Hannah gathered together a considerable amount of genealogical information about his ancestors, whose name has also been spelt "Hanna" and "Hannay". A major concentration of the Hannah family was established as early as the thirteenth century in the Galloway area of southwestern Scotland; a short sea passage made it easy over the course of many years for members of the Hannah clan to move to Northern Ireland and to settle there. From their bases in Scotland and Ireland, the Hannahs emigrated to many parts of the world but predominantly to Canada, the United States, and Australia.

Jason's mother, Margaret Jane, was born in 1857, one of identical female twins, to Robert Brown and Rebecca Cassidy, both children of Scottish families who had settled in the 1820-1825 period in the vicinity of Kars, a village in Carleton County some ten miles east of Munster. Margaret was a descendant of an old Scottish family by the name of Callander, whose Canadian and North American derivatives resulted from the emigration to Canada in 1820 of Alexander Callander and his wife and their settlement as homesteaders near Kars in 1823 to 1825. They had six children, whose marriage to the Browns, Wallaces, and Millars produced a large number of progeny, most of whom ceased to be farmers and established themselves in the professions throughout Canada and United States.

Samuel Hannah and Margaret Jane Brown were married in the early spring of 1874, at which time the groom was in his twenty-first year and the bride had only recently reached her eighteenth birthday. Shortly before the marriage, Samuel had acquired a plot of one hundred acres of uncleared Crown land in Carleton County. This land could be acquired by suitable and deserving applicants on their undertaking that they would settle on the land and develop it for farming purposes. The Hannah's plot, about two miles north of Munster, was heavily covered with a mixture of hardwood and evergreen trees and was not accessible, at the time, by any semblance of a road.

To this isolated and forested wilderness Samuel Hannah brought his bride. Some neighbours provided temporary accommodation for the couple, and Samuel, with some skills in carpentry, set to work to build a one-storey log cabin containing one room measuring about twenty-five by twenty feet. The second necessity was enough cleared land to permit the planting of a vegetable garden. The clearing of larger tracts of the land involved the manual removal of a multitude of trees, the stacking of logs for sale as timber, and the extraction of stumps. Fortunately, Margaret Jane had been taught how to card and spin and weave and could produce homespun clothing and blankets; any surplus product was offered for sale at the nearest market in Ottawa. As time went on, horses were acquired, as well as cattle, hogs, and chickens. The stories of these days, which are covered at some length in Dr. Hannah's memoirs as recollections of his mother and brothers and sisters, seem to be those of a typical pioneering family in Eastern Canada as it struggled with the basic problems of acquiring food, shelter, and clothing under primitive conditions while gradually expanding the farming base to achieve greater productivity along with more security and comfort.

Large families were the rule in pioneering days in Canada. The son born to the couple in March 1875 was the first of eighteen children born between that date and the end of 1899: ten boys and eight girls, including two sets of twins. One of the twins, a boy, died in infancy; one girl died of an infection at about six years of age and another at eighteen. All of the remaining fifteen survived into adulthood, married, and in turn had children. Jason Albert Hannah was the last-born. At the time of his birth his oldest brother was twenty-four years old and two other brothers were over twenty.

During the period 1874 to 1903, the family growth provided needed hands to carry on the work of the farm. While money was very limited, some cash income was received from the sale of milk, eggs, firewood, and timber, and the father worked as a carpenter at every opportunity. Nonetheless, the sandy soil, while suitable for the growing of vegetables, was not supportive of a good yield of hay or grain crops. By the early 1900s reports started to come back to Eastern Canada from the prairie provinces about the very fertile land to be had there in abundance and of the ease with which high-yielding crops of grain, particularly wheat, could be grown. Attracted by these reports, the father of the family and his two oldest sons visited Saskatchewan in the spring of 1902, and on their return it was decided that the family should move to Saskatchewan the following year.

In the spring of 1903, seventeen members of the Hannah family – one of the daughters, having married, remained in Ontario – along with their livestock, horses, and home furnishings moved by rail to Rouleau, a village with a population at that time of about 250 people located thirty-two miles southwest of Regina and about the same distance from Moose Jaw. A house was temporarily rented in Rouleau while the father and his older sons moved, along with their livestock, to the recently purchased quarter section about two miles east of Rouleau in order to put up makeshift living quarters, prepare the land for its first planting of spring wheat, and construct a large but rather primitive shelter for the animals. The rest of the family joined them late that spring.

The practically flat, treeless, and apparently endless prairies stretching to the horizon in every direction were in sharp contrast to the rolling land and forested landscape of Eastern Ontario. The large landholdings here meant that the nearest neighbour might be two or three miles distant with only primitive connecting dirt roads. Any kind of fuel for heating, cooking, or lighting was scarce and expensive, and fruit (especially apples, so abundant in Ontario) was non-existent. Once again the Hannahs had become a pioneering family; this time they had to contend over the following years with isolation, the short, hot, and dry summers, hailstorms, cyclonic winds, plagues of grasshoppers, devastating prairie grass fires, and early winters with snow in abundance, blizzards, and bitterly cold temperatures. With the coming of spring, there was feverish activity to plough and plant so that the grain crops had the longest possible growing season. In the fall came the all-out concentration on cutting and harvesting, with the assistance of the harvest hands who came in the thousands from Ontario and Quebec. If the season was favourable, almost phenomenal yields of up to fifty bushels of wheat for each acre could be expected; if unfavourable, there could be little or no crop.

For the first three years after the Hannahs' arrival, crops were quite favourable and brought a good cash return. The three older sons could thus manage the down payment on land in their own names and were soon farming independently. The father, with the assistance of two of his younger sons, kept the original family homestead in cultivation and also hired out his carpentry skills.

In the winter of 1905, Samuel Hannah decided to return for a visit to his former farm at Munster, now operated by one of his daughters and her husband, and there to locate a supply of horses for shipment to Saskatchewan, where there was a ready market for them. Jason, at that time four years old, and his sister Agnes, six years old, accompanied their parents on this journey. A railway-car load of horses was purchased and consigned to Rouleau. However, many of the horses were sick at the termination of their journey, and enough of them died to make the trip a losing proposition.

This unproductive sequel to the trip east started a series of setbacks for the Hannah family. On the trip the father had contracted a persistent bronchitis. On his return home he continued to decline in health, and by March 1906 he was confined to his bed with progressive physical weakness. From there on the progress of the illness, diagnosed as pneumonia, was steadily downhill, and he died in the presence of his family at his home on 8 April 1906. Dr. Hannah's memoirs give a poignant description of the final hours of his father's life and of the words the father expressed to his wife and to his family, who had gathered at his bedside.

The death of Samuel Hannah at the age of fifty-two left his widow, now forty-nine, with eight children still at home, the oldest being sixteen and the youngest, Jason, six.

In the following years, hard work and careful management, aided by several years of good crops and reasonable selling prices, enabled them to acquire more horses, cattle, and farm machinery and to enlarge the home and construct more outbuildings. The two oldest sons, now married, both farmed nearby and were available to assist on the family farm. Several older daughters had married. Yet there was little to spare in these years, as taxes and mortgage instalments took a large part of the cash income. In addition, one of the sons persuaded his mother and a brother to act as guarantors on a $5,000 mortgage on a land purchase. As it turned out, he defaulted and went back to Ontario, leaving his mother and his brother with the debt.

Margaret Hannah was determined that the homestead should be a gathering point for the family, which now included sons- and daughters-in-law and a steadily increasing number of grandchildren. On most Sundays, weather permitting, they came for a midday dinner following church services in Rouleau. Sometimes, with neighbours and the minister included, there were as many as thirty people.

As the youngest of the family and the last to go to school, Jason spent some of his early years as the only child at home with his mother. Then and subsequently they developed a strong attachment. His nearest playmate lived three miles away. Only one sister, Agnes, is recalled as a playmate; the others were too much older. He was a great admirer of his mother's strong and unwavering allegiance to Scottish Presbyterianism, with its strong faith in God and the conviction that such faith would prevail in all times of adversity. Her religious faith and the purpose and direction it could give in life was instilled into all of Margaret Hannah's children at an early age. Each morning started with family prayers, and before bedtime arrived there were more prayers and a scripture reading. Attendance at church, often twice on Sunday, was a family ritual.

The mother was also a firm believer in respect for authority and taught her children the importance of recognizing and accepting the authority of their elders: their parents, their teachers, and their leaders (at the time chiefly clergymen and politicians). She must have been a very busy, energetic, and active person; yet she always found time to be a confidante and adviser to her children, and to recount to them the history of both sides of the family, which was intended to give them a pride in the qualities of their ancestors.

In spite of her home commitments, Margaret Hannah had the reputation of being a good neighbour. Within a radius of about twenty miles from her home she responded to requests for help at time of childbirth or illness.

All family members were taught, often at what seems to be a rather unusually early age, to assume specified responsibilities relating to the farm, the house, and themselves. They included a variety of chores that called for daily attention and early rising. His memoirs record that Jason, by the time he was eight years old, was milking four cows night and morning. As he matured into a robust teenager, he became useful in the fields, especially during spring planting and fall harvesting.

Since the Hannahs' arrival in the area, the prairie village of Rouleau had grown in size and importance, not only because of its location on the railroad but also because of the settlement of the surrounding land. By 1910, the village had a population of about five hundred and, aside from the expected commercial stores, hotel, and blacksmith shop, a two-storey school that offered primary and limited secondary education. There were five churches, each part of a two- or three-village "charge" for an itinerant clergyman. The predominant denominations at the time, recognized by the size of their church, were the Anglican, Methodist, Presbyterian, and Roman Catholic. The Hannah family were sustaining members of the Presbyterian church, although the father, during the years preceding his death, had embraced several denominations and eventually became a Methodist. This religious division was resolved by the family attending the Presbyterian service on Sunday morning and the Methodist service in the afternoon.

Jason began his schooling in the fall of 1907. His memoirs

reveal an average student who enjoyed the companionship of other students, which helped him in partially overcoming an innate shyness. He developed a few school friendships, some of which continued into adult life. He recalls both with approval and disapproval the quality of the several teachers, his main complaint being their inability to maintain discipline. For the first time he became interested in sports, and as he grew older he came to enjoy baseball, although he admitted that some awkwardness prevented him from becoming other than an average player.

When the war broke out in 1914, the patriotic reaction for many Canadians was to enlist in the Canadian Expeditionary Force. One of the enlistment centres established was in Rouleau. The only experience Jason had in military matters was as a voluntary member of the local school cadet group, who were provided with uniforms and rifles and practised marching and rifle handling during a short part of the school year. He saw the enlistment and departure of several young men from the Rouleau area, and later the names of some among the casualties. He himself attempted to enlist at age fifteen as a "bugle boy", only to find that there was no such category in the Canadian army. He was determined to enlist when he became sixteen in November 1915, but enlistment at this age required the approval of the parents. His mother most reluctantly endorsed the application, feeling that she had to support him and to accept the consequences. In the discussions on this matter between them, Jason learned that she had always hoped he would become a minister and hoped still that his present decision would not dissuade him from the possibility. In February 1916 he became a private soldier in the Canadian army.

Along with his brother Wesley and some twenty others who had been recruited in the Rouleau area, most of them older than Jason, he was quartered in a hotel at Rouleau. By June 1916 the "Rouleau detachment" had about seventy recruits in uniform and issued with full equipment. The days were occupied with "hardening programs" of drills and marchings, with rifles training, and with indoctrination in the procedures of army life. By this time Jason had acquired a liking for a local girl, and most of his spare time was spent in her company.

The Rouleau detachment was part of the 229th Battalion

based in Moose Jaw, and in June 1916 it joined the battalion to spend the summer under canvas at Camp Hughes near Brandon, Manitoba. Jason shared a tent with his brother. He recalled the summer as a time of repetitious army manoeuvres – foot drill, rifle drill, instruction in army procedures, guard duty, orderly room assignments – all familiar to the foot soldier. The local sand was carried by frequent strong winds and deposited into food and personal possessions to the point where it became an enemy to cleanliness and comfort. As might be expected, Jason at first complained about the food and the way it was served, but eventually he accepted army fare as a necessary evil and sought periodic relief in occasional visits to local restaurants. The highlight of the summer came on 1 July, when Jason's romantic interest from Rouleau arrived at the camp accompanied by her mother. Jason in his recollections reflected that his attachment might have led to engagement and matrimony but for the exigencies of war and his mother's admonition that a man should be able to support a wife before he thinks of marriage. Since he was still only sixteen, however, the seriousness of his intent must be considered in perspective.

Given the urgent need for grain crops to support the war effort, it was government policy that enlisted soldiers from the prairie provinces would be granted "harvest leave". Jason, along with most of the Rouleau detachment, returned home to work in the fields and to obtain some needed money to supplement the army pay of $1.10 per day. This "harvest leave" lasted from 15 August until 1 October and was followed by a return to Camp Hughes. Late in November 1916, the 229th Battalion moved into barracks in Moose Jaw, and training continued during a bitterly cold winter.

In March 1917, all ranks in the battalion were listed for movement overseas. Late in March they were crowded into uncomfortable colonist-type railroad cars for the ten-day trip to Halifax. After a few days of impatient waiting in that city, they embarked for Britain in an old Great Lakes grain carrier converted into a troop carrier, with crowded quarters and three-level sleeping bunks. It was a slow but uneventful trip aside from a prevalence of sea-sickness, and the ship arrived in Liverpool on 16

April. From there the battalion was moved by train to barracks at Bramshott in the south of England some fifteen miles from Aldershot. At Bramshott they were settled into long lines of military huts, which offered little in the way of comfort, and persistent rains turned the whole area into a sea of mud. A quarantine and confinement to barracks due to an outbreak of scarlet fever lasted some six weeks, during which time the weather had improved to the point where dust replaced mud. About this time the Canadian soldiers were told that one-half of their $1.10 a day would be deducted and remitted to a chosen assignee in Canada.

In early May 1917, Jason learned that recent army regulations stipulated that no Canadian soldier under the age of nineteen years would be permitted to serve with the fighting forces in France, and that starting immediately all Canadian soldiers under nineteen serving in France would be returned to England. This was a severe blow to Jason because it destroyed any early expectation of seeing action and left him behind in England when most of his friends in the platoon were sent to France as reinforcements. A seven-day leave to soften the blow was of some help. He used it to visit Edinburgh, a city that intrigued him and drew him back on later leaves.

The "under nineteens", numbering about eight hundred, many of whom had been fighting soldiers in France, were returned to Bramshott. As there was no systematic training program for them, most days were spent in idleness, which in turn led to absences without leave and to other military offences. Jason slowly settled down and stayed out of trouble, but like most of his soldier associates he felt useless and unwanted.

It was known that the Royal Naval Air Service would accept "youngsters", particularly those who were adventurous and learned quickly. Probably because promotion to officer status occurred more quickly in the Air Service than in the army, Jason applied for admission; but the processing of his application was slow, partly because of a merging in 1918 of the Air Service and the Royal Flying Corps to become the Royal Air Force. Dr. Hannah's memoirs record that he eventually received notice to report to Royal Flying Corps headquarters in London on 11 November 1918. Two days before this date, he received orders through

Canadian army channels not to report.

In the summer of 1917, it was decided to bring the Canadian soldiers in England under eighteen years of age into a "demonstration unit". This decision was made because of the increasing difficulty in finding something for these "boy soldiers" to do. To initiate this effort, they were moved to Bexhill-on-Sea. As a start, they were put on special rations that included bacon and eggs for breakfast, and in the following days were encouraged – or enticed – to improve their appearance and their military conduct. They were shown movies of a squad of cadets engaged in precision foot and rifle drill, and then the actual drill squad performed in front of them. The young soldiers were amazed by the precision performance, and it became more apparent what a "demonstration unit" was all about when a sergeant-major, whom they all came to respect and admire, challenged them to do better than the squad of cadets. In the ensuing weeks the young soldiers practised precision foot and rifle drill to the point where they were practically faultless and were despatched as "demonstration units" to numerous locations in England where they displayed their special abilities. Later, the members of the units were given their own red shoulder patches with the insignia YSB on them, for Young Soldiers' Battalion. In time the units had their own non-commissioned officers, a source of great pride to them. Among the NCOs was Lance-Corporal and later Corporal Jason A. Hannah. Frequently he acted as orderly sergeant in the company commander's office. Although he never did achieve the confirmed third stripe of a sergeant, he found the acting duties and their responsibilities to his liking, this being his first real taste of army administration.

The remaining days of the Young Soldiers' Battalion passed in England more quickly and with satisfaction in doing something challenging and worthwhile. The Young Soldiers' Battalion continued to receive some favoured treatment in terms of rations, leave, and recreational facilities. The memoirs record that Corporal Hannah was detailed to form a battalion baseball team, on which he played on first base or, if he had an off day in that position, in right field, while at the same time acting as coach and manager.

Armistice was signed on Jason's nineteenth birthday. By that time he had served two years and nine months in the Canadian Expeditionary Force, with twenty months being spent overseas. Movement back to Canada went ahead quickly, and he arrived in the railway station at Rouleau on the morning of 23 December 1918 to start a fifteen-day leave.

There had been several changes since his departure for overseas. His mother, still in good health and active, now lived in a small house in Rouleau with his unmarried sister Agnes. The home farm was now being operated by his brother Allan, who met Jason at the train station in his new Gray Dort. It was obvious that the war had been helpful to many of the farmers: crops had been good, and wheat had risen to the unprecedented price of $2.50 a bushel. Automobiles, a rarity two years previously, were now becoming commonplace. Practically all of the land in the vicinity of Rouleau and throughout most of southern Saskatchewan was now under cultivation. The more successful prairie farmers were now able to afford winter vacations in Texas, California, and British Columbia.

Jason moved into his mother's home in Rouleau and was joined there by his brother Wesley, who had been seriously wounded and did not believe that he was physically capable of returning to farming. Several members of the family came on Christmas Day to carry on a family tradition and to welcome them home. One of his sisters, however, had died of the Spanish Flu, outbreaks of which had struck southern Saskatchewan in September.

A more widespread and serious outbreak of the influenza started early in January 1919, and more than half of the residents of the Rouleau community were stricken at one time. The doctors in Rouleau, Dr. Singleton and Dr. McKean, were kept going day and night; community volunteers drove them to and from their patients. The Arlington Hotel in Rouleau was converted into a temporary hospital, with patients attended by volunteer women many of whom themselves fell ill. Men who were still healthy organized themselves to visit all farms in the area daily to look after the livestock and to deal as best they could with the stricken families. Deaths, often two or more in a family, were frequent.

Jason, still in uniform, spent his leave using his brother's Gray Dort to deliver quart sealers of soup, custard, and other foods to stricken homes. His sister Agnes was preparing these meals for as many as eight to ten families. His mother, as would be expected, moved about the neighbourhood doing what she could; she would be absent from her own home for periods of several days on these missions.

By the end of January 1919, the incidence of new cases had declined sharply, and affairs in the community started to adjust to the consequences of the epidemic. On 10 January, Jason's leave was up and he dutifully reported to Regina. There he was offered a sergeant's stripes if he were to remain in the army. However, he refused: he had become tired of army life and its regimentation, and he felt he should return to Rouleau where he was needed. His request for a discharge was granted, but he lost a month's gratuity allowance because he was exactly one month short of the three years' service needed to qualify for the full allowance.

Returning to the comfort and security of his mother's home in Rouleau, Jason had time to reflect upon his present and his future. While getting his bearings, he spent a few days or a few weeks at the homes of his various brothers and sisters. However, he soon returned to his mother's home, where he had complete freedom as well as her advice and counsel. A period of restlessness and indecision followed, during which he frequented the local pool hall and bowling alley without receiving much return in the way of pleasure or satisfaction. During this period of idleness and dependence on his mother, she never indicated any impatience that she was supporting an able-bodied man.

What follows in Dr. Hannah's memoirs of these times can be interpreted as the efforts of a mother genuinely concerned about the welfare of her youngest son. She contrived to have him reconciled, after almost two years, with his school-day sweetheart, Mildred, the same girl who had visited Camp Hughes in the summer of 1917. What follows in the memoirs are several pages on the delight of the young couple in being together again, attending skating parties, walking home from church, and being at their family homes.

During his army service, Jason had become aware that promotion was often based on education, and he had concluded that whatever he might do in the future would be aided by completion of at least high school. He therefore decided to return to the Rouleau school in February 1919. He found it difficult to adjust, for he was some three years older than his classmates and accustomed to the discipline of the army. About three months later he decided to leave school and to help one of his brothers on his farm. His brother paid him $100 monthly including room and board, a decided contrast to his army pay of about $33 monthly. His experiences as a farmhand gave him ample opportunity to reflect on his future. He even seriously considered accepting the Soldiers Re-Establishment Board's generous grant of farming land available to him as a veteran.

At this time, as on so many previous occasions, he sought advice from his mother. She urged him to complete his university entrance and did not encourage him to become a farmer, feeling that he would become weary of farm life.

By October 1919 Jason had made up his mind about his future, his goal being entry to the medical school at Queen's University in Kingston, Ontario. He returned to school in Rouleau with the intention of completing his matriculation so as to start university in the fall of 1920. He shared a room in his mother's home with his older brother Wesley, who had also decided to return to school, and paid a small weekly amount for room and board. As a veteran he received an allowance of $48 a month during his school attendance, for a stipulated period of ten months. Tending the furnace at the local Methodist church brought another $10 monthly. Working as a clerk in the village's general store each Saturday brought him $5 more, and he managed to give some time to assist a painter in the village at a rate of 50 cents an hour.

While the matriculation course required steady application, he seemed to have developed good study habits and the ability to concentrate his mind on the subject, which served him well during his education and in later life. All was not study, however, and the memoirs describe times of fun and relaxation aided by a bit of money in his pocket, congenial female company, and the availability of Wesley and his automobile. Aside from local diversions such as picnics, skating, sleigh rides, and baseball games, there were periodic trips to Regina to attend plays and other attractions.

In the 1920 spring examinations, Jason had a good pass mark in all of his subjects except Latin and geometry. At about the same time as the examination results were reported, he was advised that Queen's University had no space for him in the fall of 1920 but that he could be accepted into the entry class in 1921. He decided to return to school in Rouleau during the next year to get the necessary standing in Latin and geometry and improve his standing in several other subjects required for university entrance. The summer of 1920 and the following school year passed quickly and uneventfully, and Jason had no difficulty in passing all his examinations.

In deciding to enter medicine and to attend Queen's University, Jason was influenced by his high regard for Dr. Singleton, who was a graduate of Queen's medical school and had practised for several years in Rouleau. Contemplating his financial resources in the late summer of 1921 before his departure for Kingston, Jason concluded that he would be on his own without any possibility of financial assistance from his mother or any members of his family. One of his major assets was a strong physique, which would permit him to work each summer on the farms in Saskatchewan; another was his skill as a painter. Adding up his resources, he found about $2,000 in cash. He calculated that with this amount as a starter and a reserve, and with his anticipated earnings as a farmhand and painter during vacation months, he should be able to give his full time to his studies without there being any necessity for seeking additional income during the university year. In all these deliberations about how he should become a physician, he had the support and encouragement of his mother. She was convinced that he would succeed in whatever endeavour he followed and came to accept that having her son a physician was almost as good as having him a minister.

At the time of his entry into medicine, Jason had two options: the most popular and shortest course, leading to the degree of Doctor of Medicine (M.D.) at the end of six academic years (each of about eight and one-half months in duration); or the Biological and Medical Sciences course, leading to an honours Baccalaureate degree (B.A.) at the end of four years and the Doctor of Medicine (M.D.) and Master of Surgery (C.M.) at the end of seven years. Jason's comment on his selection of the latter course was that seven years would give him the B.A. and M.D., whereas the two degrees in any other university course would require ten years.

In mid-September 1921, Jason travelled by train from Regina to Kingston to enter the medical school at Queen's University. Dr. Hannah's memoirs devote some seventy typewritten pages to his university days. There are several references to his "love life" while at the university along with reflections on the more open relationship between the sexes that was developing during the 1920s. While opportunities for attendance at social functions presented themselves, Jason admitted to a sense of unease when women were present, accompanied by an inability to engage in small talk that gave a female companion the idea that he was a "serious" person. In all of these situations, Jason heeded the admonition of his mother that he should not enter into any involvement with marriage in view until he was in a position to provide for a wife.

At the commencement of his course in Biological and Medical Sciences, Jason soon found that his education at Rouleau had not given him the background to contend with chemistry, physics, and French, which were compulsory subjects in the university. At the Christmas examinations, he failed in these subjects, placing his continuation in the course in jeopardy. With some tutorial assistance and the help of textbooks he had not had available at Rouleau, he was able to pass the examinations at the end of the academic year.

The memoirs are replete with references, some complimentary and some otherwise, to his teaching professors and their idiosyncracies. He spoke highly of the quality of most of them, but he was critical of the administrative abilities and personal relations of some. He was particularly impressed with Dr. James Miller, the Professor of Pathology, who had considerable influence on his future, and with Dr. Ford Connell, the Professor of Medicine, whom he visited in later years on periodic visits to Queen's University.

Jason's non-participation in sports he attributed to a lack of physical aptitude, which he realized he could not change. In Rouleau he had managed a hockey team that had some success in competition; at Queen's he became one of the many who gave their vocal support to the Queen's football team. Even with a relatively small student enrolment, Queen's was able to field strong football teams, which in the 1920s won several intercollegiate championships and the Grey Cup for four successive years. In his later years, he attended many Queen's games.

In the memoirs Jason records that his experience at medical school confirmed his choice of medicine as a career, but in his undergraduate years his principal concern was simply to pass the necessary examinations. The first four years of Biological and Medical Sciences led him into subjects rather removed from medicine, and he had difficulty with some of them – chemistry, physics, French, and Latin being noted – but he did attain his B.A. degree in June 1925. He then entered into a three-year period devoted entirely to medicine, predominantly in its clinical aspects.

In the summer vacation each year he returned to his mother's home in Rouleau and spent the summer working in the fields and as a painter, and accepting whatever other jobs offered some remuneration. Jason made no reference to any financial difficulties encountered during these years and, as far as can be gathered, met the costs of his university education without any help.

For the summer of 1927, Jason decided that it would be helpful to him to spend the vacation as a "junior interne" in a hospital to gain practical experience. His application for such an internship at the Grey Nuns Hospital in Regina was accepted, and he reported there late in May 1927. An advantage of the internship was that it provided room and board and $75 a month, although that hardly compared with what he could have earned as a harvest hand or a painter in Rouleau.

Fifty typewritten pages of Dr. Hannah's memoirs describe some of his experiences at the Grey Nuns Hospital. Aside from many routine duties an intern was required to perform, Jason recorded that he administered about 250 ether anaesthetics, delivered some twenty-five babies, and assisted at numerous operations. It was a busy summer with little time for rest and relaxation, but it did give him useful experience in the actual practice of medicine, and he was pleased that at the end of the summer he was offered an internship by the hospital on the conclusion of his university course.

In his final year at the university in the academic year 1927/28, Jason became involved in a students' strike, which lasted for two days in March 1928. His involvement was as a member of the executive of the medical students' representative body, known as the "Aesculapian Court". According to the memoirs, three medical students, supported by the medical class in general, considered that they had been unfairly disciplined by the university Senate. Jason appeared as the principal spokesman for the students. After negotiations reached a stalemate he called in the President of the Alumni Association, and the subsequent three-sided negotiations produced sufficient agreement for the students to be able to return to their classes. Subsequently the Senate conceded most of the students' points, and students and the university administration got on a better footing than before. The record of these events, as written many years later by Dr. Hannah, suggests that in 1928 he already showed a determination that continued in later years – to defend principles in which he believed, to prepare written or verbal arguments in support of the principles in a logical manner, and to present them clearly and concisely. At times, however, then and later, his language was rather more elaborate than the situation merited.

As a medical student Jason had no difficulty in passing his examinations, and his ranking was described as "average", being in the middle third of his class. On his graduation in June 1928, he had reached no conclusions about the direction of his future in medicine. At that time there was no stipulation that he serve a minimal period of one year as an intern in an approved hospital before becoming eligible for a licence to practise medicine in a province of his choice. The summer internship at the Grey Nuns Hospital in Regina had stimulated his interest in clinical medicine, but with a greater interest in the diagnosis of disease than in its treatment. During his years as a medical student he had become an admirer, and later a friend, of Dr. James Miller, a graduate of the University of Edinburgh who had come to Queen's University as Professor of Pathology in 1920. As a student Jason had discussed his future with Dr. Miller and was persuaded that at least a year of postgraduate work in pathology would be useful to him in whatever choice he might make, whether medical practice or research. Dr. Miller was able to offer him a one-year appointment as a Richardson Fellow in Clinical Pathology at the Kingston General Hospital. This appointment was accepted, to take effect from 1 July 1928. This year gave him a good opportunity to gain experience in anatomical pathology by the examination of surgical specimens and by the performance of autopsies.

He kept in touch with clinical medicine by accepting evening and weekend rotations as an intern on the hospital wards and by attendance at clinical rounds, where he was able to contribute to the presentations of a variety of diseases from the viewpoint of a pathologist. As a research project he undertook a study of the factors influencing and causing "false positive" results on the Wasserman test for syphilis. With Dr. Miller readily available as a teacher, critic, and preceptor, it was a most satisfactory year in general pathology.

As he faced the following year, Dr. Hannah had developed his interest in pathology and particularly its research aspects. He again sought the advice of Dr. Miller, and through the latter's influence was offered a George Christian Hoffman fellowship in pathology at the University of Edinburgh. He decided to accept this fellowship and its stipend of $1,000 for one year.

During his year at the Kingston General Hospital, Dr. Hannah had met Ruth Lyons, a graduate nurse of the hospital and a member of its staff. They became engaged and planned on being married late in 1929. However, on his receiving the Edinburgh appointment, they decided to be married early in September and to have the sea voyage to Scotland as their honeymoon. They arrived in Edinburgh on 21 September 1929.

At the university, Dr. Hannah was not impressed with the Professor of Pathology to whom he was assigned, whose arrogance was disturbing and whose welcome was rather chilly. He found difficulty in fitting into the division of general pathology and believed that the four months he spent there would not be of any real value to him. He came to hear about Professor Reynolds, a neuropathologist who, with his associates in neurology, was putting on a course in neurology and neuropathology. He attended this course, found it most interesting, and with the help of Professor Reynolds moved from general pathology into neuropathology. During the following eight months, he had a wide exposure to neuropathology under the direction of excellent teachers. His interest in research was stimulated and encouraged by the assignment to study the techniques developed by a Spanish neuropathologist, Dr. Ramon Y Cajal, for demonstrating neurological tissue by silver and gold impregnation methods.

While in Edinburgh, Dr. Hannah met Dr. Ambrose McGhie, who was in charge of the medical division of the McGregor-Mowbray Clinic in Hamilton, Ontario, and was visiting several medical centres in Great Britain and Europe seeking the latest information on advances in medicine. His visit to Edinburgh was in order to attend a course of lectures in neurology and to sit for his membership in the Royal College of Physicians. Dr. McGhie and Dr. Hannah developed a close friendship, and during their time together Dr. McGhie inquired about Dr. Hannah's plans for the future. Since at that time they were indefinite, Dr. McGhie suggested that Dr. Hannah might investigate opportunities in the Ontario Civil Service by writing to his brother, Dr. B.T. McGhie, a psychiatrist who would shortly be assuming charge of the direction of the Ontario psychiatric hospitals. Correspondence with Dr. B.T. McGhie ensued, and when Dr. Hannah and his wife returned to Kingston in early September 1930, Dr. Hannah and Dr. McGhie met in Toronto. Although no definite offer of a position was made, Dr. McGhie revealed that he was hoping to set up a division of neuropathology under government auspices, to be devoted largely to research into the pathology of neurological diseases and psychiatric illnesses. It was agreed that Dr. Hannah would not accept another position without prior discussion with Dr. McGhie.

Shortly thereafter, Dr. Hannah was offered a position as pathologist at the Royal Jubilee Hospital in Victoria, British Columbia. He reported the offer to Dr. McGhie, who in early

October 1930 arranged a meeting in Toronto between Dr. Hannah and Dr. Farrar, Professor of Psychiatry at the University of Toronto, and Dr. Klotz, Professor of Pathology. The proposal by Dr. McGhie to have Dr. Hannah offered an appointment on the staff of the Department of Health as neuropathologist was discussed. The proposal was most acceptable to Dr. Farrar, but Dr. Klotz was only lukewarm, although he did offer some office space for Dr. Hannah in the Banting Institute if he were appointed.

Although the offered position in Victoria provided a larger salary, Dr. Hannah was impressed with the opportunities, including research, in the field of neuropathology and the possibility of a close relationship with the university departments of Pathology and Psychiatry and with the psychiatric hospitals in Ontario. He decided to accept the position in Toronto. The starting salary in October 1930 was agreed upon as $4,500 annually, with assurances that increases of at least $500 annually would be provided until the salary reached about $7,000. As events proved, the verbal agreement on salary increases was not honoured.

Pending the later rental of a house in Toronto, Dr. and Mrs. Hannah were installed in an apartment in the Toronto Psychiatric Hospital. He endeavoured to understand clinical psychiatry better, reading widely on the subject, attending ward rounds in the hospital, and functioning as a physician in the Outpatient Clinic. There and at the psychiatric hospital in Whitby he did autopsies and developed an increasing number of neuropathological specimens. All of these activities, which he carried on from a small office in the Toronto Psychiatric Hospital, kept him reasonably busy but did little to advance neuropathology, and it was only by constant pressure to the point of unpleasantness that he was able to acquire a small office and limited research space in the basement of the Banting Institute. He moved into the space in March 1932, almost a year and a half after his appointment; and further delay occurred in obtaining laboratory equipment and a research assistant – in this instance, a graduate physician with technical experience – until July.

Dr. Hannah attributed all of this delay in getting established to the endeavour of the university, which wanted any provincial funding of neuropathology for its own purpose of establishing a division of Neuropathology in the Department of Pathology. He blamed the delay on Dr. Klotz, who was determined that neuropathology at the University of Toronto would not follow the pattern established and functioning under Dr. Penfield at McGill University. Evidently Dr. Klotz was a person of strong likes and dislikes, and among those he disliked were Dr. Penfield and surgeons generally. Though at times he showed some friendliness to Dr. Hannah, he considered that Dr. Hannah had not had sufficient training and experience to associate on an equal footing with his academic confreres. Otherwise Dr. Hannah found most of the staff of the Department of Pathology friendly and helpful. To add to his frustration, however, his promised salary increases did not materialize, because (as reported to him) of a general cutting back in government expenditures – the result of the economic depression. At that time he seriously considered accepting a position as a hospital pathologist, at a salary of $2,000 more annually than he was receiving.

On 16 October 1931, the Hannahs' only son was born in the Wellesley Hospital in Toronto and was christened Stanley Albert.

Once his research laboratory was set up and a technician engaged, Dr. Hannah was able to use a new technique for staining peripheral nerves that he had learned at Edinburgh. The demonstration on slides excited a very favourable response among his confreres, especially Dr. Eric Linell, the Professor of Neuroanatomy and a contender for appointment as the first Professor of Neuropathology at the University of Toronto. At that time, as neuropathology was in a primitive stage at the university, Dr. Hannah had something new to offer.

In the years from 1932 until the end of 1936, Dr. Hannah initiated several research projects, the results of most of which were published. The following is a partial listing of these:

"The Aetiology of Subdural Haematoma", *Journal of Nervous and Mental Disease*, 84, 169-186 (1936).

"A Case of Alzheimer's Disease with Neuropathological Findings", *Canadian Medical Association Journal*, 35, 361-366 (1936).

"A Case of Congenital Malformations of Vessels of the Brain and Spinal Cord", *Canadian Medical Association Journal*, 36, 588-591 (1937).

In addition to the above, he was also the author of a research study while in Edinburgh, entitled "Regeneration of Peripheral Nerves – an Experimental Study"; this was published in the *Edinburgh Medical Journal* in February 1931.

Aside from his research projects in neuropathology, he carried out autopsies on many patients who died in Ontario psychiatric hospitals and examined many surgical and autopsy specimens sent to him. These activities were recognized by the title of Provincial Neuropathologist.

In 1935, he presented a display of slides and sections of the brain and spinal cord by invitation at the annual meeting of the American Medical Association in Atlantic City, and in 1936 at the annual meeting of the Ontario Medical Association in London he was awarded the silver medal for the best exhibit out of forty-nine displayed.

It may have been tough economic times during the 1930s that prevented Dr. Hannah from receiving all of what he considered necessary to develop his research in neuropathology. He recorded in diary entries the difficulties he had in obtaining a telephone, a secretary, and other staff, especially residents and fellows, all of which would have permitted him to be more productive. He notes several instances of what he considered government waste of money while he repeatedly tried to get some item of minor cost. During these times he developed a very critical attitude to the government bureaucracy, which he considered to be unreasonably slow in action, encumbered by political patronage appointments, and obsessed by administrative red tape. Additionally he was critical of the university organization, its inability to react to change, and the selection for responsible academic positions of persons who, in his opinion, lacked ability.

In 1936 Dr. Hannah had convened meetings of pathologists in Ontario, the majority of whom were located in hospitals, with the object of developing a provincial association of pathologists. Although he met with little encouragement initially, the Association of Ontario Pathologists was formed in 1938 with Dr. Hannah as one of its founding members. His continuing interest in pathology beyond 1937 led to his ongoing membership in the association and attendance at its annual meetings.

It is not difficult to identify why Dr. Hannah gave up his position as Provincial Neuropathologist in 1937. Some of the reasons have been suggested earlier; others he set forth in considerable detail in his writings. Although he did act as a demonstrator of neuropathological specimens to medical students, he was never offered a more advanced academic appointment. His acceptance into the university's Department of Pathology rested with Professor Klotz, who had communicated to Dr. Hannah that his training in neuropathology and related research was not sufficient to qualify him. Further, Dr. Klotz and his senior staff had never accepted the creation of the position of Provincial Neuropathologist; what they wanted was to develop neuropathology as a university, not a government, activity. Nor had Dr. Hannah endeared himself to his university confreres by his voiced and written criticism of the "politics" of university activity, which he represented as being largely directed towards obtaining government funds for the university. He reports in his memoirs one confrere's assertion that Dr. Hannah had a "belligerent" and "irritating" manner.

Dr. B.T. McGhie, who had been responsible for Dr. Hannah's appointment, became the Deputy Minister of Health and, in the words of Dr. Hannah, less accessible. His numerous responsibilities almost inevitably meant that he had limited time to devote to his original views about the position of Provincial Neuropathologist. The correspondence of the time between Dr. McGhie and Dr. Hannah shows that Dr. McGhie's enthusiasm for the position itself had waned with the passing years, although there was no direct statement that Dr. McGhie considered Dr. Hannah not suited for it.

By 1936 Dr. Hannah had come to be recognized by both the university and the Department of Health as a malcontent. When he tendered his resignation in 1937, no effort was made to ask him to reconsider. Since he was not replaced as Provincial Neuropathologist, the controversy was ended between the Department of Health and the University of Toronto about the real need for such a position. In the next few years Neuropathology became an increasingly important division of the university Department of Pathology.

Two additional factors must have been considered in Dr. Hannah's decision to retire from neuropathology. The first of these was that in 1937 he was thirty-eight years of age with a small family to support (a daughter, Katherine Anne, was born in 1936). The second factor was his interest in "medical care by prepayment". The decision he made led him to a future of interest, innovation, and financial activity.

The research activities of Dr. Hannah in the specialized field of neuropathology are now almost fifty years old, and their relevance to "modern" neuropathology is not within the competence of this writer to judge. His published articles, in the light of 1986 neuropathology, may be considered rudimentary. Yet, as one reads "The Aetiology of Subdural Haematoma", the conviction grows that if Dr. Hannah had continued as a neuropathologist he could have made significant contributions to the specialty. Whether he would have been able to achieve career satisfaction is another matter, one that can only be left to conjecture.

CHAPTER II

The Birth of an Idea

In April 1937, Dr. Hannah requested and received approval of a three months' leave of absence from the Department of Health to permit his full-time attention to bringing into operation Associated Medical Services, Incorporated, which had received its provincial charter under the Companies Act of Ontario on 7 April 1937. He submitted his resignation before the leave was completed. What turned out to be the next thirty-eight years of his life was spent as Managing Director, and later President and Managing Director, of AMS.

In reaching his decision to venture into the relatively new and uncharted area of medical care by prepayment, the immediate determining factor was his increasing discontent with the circumstances of his position as Provincial Neuropathologist. But other events in which he was a participant from the year 1931 onward were major factors. By 1936, he had become convinced that his ideas on the planning and operation of a scheme for providing medical care by prepayment were feasible and that he could make the scheme a reality.

Before his appointment as neuropathologist in September 1930, there is no evidence that Dr. Hannah had any special interest in health insurance and health economics. However, as a civil servant, he became a member of the Civil Service Association, whose primary role at that time was one of representation to the provincial government on behalf of its members, who numbered approximately 2,500. While waiting for office space and research equipment, which were very slow in materializing, he acted for several weeks as a physician to other civil servants. In these contacts, he became aware of the concern many of them had about their ability to meet the cost of unexpected and unpredictable illness. Their concern was accentuated by the deepening economic depression. Throughout the 1930s there were persistent high levels of unemployment, lack of job security, and low and fixed wages. On a personal note, in July 1932 Ruth Hannah contracted a febrile illness that required her to stay in hospital for almost six weeks. She then spent almost six months confined to her home, most of the time in bed, so that assistance was needed in the home. The hospital charge was $49 a week (his earnings at that time were about $86 weekly), and he was fortunate in that he did not have to pay any fees to physicians. This sickness episode, he remarked, "upset the family finances for the next two years", and he added that very few civil servants had his income and for most of them a similar episode could have been a financial catastrophe. This experience was an additional reason for his developing interest in how illness and its costs might be planned for within the family budget.

The Civil Service Association in response to a request from its members set up in 1931 a committee to determine what might be done to permit civil servants to meet the costs of illness. The committee came to favour an arrangement in which a number of physicians would be engaged on salary to look after all the medical care requirements of the members of the association. To meet the cost of the physicians' salaries, the committee proposed that each civil servant pay a monthly "subscriber's fee". However, when the committee sought advice from Dr. Hannah, then one of the few physicians in the civil service, he persuaded them not to consider further the hiring of physicians but to develop a plan that would permit each member to have a free choice of physician. He claimed that such a procedure was an essential first step in ensuring the support of the medical profession for any such plan. At that time Dr. Hannah agreed to act as an unpaid adviser to the committee, and this role led ultimately, early in 1936, to his formulation of a prepaid medical care plan that met with the approval of the members of the association.

During the period 1931 to 1936, stimulated by his activities to assist the Civil Service Association, Dr. Hannah developed an intense interest in health insurance and medical economics. He read widely, beginning with reports on several health insurance plans that had been in operation in European countries for twenty to fifty years. The plans he found to be of particular interest and help were those in Great Britain, Sweden, and Denmark. He became familiar with the history of health insurance in Canada and the United States, where a variety of prepayment plans had been established on a small scale.

He found a few prepayment plans in the eastern United States in which physicians cooperated with industries that subsidized medical care for their employees. At the expense of holiday time, Dr. Hannah visited several of these sites and others, both in Canada and the United States, obtaining valuable information especially on the use of the plans by their subscribers and on their operating costs.

From these studies and experiences, Dr. Hannah gradually brought together his ideas on what he considered would be needed to set up and operate a successful plan. These ideas were translated into what he thought should be the essential components: how physicians and subscribers should participate in it, the benefits to be supplied, the limitations and controls on benefits, and the costs involved. These and related considerations, identified almost solely through Dr. Hannah's initiative, were made part of a preliminary plan developed for study by the Civil Service Association. He also proposed in some detail the organizational and administrative arrangements that he believed would be needed to operate the plan, to support its almost inevitable growth, and to maintain it as a financially solvent organization. These matters of organization and administration were later dealt with in the charter of AMS and in its related by-laws and regulations. The thoroughness of Dr. Hannah's work and the general validity of the arguments he presented to support his opinions and proposed policies were impressive. He consistently emphasized that prepayment for medical services was a new and little-explored field and that his plan should be considered as requiring continuing and intensive research so that improvements could be made to keep it in touch with changing medical practice and economic developments.

The preliminary plan developed by Dr. Hannah and approved by the members of the Civil Service Association early in 1936 provided for a free choice of physician. Since most of the civil servants resided in Toronto, and the chosen physicians would thus most probably practise in Toronto, it was therefore agreed that the support and cooperation of Toronto physicians should be assured before the plan was initiated. Dr. Hannah was asked to make a report to a meeting in March 1936 of the Academy of Medicine, Toronto, of which physicians in Toronto were members. The report was so well received that Academy members decided to recommend to the Ontario Medical Association that it explore the possibility of having the plan instituted not only in Toronto but province-wide. OMA accepted this recommendation, and there followed a series of meetings involving Dr. Hannah and others who at first represented the Civil Service Association and later AMS.

To give some historical perspective to events in Canada and in Ontario at the time AMS was in its developmental stages, a brief review is necessary. "State medicine", as it was originally called, was a subject for discussion in its application to Canada by the federal government as far back as 1911. It was conceived at that time as a form of national health insurance, sponsored by the federal government but administered by the provinces, with federal-provincial sharing of costs. Nothing aside from general discussion occurred then, but in the following years the subject came up for review and discussion periodically, and the concept of a national plan came to have the endorsation of all political parties.

Between 1943 and 1945 a series of meetings, initiated by the federal government, brought federal and provincial representatives together to examine written proposals for a comprehensive form of national health insurance as prepared by the federal government. This plan came very close to enactment in federal legislation; however, there were differences between the two levels of government about how it should be funded, and differences of opinion on the interpretation to be applied to the British North America Act and its designation of matters of health as a provincial responsibility.

The movement towards a national health insurance plan continued nevertheless. Further initiatives were taken by the governments of Saskatchewan and British Columbia and by the federal government. As the result of a continuing series of federal-provincial discussions initiated by Ontario, the first step in a national plan was taken by the passing, in 1958, of the Hospital Insurance and Diagnostic Services Act. By 1961 all provinces were participants in a hospital insurance plan providing hospital benefits for all residents, with the cost being shared between the federal and provincial governments. In 1969, a full national health insurance plan was completed in Canada with the enactment of the federal Medical Care Insurance Act, which provided for the payment of medical and related services in all provinces, again on a cost-sharing basis.

During many years of discussion and debate, the Canadian Medical Association, as the representative body of organized medicine in Canada, and with the support of its affiliated provincial medical associations, came to accept the inevitability of a national, government-sponsored health insurance system. Among the many questions brought forward were those that related to the role of the provincial associations, to how the practitioner of medicine should function, and to how his or her services should be paid for. Generally, CMA was opposed to the operation of the medical care portion of the plan by a government or its agency. In 1934, CMA published a report that enunciated nineteen clauses considered by its associated members to be necessary principles applicable to any health insurance plan. The report also expressed the members' views on the basic rights to which a physician should be entitled. The principles were expanded and clarified in a submission CMA made in 1937 to the Royal Commission on Dominion-Provincial Relations and they were supplemented in 1938 by a series of articles in the *Canadian Medical Association Journal* on the problems of medical economics.

In Ontario, OMA showed little interest prior to 1920 in health economics or health insurance and the implications for physicians, although it did try to keep its members informed by editorial or articles on developments in health insurance, then largely confined to Europe. During the 1920s, minimal interest was shown in so-called "socialist medicine". In 1929, however, a report of a Special Committee on Industrial and International

Relations of the Parliament of Canada proposed among its recommendations the acceptance "of the principle of insurance against unemployment, sickness and invalidity". In a reaction to this recommendation, OMA asked that CMA request the federal government to study the whole subject of "sickness insurance" and to prepare some specific comments and recommendations. Action on this request seems to have been set aside as the developing economic depression diverted government attention to more urgent matters.

At the June 1929 annual meeting of OMA and at its annual meetings in the three following years, the spectre of some form of health insurance led to the convening of periodic "round table" conferences on health insurance. These conferences, which were well attended, featured speakers with experience in the broad field of health insurance from centres in Canada and the United States. Discussion of "medical economics" in the conferences showed that a considerable number of physicians thought that organized medicine should not be involved in sponsoring or operating plans. Their belief was that such a procedure could hasten the coming of a system of state medicine. The conferences did show that many physicians had a distrust of health insurance in any form; but if it became inevitable, it should preferably be in the form of a prepayment method sponsored by the profession.

In 1932, an additional factor came into prominence that became of serious concern to OMA. The economic depression was making it difficult, and frequently impossible, for many residents of Ontario to afford the necessities of life. Increasing numbers of people were forced to seek public welfare and to be classified as indigent. Initially, indigents were treated by physicians without any payment for their services. As the number of indigents increased, however, the income of many physicians suffered to the point that some had to seek welfare relief or income from other sources. In 1932, it was decided by government to pay the costs of medical services to welfare recipients on a stipulated basis of about fifty per cent of the amount billed for the services, the costs to be apportioned equally between the federal, provincial, and municipal governments. Initially this Medical Welfare Plan was administered by municipal and county welfare departments.

As time went on the federal Department of Welfare threatened to withdraw its support from the plan, claiming that no serious efforts were being made to contain its costs.

In 1935, after long deliberations in several of its committees, OMA volunteered to administer the plan. At the time, there were about 400,000 recipients of public welfare in Ontario. OMA assumed the responsibility for seeing that they received the medical services they required – home and office visits, and hospital treatment as in-patients or out-patients. The payments made by the plan to physicians averaged about fifty per cent of the billed amounts; if the total amount available to the plan from government sources was not sufficient to pay fifty per cent, the payment was determined on a pro-rata basis.

The Medical Welfare Plan was operated efficiently and well through a central office maintained by the OMA, and with the cooperation of physicians and OMA regional branches an acceptable quality of medical care was provided to a sizeable portion of the population. This experience was a source of satisfaction and encouragement to the members of the Association and strengthened their belief that OMA could have a role in sponsoring and supporting medical care payment plans. An additional result of the Medical Welfare Plan, highly useful to health care planners, was the compilation of extensive statistics on the utilization and costs of physicians' services to indigents. It should be noted that the medical care provided under the Medical Welfare Plan was not "contract medicine", which had existed particularly in Europe for many years, but was a pro-rata payment of fee for service.

Commencing in 1933 and continuing until 1947, OMA followed a practice of appointing a number of committees from its own membership to study and report on numerous designated aspects of the subject of medical care insurance. A recital of the names of these committees, their terms of reference, and the substances of their reports is peripheral to this treatise on AMS. Of importance to our record is the relationship between OMA and AMS that developed over the years and the decisions ultimately reached by OMA about its role in providing medical care insurance. What follows is therefore in summary form. Much more detailed information is contained in the archives of OMA, AMS, Windsor

Medical Services, and Physicians Services Incorporated and in the writings of authors whose contributions are identified in the Acknowledgements.

In the 1933-1936 period, an OMA committee circulated a questionnaire to all members requesting their views on the general question of "health insurance". The replies received and reported to the 1936 annual meeting "constituted a distinct mandate for the profession to develop an Ontario Medical Association plan on medical care insurance for the Province of Ontario". The committee report on its questionnaire and related matters was debated at length. There was no clear majority support for the committee's recommendation: many members reiterated their view that OMA should not be in the "insurance business" and that there were legal and "constitutional" implications if OMA should embark on the development of a medical care insurance plan. Although a general air of caution about how to proceed with the committee recommendation pervaded the meeting, a resolution was finally passed that was reasonably clear in its intent, but not in how it might be implemented. It read as follows:

[That] the Association go on record as in accord with any affiliated society making the effort to demonstrate, on a voluntary basis, the value of health insurance and, further, that the Association be prepared to render any support within its power to any affiliate society determining to undertake such an experiment.

With regard to this resolution, G. Howard Shillington, who had wide experience in prepaid medical care plans, appropriately commented:

In looking at this resolution in terms of the pattern of development in the years following, it must be recognized as one of the major decisions taken by the profession in its future involvement in the voluntary health insurance field. Whether it was the best decision or not, there were many who in later years wondered. [1]

---

[1] G.H. Shillington, "Prepayment and the Medical Profession – The Evolution of an Idea", Unpublished manuscript, prepared for AMS, Ch. 1, p. 19 (1974).

At the same meeting, OMA also accepted the recommendation of the committee to establish a new committee to continue its work on a province-wide plan. To this Health Insurance Committee, OMA appointed as its representatives Dr. W.K. Colbeck and Dr. W. Caldwell with the later addition of Dr. W.O. Stephenson. Dr. E.A. Broughton and Dr. J.A. Hannah of Toronto were appointed as representatives of the Ontario Health Association, the precursor of AMS. Windsor Medical Services was later asked to name representatives to the committee, and five were subsequently appointed.

"Sitting in the wings" during the deliberations and decisions of the 1936 meeting of OMA were representatives of two organizing bodies who believed they could meet the definition of an "affiliate society" as used in the resolution quoted above: Windsor Medical Services and Dr. Hannah's Ontario Health Association.

Windsor Medical Services developed as a response to the economic depression of the 1930s and its substantial effects on the automotive industry, Windsor's major employer. Conditions had directed attention towards the problems of providing medical services to residents of Windsor, the rest of Essex County, and Lambton County, increasing numbers of whom were receiving welfare assistance. The Ontario Medical Welfare Plan came as welcomed relief and led the members of the Windsor and Essex County medical societies to study the utilization of medical services and their costs. The studies were based initially on experiences with the operation of the Medical Welfare Plan and were assisted by a grant of $23,000 from the Rockefeller Foundation. The outcome of the studies was a decision by the Essex County Medical Society to set up, under sponsorship of physicians practising in Essex County and Windsor, and later in portions of Lambton County, a medical care prepayment plan known as Windsor Medical Services and available to residents of the two counties. The plan was a comprehensive one; it was available to both groups and individuals; and it provided for physicians to be paid on a fee-for-service basis. To give some financial stability to the plan, each participating physician was required to purchase participating membership shares in the Windsor Medical Society Corporation. The sponsors of WMS believed that a province-wide medical prepayment plan should ultimately be developed and recommended that OMA obtain a charter for such a plan with special provision for the establishment and operation of local self-governing subsidiaries.

WMS was granted a provincial charter practically identical to that of AMS on 3 May 1937, but another twenty-six months elapsed before the organization brought its plan into operation.

The second "affiliate society" to seek OMA approval was the Ontario Health Association. With some anticipation of this turn of events in OMA's struggle to determine its role in medical care insurance, Dr. Hannah had decided that some attention had to be given to how such a plan should be administered and brought into operation. During the period 1934 to 1936, he had with the assistance of the Civil Service Association set up an organization known as the Ontario Health Association. Its directors, in addition to himself, were five senior officials in government departments and in the Civil Service Association; one of them was Dr. B.T. McGhie, Deputy Minister of Health and Hospitals. Available to them as advisers were representatives of the Department of the Attorney General. All members of the association being convinced of the need for a medical prepayment plan, a series of meetings were held to consider the legal status of the proposed plan, its stated objects, and how it should be administered. On the advice of the provincial legal authority, the name Ontario Health Association was changed in 1936 to "Associated Medical Services". Dr. Hannah maintained that the plan he proposed should not be considered as "insurance" as defined in the provincial Companies Act, which dealt with provincial requirements for the regulation and control of insurance companies. His views were accepted: when AMS received its charter a year later in April 1937, it was granted under the provincial Companies Act.

During 1936, the Health Insurance Committee of OMA held several meetings to prepare a report for submission to the meeting of the Council of OMA in February 1937. During this period AMS, under the guidance of Dr. Hannah, studied and refined its plan and its administrative arrangements and prepared a schedule of payments for subscribers. By the end of January 1937, AMS had ready for distribution its constitution and by-laws.

When the Council of OMA met on 23 and 24 February 1937, representatives of AMS and WMS were asked to appear before it along with members of the OMA Committee on Health Insurance. Dr. Hannah was able to give a clear and concise description of the proposed AMS medical prepayment plan, noting that it could be put into operation at an early date. He added that to start the plan some financial assistance was required from OMA and requested this in the form of a loan.

While there was discussion about some aspects of the AMS plan by Council members, the only major point was the decision of the AMS plan, as distinct from that of the WMS plan, not to establish an "income limit" for plan subscribers. Several OMA members favoured an income limit of about $3,500 annually, on the premise that those at or above that level were quite able to pay their physicians' bills and should be excluded from the plan. Dr. Hannah argued that there should be no income limit, and the subject was not raised subsequently. At no time in the future did AMS have an income limit, although WMS maintained one for several years.

Representatives of WMS presented a progress report on their plan to the meeting and indicated that they expected to receive their provincial charter in April 1937. They also requested a loan from OMA to assist in getting their plan under way.

Then Dr. R.P. Smith, Medical Supervisor, Hollinger Employees Medical Services Association, described the compulsory medical care prepayment plan that was being initiated in June 1937 for employees of Hollinger Consolidated Gold Mines in Timmins, Ontario. This plan, replacing a former contract plan for medical services to employees only, was designed to give wide coverage for hospital and medical services to about 10,000 employees of the mining companies and their dependants. The cost of the plan was to be met by monthly contributions from the employee and the employer. The plan was described as the first of its kind, size, and scope in Canada. Subsequent reports prepared in 1943 described it as quite successful and beneficial to the employees, their dependants, and the mining company.

Reporting to the Council of OMA, the Health Insurance Committee gave its opinion that to gain actual experience about medical care insurance, the OMA should support the initiation of plans designed to provide statistical and other operational information on which wider decisions could be based. The committee therefore recommended financial support from OMA in starting AMS and WMS and also for a plan in Norfolk County that was in its early formative stages.

The Council finally approved a resolution reading:

> That this Council approve of the project of instituting a Voluntary Health Service Corporation in Toronto, Norfolk County and Essex County districts:
>
> That the Board of Directors of the OMA be authorized to advance on loan to the Health Insurance Committee of the OMA
>
> (a) such sums as are legally available from income,
> (b) such sums as are legally available from assets,
>
> for the purpose of aiding these voluntary medical service units in commencing operations.

At the meeting of the Board of Directors of OMA held on 6 March 1937, the Health Insurance Committee supported the resolution from Council as quoted above and requested payment of such sums as were available under the terms of the resolution. By direction of the Board the Finance Committee, with legal advice, approved an initial grant of $1,500 to be followed by further sums over the next twelve months up to a maximum of $5,000, the payments to be made to AMS and WMS. A requirement of payment was that it be advanced by OMA "as a loan repayable to the Association out of profits or, in the event of winding up proceedings, as a first charge against assets".

Left unanswered, and for spirited discussion at subsequent meetings of OMA, was the question of whether or not OMA should "support" or "sponsor" or "operate" medical care prepayment plans. The "loan" approval was interpreted as an approach of caution, with OMA not being too sure of its ground and seeking assurance that if the supported plans failed, OMA could not be held to account for the failure.

A later meeting of the directors of OMA in June 1937 was important primarily because of the report made to it by the Health Insurance Committee. Faced with the imminence of what many physicians believed would be compulsion by the state to participate in some form of national health insurance, the directors evinced more than their usual interest in the report. In a preliminary outline to its recommendations, the committee stressed its view that some province-wide experience with OMA-supported medical prepayment plans was essential. The report went as follows:

> Following numerous meetings, the Committee has now agreed upon, for establishing, in cooperation with the laity, a voluntary non-profit plan of prepayment of medical services which includes:
>
> 1) Central control
> 2) Local administration
> 3) A pooling of 10% of the funds
> 4) A maximum income level at the discretion of each local group
> 5) Various measures respecting services, participants and costs.

This report, in its vagueness characteristic of many reports coming to or emanating from OMA on this subject, shows the general indecision by OMA about what it should do to meet the increasing public and governmental demands on the medical profession for some acceptable method of meeting, or budgeting for, the costs of medical services. The OMA members, with their usual cautious approach, decided to defer any immediate action on these recommendations and to leave their subject for further study.

Dr. Hannah was quite conversant with these developments, primarily through his membership on the OMA Health Insurance Committee and his regular attendance at meetings of OMA. He supported the view of the committee that much more information was needed about the nature, scope, and extent of medical services in Ontario, which he assigned as part of the "research" function of AMS. He believed that a province-wide plan for gaining such information was necessary; nonetheless, he favoured confining the activities of AMS to the largest centres of population in Ontario. He did not subscribe to the committee's recommendation that there be a pooling, presumably for the purpose of developing a financial reserve, of "10% of the funds" paid as fees to physicians. Nor did he agree that there should be a maximum income level applicable to plan subscribers.

Following the March 1937 meeting of the OMA directors, AMS and its directors believed that they had assurance of a loan, considered at the time to be between $5,000 and $10,000, from OMA to assist in bringing the AMS plan into operation. Acting on this assurance, AMS decided to launch its plan on 1 June 1937. The Norfolk Medical Society decided not to initiate a prepayment plan; and WMS, although accepting the loan, did not bring its plan into operation until about two years later. No loan to the Hollinger Medical Services was proposed, on the premise that Hollinger Mines would fund the plan.

The new Board of Directors of AMS received the approval of the Civil Service Association to also make the plan available to residents of Toronto who were not members and to all residents of Ontario as the scope of the plan could be expanded. On application to the Provincial Secretary, a charter for the corporation was received on 7 April 1937 along with approval of its constitution and by-laws. Regulations relating to its operation were completed soon after. Through his connections with senior government officials and especially those in the Department of Health, who supported his plan, Dr. Hannah was able to procure, for a three-year term and rent-free, a government-owned house at 11 Queen's Park in Toronto. Having resigned his position as Provincial Neuropathologist, Dr. Hannah moved into this building in late April 1937 together with a recently hired secretary. There AMS opened for business on 1 June 1937.

Dr. Hannah refers in his writings on these days to his expectation of $10,000 from OMA, which would have made the capital funding of AMS much easier. But for some reasons not identified, the expected amount was reduced to $3,800. The

Civil Service Association, however, provided a loan of $1,200. Thus AMS began operations with only $5,000 in capital.

Associated Medical Services and Its Prepayment Plan

Dr. Hannah set out the details of the AMS plan in as many as forty articles, which appeared in the *Canadian Medical Association Journal*, the *Ontario Medical Review*, and other journals and in numerous speeches between 1936 and 1950. In addition, there are copies of reports prepared by Dr. Hannah for meetings of the Board of Directors of AMS and its Executive and Management Committee. All of these details about the plan may be summarized under the following headings:

1. The Beliefs and Attitudes Underlying AMS.

Dr. Hannah wrote and spoke on this subject on many occasions. His belief was that the individual should have responsibility for his or her own welfare. Included in this responsibility was providing for the costs of illness and disability before their occurrence. He believed that most people wanted to be responsible and not dependent on government for what they could provide for themselves, and that non-governmental organizations should be developed to help people exercise this responsibility.

He also believed that, as voluntary action on the part of the private sector was preferable to compulsory action initiated by government, there was thus a place for AMS as a voluntary plan. If the opportunity were offered, he was convinced, large numbers of individuals and families would budget for the cost of illness in the same way as they were budgeting for the purchase of homes, automobiles, furniture, and other items. He frequently stated that the annual cost of a medical care prepayment plan was generally less than the amount expended by a cigarette smoker.

There was also a responsibility resting on employers either to provide their employees with wages that would permit their participation in such a plan or to make direct payments to a plan on behalf of their employees.

It was admitted that there were people in society who were indigent. The responsibility for meeting the costs of medical services to the indigent clearly rested with government, which had to deal with the problem by consultation and arrangement with the medical profession, but with AMS offering whatever advice and assistance it might be asked to give.

To make the AMS prepayment plan work and to keep it solvent, there was the obvious necessity of a close cooperation with physicians and OMA. The clear demonstration that a non-governmental plan such as AMS could succeed was the best method available to OMA to show that medical care could be provided without government intervention.

Finally, the AMS plan must be considered as being in its early stages and for a period of several years would be experimental. An ongoing research element must be included, with the assurance that all information on the use of the plan would be made public.

2. The Organizational Beginnings.

In discussing the nature and structure of AMS, Dr. Hannah argued that the proposed prepayment plan was not "insurance" as the word is generally interpreted. He persistently affirmed that "health insurance" is a misnomer because health cannot be achieved by use of insurance. While admitting that the AMS plan would operate on insurance principles, he insisted that the prepayment principle was distinctive in its concept. These arguments about the AMS plan not being "insurance" – whether valid or not – nevertheless led to AMS's gaining its charter under the terms of the Companies Act for the province of Ontario as a non-profit corporation without share capital. The principal advantage to AMS in becoming a corporation and not an "insurance agency" was that it did not come directly under the surveillance of the Provincial Superintendent of Insurance. (At a later date the province decided to set up a separate Act to deal with AMS, WMS, and other organizations such as Blue Cross and Physicians Services Incorporated, and AMS was brought under the provisions of that Act.)

Dr. Hannah believed that AMS should not be a profit-making organization since its principal object was to provide quality medical services at the lowest possible cost.

While more attention will be given later to the corporate structure of AMS, it may be noted here that a strong element in OMA believed that since AMS was dealing directly with physicians in the delicate area of payments to them, the direction of AMS should be predominantly in the hands of physicians. Dr. Hannah and his associates did not accept this view, and the Board of Directors of AMS when constituted included lay members, as representatives of the subscribers, as well as medical members. AMS decided, however, that of the total number of its directors the "medical" would outnumber the "lay" directors by one, so that on a close vote the medical members could prevail.

AMS decided to confine its initial activities to its head office in Toronto, and to southwestern and southeastern Ontario, setting up branch offices in London, Woodstock, Hamilton, Peterborough, Kingston, and Ottawa. The location of the branch offices was based on the assurance that each would be financially self-sustaining. (As time went on the operations of AMS were concentrated in Toronto, and all branch offices except those in Ottawa and Hamilton were closed.)

Dr. Hannah was assigned the title of Chief Medical Officer at a salary of approximately $6,000 a year. As there were no funds available for advertising purposes, advantage had to be taken of Dr. Hannah's contacts with the Civil Service Association and OMA through monthly publications sent to their members. With what seemed to be almost unlimited enthusiasm and energy, Dr. Hannah accepted every opportunity to speak about AMS to service clubs, medical societies, and numerous other organizations having some influence on public opinion. He was also readily available for interviews by newspaper and radio reporters. He did recognize and emphasize that the success of AMS could, in large part, depend on "word-of-mouth" support from its subscribers.

3. Description of the AMS Prepayment Plan.

The plan can be described under several headings.

(a) Policy on Subscribers to the Plan. Initially the membership in the plan was restricted to single individuals and to family units consisting of husband, wife, and dependent children under the age of seventeen years. Certain exceptions could be made for including children over seventeen in the family unit – an example being children in attendance at university. Group memberships were excluded. The following is from a report prepared in 1940 by Dr. Hannah on AMS development:

Although we had hoped to get subscribers in groups, AMS has always felt that the majority of the population of the province does not fall into groups and, therefore, our organization must be so constituted that it can accept individuals. Shopkeepers, farmers and others will have to be cared for and they would find it difficult to be in groups. These must be included if our solution to the problem is to be effective . . .

Nor do we believe that we should be entirely dependent upon industry for our progress. Industry can offer us a very great deal of security either by assuming the cost in part or in whole for their employees, or by collecting the fees for them. There is, however, an inherent tendency on the part of industry to barter for a price, and even, if possible, to dictate. No one element of the community should ever be allowed to get into the position where it exercises too great an influence. If the profession wants the security which any other body can give, they can buy it, but usually such bargains result in a mess of pottage far from palatable. It is our firm conviction that the profession must never barter its birth-right, whatever the prize offered.

It is of interest to note that the policy remained in effect until 1945, at which time AMS offered its first group contract. By 1951, the number of individual and family contracts had decreased by about thirty per cent, and the group contracts were about three times the number of individual and family contracts.

(b) Procedure for Enrolment as a Subscriber. Any single or married person could apply for enrolment in the plan. The application required completion of a form giving information about the age, sex, and health history of the applicant. In the case of a married man the name, age, and health history of his wife and their children were required.

(c) Selection of Physician. Every applicant for enrolment was required in the application form to name his or her physician who would provide medical attendance as required. The physician so named was required to be a general practitioner, and only one could be named. The applicant agreed to not change the physician named without notification to AMS and the acceptance of the change by AMS.

(d) Processing of the Application. AMS staff reviewed the application information. If the form indicated a "pre-existing" health condition, its nature would be examined by a "medical referee", paid by AMS usually on a part-time basis, and in questionable circumstances the physician attending the patient for the pre-existing condition would be asked for comments and advice. Depending on such information, and also depending on the agreement of the selected physician, a decision might be made to accept the application – either without any conditions or limitations, or excluding the cost of services for any pre-existing condition. An applicant whose application was rejected for whatever reason was notified in writing of the rejection; an accepted applicant was also notified in writing and provided with a "notification card", as well as being informed about the inclusion or exclusion of pre-existing conditions. Final acceptance was dependent on the payment by the subscriber of the appropriate fee. The selected physician was also notified of the decision; acceptance of the subscriber by the physician was required in writing or by telephone.

(e) Specifically Excluded Services. Aside from the judgement factor exercised by AMS in dealing with pre-existing health conditions, AMS specifically excluded from the scope of services it covered in its plan the following:

— services in an institution available to residents of Ontario where treatment for illness, predominantly of the psychiatric type, but also for tuberculosis, is a responsibility of the Province.

— injuries and illnesses which are the responsibility of the Workmen's Compensation Board.
— the costs of treatment of venereal diseases
— the costs of "annual health examinations"
— the costs of medicines prescribed for patients receiving such medicines outside hospitals
— such other exclusions as may be defined by AMS from time to time to protect the integrity of the prepayment plan.

(f) Benefits Included. A subscriber to the Plan with no restriction or limitation on the benefits offered would be entitled to the following services:

— attendance by the selected physician at the home of the subscriber and his dependants to render necessary medical care and for attending a subscriber while in hospital
— attendance of the subscriber at the office of the selected physician to receive necessary medical care
— surgical operations performed by a qualified surgeon upon the subscriber and including the cost of the services of an anaesthetist
— approved consultations by qualified physicians as required by the subscriber and including the necessary services of a medical or surgical "specialist"
— attendance of a physician at the time of childbirth and the subsequent care of the newborn child
— X-ray and laboratory services provided to a patient admitted to hospital
— services rendered to a subscriber admitted to hospital and including hospital charges, in the form of a daily room rate for care of the patient, for drugs administered in hospital and charges for use of the operating room
— nursing services, defined as the cost of special services by a registered nurse required in hospital on the specific request of the selected physician or a specialist physician.

4. The Financial Aspects of the AMS Plan.

(a) Cost Estimates. Dr. Hannah realized that any plan he developed must be solvent and capable of adjustment to changes in economic circumstances and consumer demand. He sought and studied information on the costs of medical care insurance plans in North America and Europe, and from the information he gathered in 1937 he developed the following cost figures.

Home Calls by a Physician – These were reckoned to be one home call each year for each subscriber at $3 per call. The total for the year of this item was therefore $3.

Visits to a Physician's Office – These were reckoned to be 1.5 visits per subscriber per year at a cost of $2 per visit with the total for the year being $3.

Consultations and Services of Specialists – It was difficult to find any definite information about the frequency and cost of consultative services; but with the information available, a cost of $4 each year for each subscriber was assigned for estimation purposes.

Surgical Operations – The information available indicated that surgery would be required by eight per cent of subscribers each year. At an estimated cost of $50 for each procedure, the amount to be paid out each year would be eight per cent of $50, or $4 per subscriber, these including costs related to childbirth.

X-Ray and Laboratory Examinations – Again there was little precise information about the cost of these services as provided to hospitalized patients, and an estimate of $1 per subscriber each year was made.

Hospital Services – The expectation was that each subscriber would require an average of 1.3 days of hospital care per year. Calculated at the hospital rates in effect at that time ($3.50 per day), the cost for each subscriber for hospital services in a year was set at $4.55.

Nursing Services – The estimate of the cost of these services was made at a time when private nursing services were provided in two twelve-hour shifts each day. The going rate at the time was $5 for each shift, and it was calculated that on average each subscriber would require one half-shift of nursing services at a yearly cost of $2.50.

Administrative Services – The cost of administration of the plan was estimated to be $2 per subscriber per year.

(b) Subscriber's Fees. The sum of the above calculations gave the average cost of providing benefits to an individual subscriber for a year as $24. The fee payable was thus $2.00 per month.

With the above calculations and data from Ontario sources on "family size", the monthly subscription fees payable by families were derived. These were established effective 1 June 1937 as follows:

For the husband and wife	$3.75
For a family with one dependent child	$5.25
For a family with two dependent children	$6.50
For each additional dependent child (to be added to the $6.50 fee)	$1.00

At the inception of the plan each subscriber was required, as his or her personal responsibility, to pay the fee on a monthly basis and on its due date. If the fee was not paid, the subscriber's contract was cancelled. AMS did not undertake to give any notice to the subscriber of the due date and the amount of the payment. Some consideration could be given to delinquent subscribers when there was some justifiable cause for delay in remittance of the fee. Subscribers of some standing and without undue claims on the plan were usually dealt with leniently if the delay was not too long.

In the case of first-time subscribers, the required initial payment was for a three-month period. The benefits under the plan only became effective two months following receipt of the initial payment. The fee for the two-month period was considered "administrative" or "acquisition" costs incurred by AMS in enrolling the subscriber.

By contractual agreement the subscriber was required to notify AMS of any change in his or her marital status and, in the case of a married couple, the addition of each child to the family.

(c) **Payments for Services.** The document provided by AMS to its subscribers detailed the services to be paid for under the terms of the agreement:

Physicians' Services

— For each attendance of a participating physician at the subscriber's home (a "home call"), $3.
— For each visit to the physician's office (an "office visit"), $2.
— For the consultant services of a "specialist" physician or surgeon, requested by the subscriber's participating physician, the need for such consultant services requiring approval by a "medical officer" on the staff of an AMS office. (The consultant services of otolaryngologists and ophthalmologists were frequently requested.)
— For the professional care of a female subscriber during her pregnancy, confinement, and post-partum care and including the care of the newborn infant.

All of the above fees for services of physicians were those listed in the fee schedule of the OMA. The fee paid by AMS was the minimum set down in the schedule, this fee usually being that for an uncomplicated illness or surgical procedure. There was no prohibition on a participating physician from billing a subscriber more than the minimum fee; the subscriber was responsible for payment of the additional charges.

While the OMA schedule of fees provided for payment of travel costs incurred by a physician in attending a patient located at a distance from his or her office, no payments for travel costs were provided by AMS.

Hospital Services – An AMS subscriber admitted to hospital had the cost of most services rendered by the hospital paid by AMS to the hospital. They included accommodation in the standard ward, meals, nursing services, and use of the operating room, as required. The cost of these hospital services in 1937 in Ontario averaged $3.50 per day, and AMS paid up to this amount. The subscriber who elected a semi-private or private room would have to pay the difference.

X-Ray and Laboratory Services – The cost of these services was paid by AMS only when the subscriber was a hospital patient. The charges for the service were those established in the OMA fee schedule and were, in most circumstances, paid to the hospital.

Nursing Services – These services were interpreted as special or additional nursing care beyond that normally rendered by hospital nursing staff. The cost of providing this additional nursing care was accepted by AMS only if ordered by the subscriber's physician with a clear indication for its necessity.

Limitations and Exclusions – In addition to some of these that have been mentioned previously, the AMS plan regulations provided that:

— To be eligible for maternity benefits the subscriber had to be a member of the plan for a minimal period of ten months ("the waiting period").
— No person over fifty-five years of age would be accepted as an initial subscriber to the plan.
— The contract between the subscriber and AMS could be terminated when the subscriber attained the age of fifty-five years.
— The total amount payable by AMS on behalf of a subscriber would not exceed $800 in any twelve-month period.

(d) Administrative Arrangements. To facilitate processing and payment of benefits, AMS adopted the following procedures:

Physicians were asked to accumulate the required records on services rendered to subscribers – home and office calls, consultations, maternity care, surgical procedures, and any other services – and to submit these to AMS at the end of each month. For all claims that were "in order" and not subject to any questioning, payment by cheque would be made by the tenth day of the succeeding month.

Any claims that were questioned by AMS medical officers on whatever grounds would be held for payment until the matter was resolved, if necessary by decision of the Board of Directors of AMS.

Claims from hospitals, including requested payments for X-ray and laboratory services, were to be submitted to AMS as soon as possible; AMS undertook to make payment before the end of the month in which the claim was received.

Claims for the services of private nurses were accepted by AMS and were paid to the nurses as quickly as possible.

CHAPTER III

The Experimental Years – 1937 to 1947

This period in the operation of AMS requires special attention, since it saw the development of what proved to be, in the words of Dr. Hannah, "a successful experiment in the field of medical services".

The most important matter for AMS – the growth of the plan – may be traced in a summary manner for this ten-year period in terms of enrolment statistics. In the seven-month period 1 June to 31 December 1937, AMS had enrolled 737 subscribers, and the fees paid by them had been sufficient to meet all current expenses. By the end of 1938 the number of subscribers had become 4,020, and steady increases followed: 20,000 at the end of 1940 and 30,000 at the end of 1941.

By 1 June 1947, the number of subscribers was approximately 43,000. At that time, in his report "The First Ten Years of Progress", Dr. Hannah noted that the primary criterion of success had not been the achievement of a rapid increase in the number of subscribers but rather soundness of operation, solvency, and the degree of benefit and satisfaction to those who received and those who rendered the services provided by the plan. He pointed out that during the 1939-45 period, large numbers of potential subscribers had become members of the armed forces in the Second World War, receiving medical services through the medical corps; AMS had offered them special rates so that they could enrol their wives and children. As an indication of the continuing acceptance of the plan, he reported that seventy-five per cent of the first 1,800 subscribers to the plan were still subscribers. AMS had paid some $4,400,000 for the medical and hospital services rendered to its subscribers and had an accumulated reserve of $625,000 to meet contingencies. At June 1947 approximately

2,400 physicians in Ontario were participants in the plan; fifty per cent of them were located in Toronto.

The by-laws provided that an unlimited number of members of the corporation could be elected for terms of one to three years. The members, one physician and one layman, were proposed for membership by a local committee formed in each of the locations in the province where AMS had offices. The number of offices, including the head office in Toronto, reached eight in the 1940s. The by-laws required that there be seven directors, elected for terms of one to three years at an annual meeting of members, with the members in turn being elected for one to three years by the directors. Of the seven directors, the by-laws required that four be physicians and three be laymen – that is, the physician directors would have a majority of one.

The custom followed was that the Board of Directors would hold at least four quarterly meetings and that one of these, held usually in the month of April or May, would be the annual meeting; that the President would be a physician; and that an effort would be made to avoid having a preponderance of directors from Toronto.

In 1940, Dr. Hannah, who acted as both Chief Medical Officer and Secretary of the Board, was given the title of Managing Director, and a full-time Secretary-Treasurer, Mr. K. Atcheson, was appointed. To assist the Board of Directors, an Executive Committee of the Board was appointed consisting of the President as chairman, a layman director, the Managing Director, and the Secretary-Treasurer. This committee met at the call of its chairman to consider and give advice to the directors on many subjects of policy. These could be in relation to benefits for subscribers, financial matters, relationships with OMA, and other subjects requiring study, as might be directed to the committee by the Managing Director.

The records of the 1937-47 period reveal the success of AMS in reaching its principal objective of initiating a workable plan. This success was not achieved without the ability of Dr. Hannah and the AMS Board to react effectively to developments of the period.

As noted previously, the number of subscribers increased

from zero in June 1937 to approximately 43,000 ten years later. This number of subscribers required an extensive administrative organization to deal with fees, claims, and payments. The physical facilities at 11 Queen's Park soon being inadequate, Dr. Hannah searched for more commodious quarters. In 1943 AMS moved to a five-storey building located at 615 Yonge Street in Toronto with 6,500 square feet of usable floor space. In the ensuing years up to 1947 its executive, administrative, and clerical staffs were gradually expanded to reach a fluctuating number of about seventy persons, the majority being full-time employees.

In giving emphasis in the AMS plan to the enrolment of individual and family-unit subscribers, Dr. Hannah recognized that there would be greater administrative costs than there would be with "group" enrolment. His opinion on the enrolment of individual and family-unit subscribers was based on his belief that these were the people who had the most need of the plan, and the AMS experience up to 1945 served to support this opinion.

During the early years of the plan, Dr. Hannah began to build his administrative organization. The first appointment was a Secretary-Treasurer of the corporation. The second appointment was a Chief Medical Officer, whose primary responsibility was to deal with the adjudication of claims and to act generally as a liaison between AMS and its participating physicians. A third senior appointment was a manager of enrolment services, who travelled widely across the province visiting the branch offices and promoting interest in the plan among potential subscribers. The steady increase in business called for the appointment of an office manager. These senior staff reported directly to Dr. Hannah.

The majority of claims submitted were for home calls and office and hospital visits. Accompanying the claims were supporting statements, summaries, and explanations. These all had to be processed, as did the monthly payments of fees from thousands of subscribers, each for a small amount. The administration of these transactions cost the plan, in its first year, approximately thirty-five per cent of the revenues received. Considering these administrative costs excessive, Dr. Hannah and his staff began an examination of available methods and those projected for the future that would lead to systems of machine accounting. By

1941 AMS had a system making extensive use of rotary wheel cards, machine-punched record cards on each subscriber, and a cheque-writing machine. Throughout the organization there were "noiseless" typewriters and dictating equipment. By these methods it became possible to decrease the number of staff and to achieve a reduction of about fifty per cent in administrative expenses by 1950. By that time, greater efficiencies became possible with the new "punch card" systems of accounting.

From the start of AMS, Dr. Hannah had stressed the importance of deriving statistical information from its operations. During the 1937-1947 period, this information was obtained showing utilization of services and their cost by sex, age group, marital status, diagnosis of disease, type of service rendered, and the branch location of the subscriber. Additionally, it was possible to track payments for each physician and each subscriber. Certain figures were computed and reported on a monthly basis. As time went on, the statistical information became more extensive and more refined and facilitated adjustments in benefits and fees.

Although AMS did not establish a research section in its staff organization, the services of a health economist and a physician having extensive experience in epidemiology were engaged on occasion to review the statistical data and to give advice about other avenues of research that could be useful to AMS.

During the ten-year period, in addition to its central office in Toronto, AMS approved the setting up and operation of "regional" offices in Hamilton, Ottawa, London, Woodstock, Peterborough, St. Catharines, and Oshawa. These were established in response to a request from the area, supported by written information signed by laymen and prospective participating physicians in the area. The Board of Directors of AMS would not approve establishment of a branch without a reasonable assurance that it would be self-supporting financially, the minimum requirement being that it could initially enrol at least 1,200 subscribers.

Each branch office required at least one full-time secretary, with additional secretarial assistance being added as needed. The office provided information about the plan, assisted subscribers with the enrolment procedures, collected and remitted to the Toronto office the subscribers' fees, and gave secretarial assistance as required. At each office, a Medical Officer, appointed on a part-time salaried basis, acted as the contact with physicians in the area and dealt with their applications as participating physicians. His additional responsibility was the examination and assessment of claims. Problem claims were referred to the Toronto office for assistance and decision, and on occasion the Board of Directors was consulted, particularly in matters of policy.

Some of the branch offices assisted in publicizing and promoting the plan and occasionally employed a person well known in the area as a salesman.

A local advisory board of laymen and physicians was set up to advise on the planning and operation of each branch office. This board also proposed the names of persons considered suitable to become members of the AMS corporation; the AMS Board usually elected one layman and one physician representing each area from among these nominations.

In the 1937-1947 period, AMS's accomplishments were watched across Canada and in several areas in the United States, as evidenced by letters of inquiry and comment and articles in Canadian medical periodicals. Even by the time of the 1938 annual meeting of OMA, the presence and influence of AMS across the province had become known to physicians, and many of them were enthusiastic supporters. The report of the OMA Health Services Committee to the annual meeting gave some favourable information about its progress. Early in 1939, in a publication of the Academy of Medicine, Toronto, Dr. Hannah noted in a summary of operations for 1938 that "subscribers increased 549% and our reserve went up 877%."

Relations with OMA

One of the first problems in the relationship between the prepayment plans and OMA appeared at the time of the OMA annual meeting in 1939. Put before the meeting was a proposal that there be a general and steep increase in the OMA schedule of fees, with the expressed intention that the prepayment plans should pay the new fees. The representatives of the three prepayment plans – AMS, WMS, and Hollinger Medical Services – protested. To meet the new fees would require a stiff increase in subscribers' payments, which could result in large numbers of subscribers withdrawing from their plans. The protesters did not object to a new schedule of fees as a voluntary guide for physicians but argued that the prepayment plans should not be required to pay it. A further review of the schedule of fees was decided upon at the meeting, and this decision was a first step towards ensuring that OMA accepted the importance of fee schedules in prepayment plans and understood that unilateral adjustments in the schedules without consultation with the plans could result in difficulties. During the following years, until Physicians Services Incorporated began to operate in 1947, representatives of the prepayment plans were invited to attend meetings of the Tariff Committee of OMA, which periodically reviewed the OMA schedules of fees.

In November 1939, Dr. Hannah repaid the loan of $3,800 advanced by OMA to AMS in 1937. His accompanying letter reviewed the steady increase in the number of AMS subscribers, which at the time was approximately 11,000. He also referred to the financial stability of AMS, which had an accumulated cash reserve sufficient to meet "double our monthly expenditures for from two to three months depending on the severity of the emergency – for example, an epidemic". AMS was eager to continue its relationship with OMA: "An even closer relationship would be beneficial to both, to which end we invite consideration of that problem." In the letter no mention was made of a "sponsorship" or "support" role for OMA in regard to AMS. Rather, since AMS had paid its debt to OMA, the directors of AMS were free to proceed with their business on a cooperative basis with OMA, which permitted a wide interpretation of the relationship between them.

By 1940, the directors of OMA were becoming disturbed about the relations that had developed with AMS. In spite of the expressed interest of OMA in having income limits for subscribers to prepayment plans (a policy followed by WMS), AMS continued to be opposed to them. Increasing numbers of physicians were complaining about what they considered to be an arbitrary adjudication by AMS on some of their claims. Many physicians believed that OMA should have some control over the operation of AMS; AMS was not ready to accept any control. Nor did AMS acknowledge that its plan was being operated as an experiment on behalf of OMA and the physicians it represented. OMA noted that there were no OMA appointees on the AMS Board, and considered the medical representation on the Board inadequate for a corporation dealing almost exclusively with "medical" business. Several OMA directors believed that, in view of the growth of AMS, the time had come, or was fast approaching, when a decision had to be reached as to whether AMS should become part of OMA or become completely separated from any OMA sponsorship.

AMS's size made it the most likely candidate for province-wide development under OMA auspices, a direction that did not fit in with Dr. Hannah's intention. However, AMS was anxious to cooperate with OMA and had suggested that a liaison committee be appointed to discuss matters of common interest and concern. Nevertheless, the above factors, along with a lack of communication between the two organizations, led to a growing coolness.

Because Windsor Medical Services did not become operative until the latter part of 1940, OMA reactions to its operation did not develop until about 1942.

In 1940, and more so in the following years, OMA became concerned about other organizations attempting to get into the field of health insurance: several insurance companies, and "friendly societies" who were engaging physicians to serve their members on a contract basis, paying them the equivalent of a retainer. Further, the Heagerty Report of 1943 prepared under federal government auspices was being intensively studied; there was apprehension that a national form of health insurance sponsored by the federal government, with the participation of the provincial governments, might become a reality in the next few years. However, as a substantial number of Canadian physicians were serving in the armed forces, there was a reluctance by physicians remaining in civilian practice to take any action on health insurance without the participation of their colleagues.

To examine all of these issues and others that might arise, the Joint Advisory Committee was revived on the initiative of OMA. As constituted at this time, the committee had representatives from OMA, the College of Physicians and Surgeons of Ontario, and the medical faculties of the universities, with the chairman being an OMA representative. The committee invited to a meeting in June 1940 Dr. J.A. Hannah of AMS, Dr. F.A. Brockenshire of WMS, and Dr. R.P. Smith of Hollinger Medical Services, along with representatives of other prospective medical schemes.

The committee met primarily in response to a resolution passed some two months previously by the College of Physicians and Surgeons of Ontario: ". . . That the whole matter of medical services be referred to the Joint Advisory Committee, for a meeting in June."

Items on the agenda for discussion included the "airing of certain complaints" and the larger question of how much regulation was going to be tolerated by the medical profession. The question in the mind of one physician attending the meeting was expressed as:

Are we going to regulate ourselves or are we going to have imposed upon us the regulations of non-members of the directorates of organizations giving a legitimate medical service to the public?

In requesting the reconvening of the Joint Advisory Committee, the College of Physicians and Surgeons was evidently seeking some clarification on how physicians were to be "regulated" in a health insurance plan. As with many committee meetings dealing with the complex subject of health insurance, discussion was lengthy, with much of it wandering from the point. Drs. Hannah, Smith, and Brockenshire expressed their surprise that such a meeting seemed necessary. They described in detail the background of the prepayment plans they represented and stressed their desire to work closely and amicably with OMA and their own participating physicians. The College said that its resolution followed on the receipt of several complaints from its members that they were being discriminated against by "certain medical services organizations", the principal one being AMS. Objections were voiced about AMS's "advertising" and the refusal of the three plans to accept the full fee schedule of OMA. These assertions led to a discussion, largely led by Dr. Hannah, about the responsibility of members of the medical profession to support prepayment plans and the necessity for an objective assessment of claims as a protection of the rights of all subscribers. In the discussion there was no general objection to the right of the prepayment plans to adjudicate claims. The committee had no solution to the problem of who should decide which physician was more deserving of a greater fee for his services than another. Nor had it any alternative to offer to the policy of the prepayment plans that the same fee be paid to all physicians for the same service rendered.

The committee reviewed in some detail what it considered to be an indiscriminate issuing of charters by the Attorney General's Department in the province to organizations offering health insurance policies. Committee members stated that if the prepayment principle in Ontario was to be supported by OMA, then OMA should do all in its power to prevent or limit insurance agencies, friendly societies, and other organizations who, to attract business, did not subscribe to the basic principles enunciated by the prepayment plans. It was urged by several committee members that the organizations represented on the committee had a duty to stand solidly behind AMS and to endeavour to have it become province-wide. Committee members also emphasized that if the insurance and other plans were permitted to develop, a competitive "hodge-podge" could result to the detriment of prepayment plans.

The committee finally decided that there was an obvious need to coordinate the thinking and activities of the organizations represented on the committee and that its members should publicly express their support for the CMA statement in the eighteen articles contained in the "Principles of Health Insurance", published in 1937. The committee also agreed to offer assistance to the government in drafting provincial legislation that would be applicable to all organizations seeking charters permitting them to offer medical care insurance. Dr. Hannah assured the committee that he was confident that government officials would welcome their advice and assistance.

At a meeting of the Council of OMA that followed shortly after, the report of the Joint Advisory Committee was received, and discussions followed on developments in other provinces in relation to medical care insurance. It was agreed that OMA should continue to be committed to the support of the three prepayment plans – AMS, WMS, and Hollinger Medical Services – and try to develop a profession-sponsored prepayment plan that could be available to all residents of the province. It was reported to the Council that in November 1940 the Ontario Hospital Association had announced its intention of seeking a provincial charter to establish a Blue Cross plan in Ontario, which would offer a prepaid hospital care plan to employee groups. The charter was later granted after the province had received OMA approval of its objectives. The Blue Cross plan was established under the Companies Act in Ontario and commenced operation in 1941.

Following on the above meeting of the OMA Council and its report to the Board of Directors of OMA, the Board decided to establish a Committee on Economics to study medical care insurance, with the object of eventually bringing about a single OMA-sponsored prepaid medical care plan in Ontario. The chairman of the committee was Dr. T.L. Fisher of Ottawa, who had been a declared supporter of the AMS plan. The Committee on Economics met with representatives of AMS, WMS, and Hollinger Medical Services to examine the objectives of their organizations and to endeavour to assess the value of their "medical care by prepayment" approach as it might apply to the contemplated OMA plan. To receive some opinion regarding the AMS plan, the committee prepared a questionnaire and, with the cooperation of the Academy of Medicine, Toronto, circulated it to all AMS participating physicians in Toronto. The replies to the questionnaire showed that most physicians in general practice were favourably disposed towards the AMS plan, but there were several complaints about the plan and its operation, which can be summarized as follows:

— frequent difficulties and delays in obtaining approval for "specialist services" requested for subscribers
— the occasional refusal by AMS to accept a "medical consultant" chosen by the subscriber or recommended by the physician
— the problem of wealthier patients, accustomed to extra medical attention, now expecting it under the plan

— undue use of pre-existing health conditions as an escape clause by AMS to support its refusal to pay claims
— AMS's endeavour to restrict the number of attendances by paediatricians on newborn infants
— the application of a "waiting period" before ophthalmologists were permitted to carry out eye examinations.

The committee reported the results of this questionnaire and related discussion with Dr. Hannah, as well as on inquiries about the relationship between AMS and OMA. The general tone of the report was critical of Dr. Hannah and AMS and his assertions that it was, and intended to be, an independent organization. In comment on the committee's report, Dr. Hannah wrote in part:

It was distinctly understood when the charter was secured for AMS with the sanction of OMA that AMS was to be an independent incorporated body with control as set out at that time. The OMA did not wish to assume either financial or administrative responsibilities to promote prepayment and could, therefore, expect only that degree of control mutually agreed upon – at no time was AMS regarded as an experiment under the direction of OMA. On the contrary it has been repeatedly stated that AMS is an independent corporation carrying on an experiment with the cooperation of the profession.

Dr. Hannah was quite emphatic in his statements that while AMS did not consider itself to be under any control by OMA, cooperation by the medical profession with the AMS prepayment plan was essential to its success. He added that AMS was quite prepared to consider the various matters raised by the committee in its report.

A cooperative attitude did serve to prevent a more direct confrontation between the two organizations. Committee members and representatives of AMS agreed to study the results of the questionnaire; they concurred that final answers must wait until AMS had more time and more experience. Research would be necessary, and the opportunity to see the operating results of WMS and Hollinger Medical Services. AMS was able to convince

OMA that it could profit from the experience and the research activities of AMS.

The question of "income limits" was one which continued to bother OMA. Many of its members persisted in their belief that such limits as were incorporated into the WMS plan should be part of the AMS plan, although the appropriate level of income remained for discussion and definition.

A remaining contentious item was that of having OMA representatives on the Board of Directors of AMS, the view of OMA being that matters of concern to both OMA and AMS could in this way be dealt with most effectively. AMS gave assurances that it would consider the matter and that the problems that had been identified could be resolved. The Committee on Economics presented its conclusions as follows:

— Further contact between OMA and Hollinger Medical Services should be through a subcommittee appointed to deal with contract practice.
— OMA should recognize and publicize that WMS was a nearly ideal scheme of health insurance, and districts in the province considering instituting health insurance should use the WMS plan as a model.
— As soon as the directors of AMS put into effect the suggestions agreed to by Dr. Hannah and included in the report, OMA should go on record as continuing its approval of AMS.

In speaking to these conclusions, and especially the third, Dr. Fisher, the chairman of the Committee on Economics, reviewed the problems the committee had encountered in the past year in reaching some understandings with AMS and with Dr. Hannah. In his view, AMS had not carried through on what had been agreed, and he recommended that the third conclusion as recorded above be withdrawn and the following substituted as a resolution:

That the official approval of the OMA be withdrawn from the AMS forthwith.

The proposal of this resolution, it is recorded, shook the

members of the OMA attending the 1941 annual meeting. After a lengthy debate, it became obvious that the members were not prepared to accept the substitute resolution in spite of its being proposed by Dr. Fisher. He had expressed strong support for AMS in the *Canadian Medical Association Journal* in 1939, as well as being a member of the local committee that had urged AMS to establish a branch office in Ottawa. His change of attitude was therefore no small matter.

In dealing with the committee report, the following motion was approved:

That the report of the Committee on Economics be referred back for further study and that the personnel of the Committee be carefully scrutinized in order that the relationship between AMS and the OMA be not terminated.

Although a majority of voting members of OMA did not support Dr. Fisher's resolution, it had become apparent that several senior and influential members were not willing to support AMS unless OMA had more direct participation in its operation.

The OMA members acknowledged that any antagonism between OMA and AMS was not going to help OMA in dealing with the practical question of its role in a prepayment mechanism. Following its usual course when faced with a problem requiring some solution, OMA decided to establish a new committee, which was given the title Voluntary Health Insurance Committee. Its purpose was described as "to enquire into the operation of the voluntary health schemes now in operation in the Province with a view to ascertaining their strength and weak points and consolidating these into a report to OMA". Since AMS was, at the time, the principal voluntary "health scheme" in Ontario, the committee directed most of its attention towards the structure and function of AMS and the examination of points of difference in viewpoint and opinion that reflected on the relationship between OMA and AMS. As expected, the committee did not find any serious differences between OMA and WMS, noting that the control of WMS was firmly in the hands of its participating physicians and was responsive to advice and suggestions from OMA.

In December 1941, this latest committee submitted an interim report that dealt largely with the results of its discussions with representatives of AMS. The major concession achieved in these discussions had been an agreement whereby AMS would accept as members on its Board of Directors two designated representatives of OMA, who would serve on the Board in a liaison, consultant, and advisory role. AMS also agreed to accept the names of two physicians put forward by each medical society in Ontario in which AMS had a significant number of participating physicians in its plan, and that these physicians would be considered by the Board of Directors of AMS for election as members of the AMS corporation. As members they would become entitled to attend the annual meeting of the corporation and any special meetings that might be convened. These concessions by AMS would result in an "OMA voice" on its Board, and could serve to establish a more understanding and cooperative relationship. The committee admitted, however, that the concessions would not establish any control by OMA over the operations of AMS. It is of interest and importance that Dr. Hannah stated his opposition to the appointment of OMA representatives to his Board but was outvoted by the other directors.

Accepting the interim report of the committee, OMA acted quickly early in 1942 to name its two representatives to the AMS Board: Dr. C.C. White, a senior member of the Board of Directors of OMA, and Dr. W. McCutcheon, the Assistant Secretary of OMA.

In the following months, the Voluntary Health Insurance Committee examined the prepayment plans of AMS and WMS and the difficulties they were experiencing in their operations. While both plans were reporting a steady increase in the number of subscribers, they both agreed that their continuing success and their solvency depended on the cooperation of the participating physicians. This cooperation included physicians' submitting claims that were reasonable, supportable on the basis of good medical practice, and sensible of the financial resources available to the plans. The committee was also made aware of the increasing number of "specialists" in the ranks of physicians and the contention of such specialists that they were entitled to additional fees for all the services they rendered to subscribers. The committee appreciated that prepayment for medical services was a new venture in Ontario and that more experience with the operation of the plans would be needed before an "ideal" plan could be developed.

In May of 1942, the Voluntary Health Insurance Committee submitted its final report to OMA. It contained thirteen recommendations and conclusions, most of which had appeared in some form in reports of other committees. The report stressed the necessity of full cooperation of physicians with the prepayment plans, and emphasized that the aim of any plan should be participation of all general practitioners and specialists. There was a recommendation that an advisory committee be appointed by OMA to act as a liaison between OMA and the two prepayment plans. Several references were made to the need to resolve several differences between OMA and AMS: the principal ones lay in their views of the objectives and methods of operation of AMS and in their views of what should constitute OMA "sponsorship".

Following some preliminary and unproductive discussion with the directors of the Ontario Blue Cross plan about the possibility of developing a jointly sponsored hospital and medical care insurance plan, the directors of OMA decided to reappoint the Voluntary Health Insurance Committee to consider how a voluntary medical care insurance plan for the province might be developed. In reporting to the OMA Council, the committee described an increasing activity on the part of commercial insurance companies, who were setting their own payment schedules for medical services without any real regard for the OMA fee schedule. These companies were devising numerous kinds of policies that offered coverage for the cost of medical and hospital services on an "indemnity" basis: that is, payment for the services was a stipulated maximum amount set down in the policy. Some medical and hospital care policies were being offered as "packages" – life insurance, accident insurance, and health insurance. With many of the policies, it was asserted, the commission payable to the insurance salesman was about thirty per cent of the premium. The committee also noted that many employers, often as the result of union activity, were seeking health insurance coverage for their employees with the employer to pay part of the premium. These employers were therefore interested in a comprehensive plan; the employees favoured a "service" plan such as that offered by AMS and Ontario Blue Cross. As well, the provincial government was moving into the medical care field by subsidizing the costs of the diagnosis and treatment of cancer in clinics across the province.

The committee reported that after several conferences with representatives of AMS and WMS, it had been unable to persuade the two plans to consider amalgamation or to expand into a provincial plan under OMA sponsorship. The expressed intent of both AMS and WMS was to continue as separate corporations. Exploring the legal position of OMA, the committee had determined that the existing letters patent of OMA would not permit its operation of a prepaid medical care plan, but little difficulty was anticipated in obtaining their amendment for that purpose.

Weighing all the above factors, the committee recommended to OMA that it abandon its endeavour to expand the existing plans to permit province-wide coverage. In the view of the committee, it was time for OMA to assert itself and make clear its commitment to prepayment of medical care by becoming directly involved in the planning, development, and operation of its own plan.

The members of OMA were not prepared to go ahead with the committee's recommendation, and at their annual meeting in 1943 decided to again examine the possibility of amalgamating AMS and WMS. In addition, further discussions were undertaken with the Ontario Hospital Association and its Blue Cross plan and with representatives of insurance companies operating in the health care field. That no definite course of action followed for almost two years was due largely to two factors. First, from mid-1943 to mid-1945 a committee of the Canadian Medical Association was actively considering a federal government scheme of compulsory health insurance patterned on the studies carried out following the report of the Heagerty Committee. The Heagerty Committee had studied intensively the whole question of health insurance in Canada and proposed a comprehensive form that would be instituted with the cooperative participation of the provinces. Largely as a result of federal government support for the recommendations of the Heagerty Committee, there were some indications that a federal-provincial plan might become a reality. CMA had gone so far as to appoint its "negotiating" committee to ensure that the voice of organized medicine was heard in any federal-provincial deliberations. In this two-year period OMA, anticipating the coming of a federally sponsored plan, decided to leave CMA to express its views, and provincial activity on the subject of health insurance was restrained. By mid-1945, however, no national health insurance plan was imminent because the federal and provincial governments were unable to reach agreement. Primarily the problem was how such a plan would be financed, although numerous other matters, such as the role of physicians in the proposed plan, were far from resolved. There seemed to be general agreement at the time that national health insurance was not a top priority for the post-war period; as it turned out, the question was set aside but not abandoned.

The second factor causing delay by OMA was the concern expressed by several members about the significant number of Ontario physicians who were then serving in the armed forces in Canada and overseas. A survey of these physicians showed that a majority of them were not in favour of a national health insurance plan in which physicians would be required to participate. The opinion of OMA was that no decision on medical care insurance in Ontario should be made until the war was concluded and the returned physicians had an opportunity to express themselves.

The spectre of a state form of health insurance, which alarmed many Ontario physicians, now appeared to recede into the future. With the end of the war imminent, OMA could be in a position to move towards establishing its province-wide plan. The Board of Directors of OMA and its General Council were still hesitant about taking action as recommended by its committees. Early in 1945, the directors of OMA decided to establish an organization to be known as Ontario Medical Services Incorporated and to provide funds to meet the expenses of its board of directors. This new organization was to have on its board of directors three representatives from OMA, six from AMS, and three from WMS, and it was proposed that this organization "be established on such terms as might be mutually agreed upon and that such organization be charged with the responsibility of administration and development of health insurance in the province of Ontario". However, when the directors of OMA approached the provincial government with an application for an amendment to its letters patent to set up Ontario Medical Services Incorporated, the application was turned down on the grounds that it had not been approved by a majority vote of the membership.

Faced with a strong element of indecision within its own ranks, OMA decided to seek some compromise short of recommending its own movement into a prepaid medical care plan. In 1945 and into early 1946 it again discussed with the Ontario Blue Cross plan the possibility of developing a combined or amalgamated Blue Cross/OMA plan to cover both hospital and medical care. Discussions were also held with representatives of the insurance companies in Ontario that offered hospital and medical care policies.

In all of these discussions, the problem was the measure of control OMA might have over the operation of plans sponsored by Blue Cross and insurance companies. By early 1946 OMA had concluded that any plan with which it might become involved must be substantially under its control.

Late in 1945, the Board of Directors of OMA approved a by-law for amending the letters patent of the corporation to permit it to legally participate in developing and supporting a prepaid medical care plan but precluding it from having ownership and full control of such a plan. When this by-law came to the General Council of OMA for approval, a variety of differing views were expressed about what should be done. A vote of those at the meeting showed a majority opposed to the by-law and in favour of deferment of any action on it at that time.

To ratify the by-law, as required by government, a general meeting of members of OMA was convened on 13 February 1946. The members divided themselves into three categories – those who believed OMA should not be in the "insurance business"; those who believed any plan in the province should be run by AMS, WMS, insurance companies, Blue Cross, or amalgamations of these; and a third group who sought delay in any OMA action on the premise that the whole subject required further study. The by-law revision was defeated in that it did not receive the required two-thirds vote of the members. During the meeting AMS, reacting to the indecision of OMA, advised OMA of its withdrawal from Ontario Medical Services Incorporated.

Probably with the hope that the passage of time would help to resolve the problems facing it, OMA decided to delay any action and to bring the controversial by-law for discussion at the May 1946 annual meeting. Again an intense debate ensued, with Dr. Hannah speaking strongly against the by-law revision. To complicate matters, WMS supported the by-law revision. When the proposed revision came to a vote, there were 109 in favour and 94 opposed; the by-law was again declared defeated because it did not receive the required two-thirds majority vote. To complicate matters even further, the Ontario Hospital Association notified OMA that it intended to seek supplementary letters patent to permit Blue Cross to offer medical care benefits along with its hospital care benefits. OHA's action was motivated by its inability to develop a joint package with OMA support.

In October 1946, the directors of OMA sought the views of members through a questionnaire mailed to 5,122 physicians in Ontario. Replies were received from about half of them. Opinions were quite decisive on two questions: eighty-two per cent were in favour in principle of voluntary prepaid medical care in Ontario; and eighty per cent were opposed to such a plan being operated by the Ontario Hospital Association. Almost sixty-five per cent were opposed to OMA's operating a plan, but some sixty per cent were in favour of OMA's sponsoring a plan – independent of the Board of Directors and Council of OMA, but in the control of physicians who were members of OMA. The directors of OMA concluded that the results made it clear that OMA now had the responsibility to organize a province-wide plan according to these criteria. A final effort was made to structure the plan with the existing plans of AMS and WMS, but without success; both AMS and WMS continued during their lifetimes to function independently.

To proceed as quickly as possible, OMA moved in February 1947 to appoint a three-man Special Committee on Voluntary

Prepaid Medical Care, chaired by Dr. M.C. Watson. It is recorded that the committee held thirty-three meetings in three months and by June 1947 presented a detailed list of recommendations to the Board of Directors of OMA. The most important one was to seek from the Provincial Secretary a charter for a new corporation, to be known as Physicians Services Incorporated (PSI). The charter, similar to those granted to AMS, WMS, and Blue Cross, effectively created one more prepaid plan. To meet the organizational and start-up costs of PSI, OMA authorized a loan of up to $25,000 at 2½ per cent interest and agreed to make available on loan such other funds as might be required. By October 1947, the corporate structure of PSI was completed, a general manager and medical officer were appointed, and a small office was acquired. PSI started business in December.

In planning PSI, great care was taken to ensure that, while it was separate from OMA, its "control" (which implied control of its operation) was in the hands of the medical profession. The governing body, known as the House of Delegates, was made up of elected representatives from the medical societies and academies across the province, with the addition of direct appointments by OMA. The directors were to consist of not more than ten persons of whom seven must be medical practitioners. The directors constituted the Board of Governors; although they could appoint carefully selected laymen to the House of Delegates, the control of the organization clearly rested with the physician appointees from the medical societies and academies in the province.

Following the pattern of AMS and WMS, each physician in Ontario could become a participating physician in PSI by signing an agreement. A physician in general practice had to accept the payment by PSI as final payment unless the patient's income exceeded a specified limit. A certified specialist physician was paid the specialist fee based on the OMA schedule of fees, but could bill a patient, regardless of income, for the difference between that fee and the usual fee applicable to his or her specialty. The PSI payment to the physician was set at ninety per cent of the OMA fee – a procedure described as "prorating"; the remaining ten per cent of the fee was retained by PSI as "reserve" funds, sometimes referred to as a contingency reserve.

Although PSI did provide coverage for single and family subscribers, it did not seek them as AMS did but concentrated on group enrolment. Its principal plan covered home and office calls, care in hospital, consultations, operations, childbirth, and X-rays and other diagnostic procedures. The initial rates established were $1.50 per month for a single subscriber, $3.50 for a subscriber and one dependant, and $5.00 for a family. Lower rates were available to those who wished coverage only for surgical and obstetrical services.

In its first year of operation, PSI acquired 2,400 participating physicians and enrolled 21,263 persons, of whom about 10,000 were subscribers and the balance dependants. Its first year of operation compared rather closely with that of AMS, but in later years it far surpassed AMS, reaching about 1,400,000 subscribers by 1961 and establishing itself as by far the largest prepaid medical care plan in Ontario.

Thus, after ten years of indecision, debate, and the appointment of many committees, in the finale it was on the basis of a questionnaire to which only approximately half its members replied that OMA decided to sponsor and create a voluntary, non-profit prepaid medical care plan. Although the growth of PSI in terms of its number of subscribers was indicative of the need for such an organization, many problems in its operation revealed that the economics of the practice of medicine are difficult to handle by any method: most physicians were inclined to practise as individuals and were often reluctant to accept any "third party" arrangement in the financial relationship with their patients.

Although it might have been possible for AMS to have become part of, or the centre of, an OMA-sponsored plan, the discussions between OMA and AMS revealed some fundamental differences in general philosophy in the operation of such plans, along with serious differences of opinion on the meaning of medical sponsorship. An additional factor was the tendency of Dr. Hannah to express publicly his criticism of OMA, primarily because, in his view, OMA was not prepared to take a firm stand on the question of maintaining control over matters that were the primary concern of physicians – the provision of medical services of quality at a price within the ability to pay of those receiving the services. If a province-wide plan were to be initiated by OMA, using existing plans, then AMS was a more natural choice because it had offices in several centres in southern Ontario. As it turned out, AMS began to broaden its service base, particularly into parts of northern Ontario. WMS, as an independent organization, confined its activities largely to Essex County and, operating in close cooperation with OMA and PSI, ultimately achieved an enrolment of approximately 300,000 subscribers.

The views of OMA are exemplified by an address by its president, Dr. W. Magner, to the Annual Dinner of AMS on 17 February 1947. He reviewed the results of the OMA poll of its members of October 1946. Anticipating the development of PSI, Dr. Magner stated the opinion of OMA that WMS and AMS should become part of the OMA plan on terms that he was sure could be worked out in a cooperative manner, the result being one plan in Ontario, sponsored and supported by OMA. This proposal met with no positive response from AMS. There ensued a long period in which there was no real cooperation between AMS and OMA-PSI, in spite of their common objectives.

Developments within AMS

The early years of operation and administration of the AMS plan presented numerous problems. Most of these problems Dr. Hannah accepted as inevitable in such a new enterprise, and he continued to stress that the AMS plan was an experiment and a research project. He reiterated that a plan acceptable to the subscriber and to the medical profession, and at the same time administratively sound and financially solvent, could be ten or twenty years away.

From the start of the plan, and throughout its whole period of operation, Dr. Hannah insisted on the compilation of a great deal of information. Rather voluminous and detailed statistics in the form of reports, tables, and graphs showed clearly the age and sex and yearly income of subscribers, utilization and morbidity data, and financial information, which included extensive cost analysis. This information was made readily available to those asking for it and was used in other Canadian provinces where similar prepayment plans were in their formative stages. For several years, Dr. Hannah served on the tariff committee of OMA, and his advice and the results of his experience were frequently sought when changes in the OMA schedule of fees were being considered. He was a popular speaker and made numerous speeches, predominantly to medical audiences, across Canada and at several locations in the United States.

The number of subscribers, as previously noted, showed a steady increase in the ten-year period, reaching approximately 43,000 by the end of 1947. Dr. Hannah concluded that this was a satisfactory rate of growth, especially since it was accompanied by financial solvency and the accumulation of a reserve fund to which additions were made almost every year. He was opposed to AMS becoming "big business" by seeking large numbers of subscribers, believing that the most important consideration was to develop the plan in the light of experience and to carry on continuous "research". From the start, the plan had offered its benefits to single and family subscribers, because Dr. Hannah believed that young and growing families were most in need of a method of budgeting for the cost of medical care and would be a source of future subscribers. The plan had been geared to appeal to middle-class earners, who, Dr. Hannah was convinced, were the ideal market for prepayment plans. Confirming that the plan was serving this middle-class group, statistics compiled on the wage groupings of applicants for membership in the plan showed that seventy-eight per cent had yearly incomes under $2,000 annually, and of these, twenty-eight per cent had yearly incomes under $1,000. Over the ten-year period, AMS became aware of the many administrative problems with single and family subscribers, such as keeping track of the number of dependants. The administrative costs came to be excessive, and experience with the utilization of benefits showed a need for spreading the risk on insurance principles.

Although WMS and later PSI offered single and family plans, their emphasis was on "group" enrolments, which were more attractive to would-be subscribers and much easier and cheaper to administer. While maintaining its single and family offering, AMS decided late in 1945 to move into the group enrolment field. The experience with this form of enrolment will be discussed later.

With regard to benefits offered under the plan, two of these were changed during the period. Most of the earlier estimates of the utilization of benefits and their cost proved to be reasonably accurate. By 1941, however, the benefits associated with childbirth had shown a remarkable increase in utilization, and a resultant increase in cost. Included in the childbirth costs were the attending physician's fee for prenatal and obstetrical care, the use of the obstetrical facilities at the hospital, the care of the newborn baby in the hospital, and the physician's fees for subsequent visits of the well baby to the physician's office. In the initial cost studies it had been estimated that in the first year after its birth, a well baby would not visit the physician more than three or four times. Experience showed that such visits were occurring much more frequently than calculated, especially when the care of the baby was in the hands of a paediatrician. Although there was a moderate increase in the birthrate in those years, the major cost factor was well-baby visits to physicians. Studies by AMS showed that if the current level of visits continued, their cost could place in jeopardy AMS's financial solvency. Further, when the war would end, a substantial increase in the birthrate could be anticipated and a concomitant increase in childbirth benefit claims. The only solution to this problem that AMS could see was to withdraw the benefit for well-baby visits; this was done with an effective date of 1 July 1942.

The belief of municipal health and welfare agencies that well babies should have periodic examination by nurses and, as might be required, by physicians led to the development across Ontario of "well-baby clinics", generally operated by municipal departments of health. To these clinics well babies could be taken for periodic health examinations without cost. It may be conjectured that AMS's decision to withdraw this plan benefit was of some importance in the development of the clinics.

The "special nursing" benefits provided by AMS, while not exceeding cost estimates in the 1937-42 period, became a problem in discrimination. By definition AMS was to pay for this benefit only when there were complications in the illness of a patient that required the attendance of a private nurse, the need being certified by a physician. But when some claims were refused and others were accepted in comparable circumstances, criticism arose against AMS. Rather than being cast as the arbitrator in disputes that involved the patient and the attending physician, AMS decided to withdraw this benefit effective 1 July 1942.

In both of the cases described, the alternative of increasing the fee of the subscriber was considered, but it was rejected as not likely to solve the problems.

Financially AMS appeared by 1940 to be on a sound footing. The corporation was debt-free, it owned a building well suited to its operations, and the steady growth in the number of subscribers was producing enough income to meet all expenses and leave some funds to establish a reserve for any "rainy days" that might be ahead. In the 1940-41 period, however, the predictions of income and expenditure showed that if some preventive action were not taken, the reserve could fall steadily through 1945 and the possibility of AMS becoming insolvent by 1946 would have to be faced. The withdrawing in 1942 of two subscriber benefits, along with continuing close attention to the costs of operation, resulted in a continuous rise in the percentage of income added to reserves until the end of 1945. In 1945, the addition to reserves was 16.9% of income, or $103,000 on an enrolment of some 33,000 subscribers.

The improvement in its financial position in terms of the reserves led the Board of Directors in 1945 to re-examine the decisions it had reached in 1942, and there were some suggestions that the withdrawn benefits should be reinstated. The concern of the Board was that a non-profit corporation might have difficulty in explaining the retention of a "profit" of $103,000. Dr. Hannah cautioned the Board that the conclusion of the Second World War would result in the return of several hundred Ontario physicians from service in the armed forces and many thousands of servicemen and women, of whom a significant number, especially those who were married, would seek membership in AMS. Although an increase in enrolment could be helpful, more physicians could mean expenses in excess of earnings at least in the 1946-50 period, and the present accumulated reserve funds could be needed in sustaining AMS through what could be a difficult five years.

The Board of Directors decided, however, that something should be done in reaction to the increase in the reserve funds. The first decision was to add as a benefit under the plan, for subscribers of at least five years' standing, the cost of treatment of pre-existing conditions that could be remedied by surgery, but with the exclusion of surgery for cosmetic reasons. The second decision was to add, for those subscribers, the treatment of pre-existing medical conditions. These decisions were reached only after long and heated debate and against the opinion of Dr. Hannah, who did not consider the reserve to be excessive.

As it turned out, the amount of money added to reserves in 1946 was about half that added in 1945, and again in 1947 it was about half that of the previous year. Expenditures exceeded income by 8.1% in 1948 and by 9.5% in 1949.

In 1946 and 1947, the AMS staff gave a great deal of study to costs. Practically all costs were showing increases; the increase in average cost per subscriber per month over the ten-year period was practically 100 per cent ($1.47 vs. $0.73). In 1947 the income from subscribers was $679,000, and the total paid out in claims was $649,000.

Of particular concern to the future of AMS were the results of a study made on the incidence and cost of home and office calls. The study showed that the cost of processing the claims for home and office calls was equal to, or greater than, the cost of the claims themselves. The conclusion expressed by Dr. Hannah is recorded as follows: "At the end of ten years' experience in this field, I personally concluded, and was supported by our administrative staff, that it is not possible to retain solvency on a fee for service basis if a plan includes home and office calls."

Other Developments

Reference may at this time be made to some other matters of interest and concern to Dr. Hannah and AMS during the ten-year period.

In the late 1930s, Dr. Hannah acquired a former summer

resort located on Lake Mazinaw near Cloyne, Ontario, about 18 miles north of Kaladar and 170 miles from Toronto. The property had several acres with a lake frontage and some cabins. Here Dr. Hannah developed an isolated weekend or holiday hideaway. Over the years, he gradually improved the property and its buildings. In the 1940s he invited, on weekends and holidays, members of the Board of Directors and representatives of the federal and provincial governments and of subscribers to AMS. Along with time for fishing, card playing, and other diversions, time was found for discussion of many aspects of health insurance. On occasion there were guests from the United States and other provinces, who presented their viewpoints on the subject. In October 1945, twelve guests were invited at AMS expense. The weekend conference was the first of what became known as the "Mazinaw conferences" and had a structured program with presentations on several selected subjects. In the following year another conference was held in October, and guests were present from British Columbia, Alberta, Manitoba, and Ontario. These conferences provided useful exchanges of information about activities across Canada in the development and operation of prepaid medical care plans.

In 1947, at the instigation of the Canadian Medical Association, representatives of all medical prepayment plans in Canada met in Winnipeg for a day during the CMA annual meeting. The program was largely designed by the leaders of AMS. The comment of Dr. Hannah on this meeting was that the results were as he had predicted – there was much talk, but not much of value was accomplished. At the meeting, Dr. Hannah presented a paper in which he emphasized the necessity of conducting prepaid medical care on a businesslike basis. He said that a primary objective of any plan must be to prove that it can provide for the costs of medical care and remain solvent. He defined the responsibility of a physician participating in a prepaid plan "to serve the interests of his patients in medical matters and to provide such reports as will enable a fair judgment to be made as to the responsibility of the plan towards the cost".

The success of AMS soon became widely known across Canada, and the consultant services of Dr. Hannah were in demand in several provinces. At his Toronto office Dr. Hannah had a rather steady stream of health care planners seeking firsthand information. For those for whom personal contact was not possible or practicable, his detailed descriptions of the plan and its experiences were reported in several journals, notably the *Canadian Medical Association Journal* and the *Ontario Medical Review*.

By the mid-1940s, most of the provinces in Canada had groups planning voluntary prepaid schemes with support and encouragement from organized medicine. At the CMA-sponsored conference held in Winnipeg in June 1947, the opinions expressed by CMA and the provincial planners were that there was an urgent need for the medical profession to develop plans as an alternative to government-sponsored medical care insurance. At that time, there were only two other medically sponsored plans in Canada aside from AMS and WMS in Ontario: one in Saskatoon was incorporated in 1946, and the other in Manitoba started to operate in 1944. Between 1947 and 1954, medically sponsored voluntary non-profit plans came into operation in Ontario (PSI), British Columbia, Alberta, and Nova Scotia. A plan under a cooperative arrangement with Blue Cross was developed in Quebec in 1946, and in 1948 a medical care plan under the auspices of the Maritime Hospital Association was organized.

Tragedy was also a part of these years for Dr. Hannah and his family. In October 1945 Dr. Hannah's only son died as the result of injuries received when his bicycle was struck by a car. The loss was a particularly hard and lasting blow to Dr. Hannah, who had seen the possibility of his son carrying on as his successor in the future of AMS.

CHAPTER IV

Growth and Development – 1947 to 1959

By 1947 AMS had accumulated much information about the utilization of plan benefits, their costs, and the effects of various types of controls on the total payments AMS would be responsible for in a specified time. On the basis of this information, the directors were able to set subscriber fees with some accuracy. The concerns about the solvency of the plan had been relieved by the accumulation of reserves of $625,000 by 1947. (AMS was apparently never called to account for these reserves as a non-profit corporation.) Branch offices were still functioning in Ottawa, Hamilton, London, and Woodstock. (The Woodstock and London offices were closed late in the 1940s.)

In Canada Dr. Hannah came to be recognized as a pioneer in the prepaid medical care movement. He visited most provinces to describe the AMS experiences and to give advice and assistance to those concerned with the planning and development of similar plans. The continuing success of AMS had considerable influence in persuading several provinces to bring into operation plans based in most instances on the AMS plan. During the period 1946 to 1954 plans were started in Saskatoon, Regina, Winnipeg, and Vancouver. Representatives of these plans and from WMS, and Dr. Hannah from AMS, met in Winnipeg in June 1947 under the auspices of the Canadian Medical Association. The intention of the meeting was to establish by some form of organization for the benefit of present and future plans, a cooperative arrangement. Further meetings continued, and by 1951 a national organization, initially called Trans-Canada Medical Services, and later, in 1953, Trans-Canada Medical Plans (TCMP), was formed with Mr. G. Howard Shillington as its executive director. This organization invited to membership all non-profit prepayment medical care service plans in Canada, each endorsed by a division of CMA. The stated purposes of the organization were described as

i) To coordinate the activities, methods, procedure, coverage and data of members plans.
ii) To promote the establishment of an operation of such other non-profit medical care plans throughout Canada as will adequately meet the health needs of the public and maintain the high quality of medical care rendered by the medical profession.
iii) To arrange for the provision of medical care on a national basis through the medium of its members plans and cooperating carriers.
iv) To provide statistical or other information, counsel or assistance on all matters pertaining to the provision of prepaid medical care.

At the time of formation of Trans-Canada Medical Services in 1951, there were six member plans: two from Ontario, one from Manitoba, two from Saskatchewan, and one from British Columbia. In the following years members from Alberta, Ontario (PSI), Quebec, and the Maritime Provinces were added to bring the total to eleven plans in 1954, the maximum number of TCMP members. In the years of its operation (it continued until 1969), TCMP showed a steady growth in the number of Canadians enrolled in the member plans: in 1951, 775,165, which represented 5.5 per cent of the population of Canada. By 1960 the enrolment had increased to 4,139,572, or 23 per cent of the population.

With regard to membership standards in TCMP, it was stipulated that:

The Plan shall be sponsored, endorsed, approved, or designated by a Provincial Medical Association as a plan acceptable to its standards in each Province and shall maintain close cooperation with members of the medical profession in the area served by it.

AMS had an active part in the formation of TCMP in the years 1947 to 1951, but it did not become a member, although both PSI and WMS in Ontario became active and influential members. Mr. Shillington has written: "The major reasons for failure [of AMS] to affiliate [with TCMP] seemingly related to differences of opinion between the [AMS] Plan and the Ontario Medical Association during the 1940s, which led to the decision by the profession in 1947 to establish Physicians Services Incorporated."[1] From the records, including the comments of AMS on this membership issue, it appears that Mr. Shillington had but part of the answer. The rest of the answer is the determination of AMS to operate as an independent organization removed from the influence or direction of OMA.

In its years of operation, TCMP became a leader in developing a common nomenclature for its member plans, in encouraging and reporting the results of research and statistical studies, and in developing procedures for inter-plan transfers of subscribers who moved from one province to another. TCMP also endeavoured to develop in cooperation with its provincial members what was described as a "national uniform contract" to be made available to groups of employees whose employer operated in more than one province. The difficulties in developing such a contract became a major concern for TCMP, and AMS came to the rescue of TCMP by developing a national uniform contract for the railways – an activity of AMS that will be described later. As it turned out, this background role with respect to TCMP was particularly valuable to AMS, but it does appear that AMS could have made an important contribution to TCMP by assuming membership.

In the late 1940s, the Ontario government decided that the three non-profit medical care plans – AMS, WMS, and PSI – as well as the hospital insurance plan, Blue Cross, should be brought under separate and specific legislation. When AMS was formed, it had been granted its charter for incorporation under the Companies Act, and similar charters were subsequently granted to WMS, PSI, and the Ontario Hospital Association for Blue Cross. In the case of the first three corporations, the Companies Act required only that they make an annual return to the Provincial Secretary

---

[1] G.H. Shillington, *The Road to Medicare in Canada* (Toronto: DEL Graphics Publishing, 1972, p. 66).

showing the names and addresses of directors and officers. The rest of the return concerning bond holdings and debenture debt was not applicable to them. The letters patent for the Blue Cross corporation required that its operations be under the supervision of the provincial Minister of Health and that "all schedules of subscription charges and schedules of hospitalization shall be subject to the approval of the Minister of Health and filed with the Provincial Secretary". This reporting requirement was withdrawn in 1951 by amendment to the letters patent.

In the spring of 1950, an Act Respecting Prepaid Hospital and Medical Services was passed by the provincial legislature. This Act transferred all four plans from under the authority of the Companies Act and the Provincial Secretary to the provincial Department of Insurance, whose Superintendent was given designated powers of supervision of the plans. These changes seemed to express the view of government that the prepaid plans were a form of insurance.

In the Act, the word "Association" was used to describe any organization that offered, on a non-profit basis, prepaid medical or hospital care or both to residents of Ontario. By the terms of the Act, all such associations had to make application to the Superintendent of Insurance to be registered to conduct their operations in Ontario. Yearly renewal of registered status was required. The granting of registration was conditional on the Superintendent of Insurance being satisfied that the contracts by the association with hospitals, physicians, and other persons for the rendering of services and the contracts with subscribers or members were fair and reasonable. An additional requirement was that the applicant association establish and maintain working capital and reserves that the Superintendent considered adequate. Each registered association had to file each year with the Department of Insurance a general report on its affairs along with a statement of income and expenditures. The Act also stated that the Superintendent might at any time inspect the books, documents, and records of any registered association.

This Act came as a shock (although not entirely as a surprise) to Dr. Hannah, who continued to maintain that prepayment for medical care as AMS pictured it, although it functioned on insurance principles, was not in fact a form of insurance. This thesis he had propounded on many occasions previously and continued to do so, but with a worrisome lack of converts. He also – and in this had some support from the other plans – expressed his belief that the Act and the supervisory authority granted to "government bureaucrats" by the Act was a prelude to more governmental control over physicians and hospitals. The Act, however, was the contact between the plans and government from 1950 to 1969, and there were very few occasions of difference or conflict. Each plan sought some support for increases in subscription rates by submitting them for approval to the Superintendent of Insurance, who often had a difficult role to fill in dealing with them.

Prior to 1947, AMS had for comparison purposes WMS. Its benefits and subscription rates were almost identical with those of AMS. By 1951, WMS had about 106,000 subscribers. Late in 1947, however, PSI became operative in Ontario. Concentrating on group enrolment, it rather quickly covered most of the province. Its benefits and subscribers' fees were usually quite similar to those of AMS. At the end of 1951, PSI had about 218,000 subscribers, and by the end of 1959 this figure had become 1,246,000, a rather remarkable growth.

During the period under review, but particularly in the 1950s, the commercial insurance companies expanded rapidly into medical and hospital insurance. By the end of 1959, their policyholders almost matched the total number insured by WMS, AMS, and PSI. The companies offering coverage for medical services fell into two categories: the first were those selling life insurance but also offering sickness and accident policies as additional coverage; the second were those offering insurance coverage for sickness and accident, the coverage usually paying varying portions of the costs of hospital and medical services. Some of the companies also offered policies that provided cash benefits for time lost from work because of accident or illness.

The protection offered by these companies was of the "indemnity" type; that is, the company undertook to reimburse the insured person a stipulated amount, known as a cash indemnity, if an insured contingency occurred such as a surgical operation or an admission to hospital. The amount paid was usually less than the charge made by a physician or a hospital, unless the policyholder had paid a higher premium for fuller coverage.

With these indemnity policies the insurance companies were able to offer a variety of health and accident insurance to both groups and individuals and to tailor insurance contracts to meet the desires of those seeking the insurance and the premiums they were prepared to pay. In contrast, the non-profit prepaid plans offered what were described as "service" contracts to their subscribers, which were designed to pay the total cost of services rendered by a physician or hospital. The non-profit plans usually had some limitations on the amounts they were obligated to pay; those providing medical care coverage offered some stipulated payments of an indemnity type for hospital services. The other apparent contrast was that the insurance companies had to make a profit, and to remain competitive with the non-profit plans they had to design their policies with considerable care and market them by salesmanship.

The 1950s were years of economic growth, unemployment was a minor problem, wages and salaries were rising, inflation was not a worrisome concern, and employers were generally pleased with their profits. As the national economy moved from the war years to the post-war period, questions of social assistance came to be considered by all political parties. Employers and employees were giving increasing attention to "employee benefits", and unions often gave prominence to benefits in bargaining.

Growth of sponsored and supported health care programs was world-wide. In such a setting, it seemed inevitable that there would be a rapid growth of medical care insurance. The post-war years came to be a period of intense competition for its provision. Employers increasingly accepted that they had an obligation to assist employees, and frequently their families, with payment of the cost of fees or premiums.

In the late 1940s and into the 1950s, employee groups, especially the larger ones, having both hospital care and medical care plans, began to seek a "package" arrangement whereby one insurer would provide both types of coverage. The non-profit medical care plans had considered this eventuality in their offering as an additional benefit a cash indemnity on admission of the subscriber to hospital, plus an amount for hospital charges not paid by Blue Cross such as for use of an operating room and for X-ray and laboratory services. Continuing demand for package arrangements in the early 1950s resulted in Blue Cross losing existing and potential subscribers, chiefly to insurance companies who were offering the packages.

Suggestions were made about a possible amalgamation between Blue Cross and AMS, both of whom would offer each other's coverage. There was also some discussion about some form of a combined hospital/medical-care insurance plan between AMS and Blue Cross, but without any tangible result – possibly because at the time Blue Cross had some one and a half million subscribers whereas AMS had about a hundred thousand. In any event, AMS seemed determined to maintain its independence. In 1952 Blue Cross obtained an amendment to its letters patent permitting it to offer contracts that would pay for the services of a physician to a hospitalized subscriber as well as for surgical and obstetrical procedures performed in a hospital. This move by Blue Cross was to its advantage; two years later about 300,000 Blue Cross subscribers were covered for the medical and surgical in-hospital benefits. However, OMA was highly critical, claiming that Blue Cross and the Ontario Hospital Association had no right or justification to be in the business of offering any form of medical care insurance. AMS entered a milder protest, noting that Blue Cross had found no answer to its problem in discussions with PSI and AMS and that there should be cooperation between the three plans since they had a common objective.

The principal cause of an increase in the cost of operating a medical care insurance plan, an increase reflected in the subscribers' fee or premium payable, is the fees payable to physicians. To deal with the difficult and contentious question of fees, OMA had had, since its inception, the authority to set its own schedule of fees and had also retained over the same period the fee-for-service principle. The Tariff Committee of OMA kept the fee schedule under constant review and made adjustments in the whole schedule at three- to five-year intervals. The principal concern was inflationary trends. As OMA-sponsored plans, PSI and WMS were frequently participants in the Tariff Committee discussions and were aware of the proposed fee changes well in advance of their announcement. These plans therefore had time to make necessary adjustments in the benefits and in the subscribers' fees. Because of its long experience, even though it was not an OMA-sponsored plan, AMS was frequently consulted by the Tariff Committee and by PSI and WMS about its interpretation of the impact of proposed fee increases. The calculations and predictions of AMS were usually proven to be remarkably accurate and reliable.

At the end of 1949, it was reported that AMS had made no general increase in its subscribers' fees since 1942, although in the period it was estimated that the costs of medical care had increased by between twenty and twenty-five per cent. This ability to maintain the same fee levels was due largely to the decision made in 1945 to establish and promote group enrolment and to give much less emphasis to enrolment on an individual basis. In June 1951, there was a general increase in subscribers' fees. The basic fee for an employee and his or her family in a group contract, which in 1946 was $2.40 monthly, was increased to $3.70 monthly and remained at that level until 1960. Over the following years fees increased significantly. Without going into more detail, it was recorded in the 1950s that the subscription rates for the three AMS plans were always competitive and usually lower than those of PSI and the insurance companies with regard to the insured benefits offered.

This competitive edge was the result of experience and careful management of all phases of the AMS operations. Many AMS subscribers had enrolled during the late 1930s, and in the 1940s, when the majority of them were transferred into the group plans, they had a continuing allegiance to AMS. Dr. Hannah and his staff operated on the basis of fairness to all and favour to none. Each group was expected to have a utilization of services within reasonable figures established over years of study. Groups who performed well and were self-supporting could expect a lower subscribers' fee or, more usually, the addition of some benefit. The groups that did not perform well could expect an increase in the subscribers' fee or some restriction on benefits.

Occasionally it became necessary to terminate a group. The same measure of scrutiny applied to individual subscribers: excessive use of services could lead to cancellation of the contract. All claims by physicians were assessed before being approved for payment, and those which appeared to involve excessive rendering of services were sent for examination by the Chief Medical Officer or Dr. Hannah. AMS could refuse to pay for the services in question as being unnecessary, and in some instances would withdraw the physician's participating status. Some of these judgements were questioned by the physicians and occasionally by lawyers acting on their behalf. Rarely would AMS withdraw or change a decision, and Dr. Hannah was not infrequently accused of being arbitrary and making decisions on claims without full command of the facts. Some of these instances led to a lasting enmity between Dr. Hannah and physicians caring for AMS subscribers. The response, by AMS, was that such judgements and decisions had to be made for the protection of all subscribers.

At the end of 1950 the total number of subscribers to AMS was approximately 80,000, which compared with about 20,000 at the end of 1940. At the end of 1959, there were about 298,000 subscribers. Part of this growth was the AMS share of the significant growth in the whole field in the 1950s, which was also experienced by PSI, WMS, and the commercial insurance companies.

A most important event for AMS enrolment, with important financial implications in the future, was its acquisition in July 1957 of the "railway contract". Reference has been made above to Trans-Canada Medical Plans (TCMP). As an organization of medically sponsored non-profit medical care plans across Canada, TCMP tried to develop in the mid-1950s a "national uniform contract" to serve companies having their employees in all or several provinces. Early in 1956, TCMP was examining the possibility of a plan for "non-operating" employees of all of Canada's railways together with their dependants. Its development involved a complicated arrangement in management-union discussions involving five railways and fifteen union groups. Many meetings with representatives of the railways, their consultants, and union representatives finally resulted in TCMP being awarded a contract to provide medical care insurance to the non-operating employees, within defined conditions, across Canada. TCMP, aware that the largest number of eligible railway employees resided in Ontario, asked PSI to develop and operate an acceptable plan that could be applied across Canada. PSI refused, stating its intention to confine its operations to Ontario. In mid-1957 TCMP then asked Dr. Hannah and AMS to take over the role proposed for PSI, even though AMS was not a member of TCMP and had previously expressed no interest in a national uniform contract. AMS accepted for several reasons: the opportunity to achieve a substantial increase in enrolment without the necessity of working for it in a competitive climate; the benefits to AMS in terms of an increase in reserves because of "built-in" profit in the plan offered to the railway representatives; and a chance to devise a plan to meet the specific requirements of the railway employees and thus demonstrate the unique capabilities of AMS. From the viewpoint of AMS, this was too good an opportunity to miss.

The primary negotiator for the railways contract was the Blue Cross Division of the Quebec Hospital Services Association in Montreal, and in that city representatives of AMS gathered in mid-1957 along with representatives of the railways and their advisers and consultants. It was understood that the contract and its dollar results would have application to railway workers in all provinces of Canada. AMS was successful in negotiating a contract to cover, for medical care insurance on a comprehensive basis, some 80,000 railway employees in Ontario, with seven railways being involved. During the following year, members of the "operating" unions of the railways were included in the contract. In 1958 and thereafter the number of covered employees grew to about 100,000. Every two years after the negotiation of the first railway contract, AMS geared itself for a negotiating session in Montreal for its renewal. Negotiations were frequently prolonged and difficult, but AMS was always successful in renewing the contract. In 1969 AMS was responsible for transferring the Ontario employees covered by the contract into the medicare plan in Ontario.

One other event of the 1950s that had important results for AMS, as well as the other providers of medical care insurance, was the coming of hospital care insurance in Ontario on 1 January

1959. This followed on, and was patterned after, the provisions for a national hospital insurance plan contained in the federal Hospital Insurance and Diagnostic Services Act, which received unanimous approval at the time of its passage in Parliament in April 1957. The government of Ontario was one of the most influential advocates of national hospital insurance to the federal government. The entry of Ontario into the national hospital insurance plan prohibited all insurers from offering coverage for any hospital services that were included in the very comprehensive plan covering such services in the province. One result was that Ontario Blue Cross ceased to provide basic hospital care insurance and became part of a new administrative agency of government, the Ontario Hospital Services Commission.

In 1952, as noted above, Blue Cross had decided to offer to its subscribers supplementary coverage for the costs of physicians' services while they were in hospital. With the coming of the national hospital insurance plan, Blue Cross withdrew this supplementary coverage, applied to some 400,000 of its subscribers in Ontario. Many of these wanted to continue their supplementary coverage, and AMS was able to transfer several thousand of them into its plan.

AMS and the other prepaid medical care plans, as well as the commercial insurance companies, were required by provincial legislation supporting the hospital insurance plan to withdraw from their subscribers' contract the indemnity component that most of them had (the stipulated payment for each day of hospital admission and for use of the operating room and X-ray and laboratory services). Removal of these hospital benefits implied either adjustments in subscribers' fees and insurance premiums or the broadening of existing medical care benefits.

In the "settling down" process following the start of national hospital insurance in Ontario, the Blue Cross plan continued to provide insurance to cover preferred hospital accommodation (private and semi-private). Later, Blue Cross expanded its coverage to include "extended health care benefits": private nursing care, out-of-province hospital care, ambulance services, and other services rendered by or in relation to hospitals.

AMS decided not to offer any coverage for non-insured

hospital services and for extended health care benefits, and to confine its coverage only to meeting the costs of medical care.

CHAPTER V

The Coming of Medicare – 1960 to 1972

Between 1960 and 1972 there was a sequence of events that ultimately required AMS to withdraw from the operation of its plan of medical care by prepayment. With the entry of Ontario on 1 January 1959 into the national hospital care insurance plan, there were predictions, not confined to political circles, that a national health insurance plan would follow: the federal government would add medical care insurance to hospital care insurance. Such a plan became a possibility with the passage by the federal government in 1966 of the Medical Care Insurance Act, which came into force in July 1968. Its provisions became known as "medicare", a descriptive term that will be used for ease of reference. By 1972 all provinces were participants in medicare.

What was described as the "imposition" of medicare was opposed with varying degrees of vehemence by the Canadian and provincial medical associations, by some provincial governments, and by numerous Canadian citizens, whose protests were given prominence in the "letters to the editor" columns of newspapers. The principal concerns expressed were that medicare was a prelude to government's taking over the control of the practice of medicine and that in time physicians would become civil servants. The deciding factor, as it had been when the hospital insurance plan was established, was the popularity of health insurance as a political issue and the conviction of all political parties that health insurance for Canadians could be established only by federal government initiative. As evidence of this political popularity, when the Hospital Insurance and Diagnostic Services Act was passed in 1957 in the House of Commons, there was unanimous approval with no dissenting votes. When the vote on the Medical Care Insurance Act was held in 1966, only two recorded votes opposed its adoption.

The most significant contribution to the ultimate debates and decisions on medicare followed on the appointment, in 1961, of a Royal Commission on Health Services by the federal government. CMA had been increasingly aware of the active public and political interest in a medical care insurance plan having national application. In 1960, CMA decided to ask the federal government to appoint a royal commission to survey the present and potential health care resources in Canada in relation to a national medical care insurance plan. It was stressed that the royal commission should give its primary attention to the adequacy of health care resources in Canada in terms of facilities and numbers of physicians, nurses, and other providers of health care – who, in the CMA view, were in short supply. CMA also stressed that the royal commission should not have as a term of reference a determination as to whether it was advisable or desirable that a medical care insurance plan should be developed in Canada.

In December 1960, Prime Minister Diefenbaker announced that the requested royal commission would be established, but it was not until March 1961 that its chairman, Mr. Justice Emmett Hall, and its six members were appointed. Several supporting staff members were also appointed to conduct several research studies on its behalf.

The Royal Commission on Health Services travelled across Canada holding public hearings and receiving many reports, briefs, and other written material from individuals, groups, and organizations. At a public hearing on 8 May 1962 in Toronto, Dr. Hannah, as the spokesman for AMS, presented a written brief. In it he reviewed in much detail the history of AMS dating back to 1937 as a demonstration that it was possible to devise and operate a plan whereby people could provide for the costs of illness by the mechanism of prepayment. The success of AMS and its continuing solvency he attributed to its practical applications of its knowledge of medical economics and a cooperative effort between physicians and subscribers. He made reference to the prevailing booming economy as a contributing factor to the success of AMS.

He stressed that AMS was the result of private initiative without any assistance from government sources, and that a wider application of medical care by prepayment, supported by physicians and administered as non-profit plans, was preferable to government-sponsored and -operated medical care insurance. He predicted that if a government plan were instituted, there would be little or no effective control over its costs, and the utilization of medical services would increase substantially. He argued that the role of government should be confined to assisting those who by reason of low income, sickness, disability, or infirmity were unable to afford a prepayment plan. In presenting this argument, of course, he supported the contentious proposition that the "poor risks" for medical care insurance should be a government responsibility while the "good risks" were available to private enterprise.

It was probably not a coincidence, given Dr. Hannah's aversion to even the possibility of government participation in health insurance, that in the April 1962 issue of the *Ontario Medical Review* there appeared a full-page article written by him. He made some very critical comments about government and its expanding role in assuming responsibilities that he thought belonged to the individual. He pictured the Royal Commission as "a most convenient tool" of government in the introduction of health insurance and as assuming responsibility for the "spiralling costs" of health insurance that would inevitably follow. No mention is made of the possibility of a national health insurance plan being beneficial to Canadians.

In late June of 1964, the Royal Commission presented its report to the federal government. In the interval since it was appointed, a federal election had resulted in the defeat of the Conservative party under Mr. Diefenbaker and the election of the Liberal party under Mr. Pearson. The disposition of the report therefore fell to the Liberal party, which had for many years not given any vigorous support to a national health insurance plan. The full report consisted of several volumes and some two hundred recommendations, but the principal, most important, and arguable recommendation was that there be established in Canada a nationwide scheme of medical care insurance available to all residents and designed to cover the cost of all services provided by physicians; that the plan be developed as a cooperative effort between the federal and provincial governments; and that a portion of the cost be paid by the federal government. There was no doubt that these recommendations created surprise, and even some measure of consternation, when they were announced at the annual meeting of the CMA, which was in session at the time the report was presented.

AMS in the person of Dr. Hannah soon made clear its response to the report. This appeared in the September 1964 issue of the *Ontario Medical Review* under the title "Report of the Royal Commission on Health Services". The comments are certainly pungent and direct and take aim at economists, civil servants, politicians, and members of the medical profession, He claimed that the approach in the report was that more money given to good health services would buy good medical care. Dr. Hannah believed such an approach to be impossible. One small paragraph that is typical of the other comments may be quoted:

The best hope now is that the political football which has been concocted will be kicked around for so long that the profession can clear the fog from their thinking and will themselves set their economic house in order. This latter is so improbable that it makes the former all but inevitable.

This assemblage of metaphors exemplifies many of Dr. Hannah's writings. Clarity of expression was not his strong suit.

Time passed all too quickly for those who were trying to develop some effective opposition or alternatives to the recommended national plan. CMA proposed a rather unexpected alliance between the physician-sponsored prepayment plans across Canada that were members of TCMP and some hundred insurance companies that offered medical care insurance. The object was to persuade the federal government that a satisfactory national plan could be devised and operated by such an alliance. There was support for this idea in Ontario.

In July 1965, the federal government convened in Ottawa a conference of federal officials and the premiers of the provinces and their advisers. The chairman of the conference was Lester Pearson, and he wasted no time in informing those gathered that it was the intention of the federal government to enact as soon as possible a national medical insurance plan. A general outline of the terms and conditions of the plan was given for the guidance of the provinces, who could enter the plan on a voluntary basis. The attraction that left the provinces with little room to even consider staying out of the plan was the offer of the federal government to pay approximately fifty per cent of its cost in each province.

The birth of a national plan was delayed for several reasons that need not be described in any detail, but they centred around the ability of the federal and provincial governments to find their share of the estimated costs of the plan. In due course, however, the Medical Care Insurance Act was passed in December 1966 and became operative on 1 July 1968. All provinces in Canada became a party to the plan during the period July 1968 to January 1971, with Ontario joining on 1 October 1969.

Development of the Ontario Plan

In Ontario, the Conservative government had, in October 1962, submitted a brief to the Royal Commission on Health Services that stated that it had no firm position on a medical care plan in the province and intended to carry out more studies before making any commitment for or against medical care insurance. The premier, Mr. John P. Robarts, noted that approximately two-thirds of the residents in the province had some measure of health care insurance in existing prepayment or insurance plans. In December 1962, the Liberal party in the province, in a statement by its leader, Mr. John Wintermeyer, in the provincial legislature, declared its support for a comprehensive plan. It was proposed that the plan be financed by a combination of personal premiums and a special medical care insurance tax and that it be administered by a medical care insurance commission that would include representatives of government and the medical profession. The New Democratic Party in Ontario had repeatedly voiced its support for a government-sponsored and -supported plan patterned on that which had come into operation in Saskatchewan in the summer of 1962.

With the intention of taking some more definite stand on the issue, the Conservative government, after several months of consultation with both the providers and clients of medical care insurance, in April 1963 presented to the provincial legislature Bill 163, which was an introduction to proposed legislation described as "An Act Respecting Medical Care Insurance." The expressed intention of the Bill was to make medical care insurance available, on a voluntary basis, to all residents of the province through government-approved providers or carriers of such insurance, which would include the existing prepaid plans and the commercial insurance companies.

The Bill proposed offering two standard contracts: a fully comprehensive medical care coverage, and a partial coverage at lower premium rates and including deductibles and co-insurance payments. Enrolment in the plan by any resident, as defined, in the province would be on a voluntary basis. All insurance contracts would be "guaranteed renewable" – that is, non-cancellable by reason of age, chronic illness, pre-existing conditions, and other factors. No waiting period for benefits would apply to applicants who joined the plan during "open" enrolment periods. The province would pay the "premium" for those who were unable to because of poverty, illness, disability, or other reasons, and would partially pay for those whose income was below a certain level, which remained to be defined.

The Bill also proposed the formation of an organization to be known as Medical Carriers Incorporated, whose members would be licensed as providers of the insurance. The description of the purpose of this organization was the subject of a considerable amount of dispute; the purpose, however, seemed to be that of a "re-insuring agent", which would review and assign payments to the insurers on an equitable basis for claims made for services to "bad risks". This procedure, which in insurance nomenclature is called "pooling", was to ensure that the cost of "bad risks" was reimbursed on a reasonable, no-loss basis to all insurers from a fund established for that purpose.

The Bill, when presented to the legislature, was immediately assailed by the opposition parties with accusations that the government was "leaning over backwards to be of assistance to the insurance companies" and that the Bill was "a 100% capitulation to the insurance companies and the medical profession". Dr. Hannah wasted little time in criticizing the Bill, claiming that its approval could mean an end for the non-profit prepaid medical care plans in Ontario. He was also very critical of the "pooling arrangement", which he claimed would guarantee substantial profits for the insurance companies by minimizing their loss on high-risk policyholders. The sparsity of comment on the Bill from OMA was accepted by the government as support for the Bill. Press comment was generally unfavourable, it being claimed that the Bill was a poor "compromise" by government between "voluntary" and "compulsory" health insurance.

The criticism of the Bill in the legislature and the imminence of the summer recess led to a decision by the government to shelve the Bill and to appoint a "public committee" to study it in detail. An investigating committee was appointed in June 1963 under the chairmanship of Dr. J.D. Hagey, President of the University of Waterloo, with its membership including representatives from OMA. The committee proceeded to have public meetings, to receive and discuss briefs, and ultimately to prepare recommendations to the government. The Hagey Committee presented its report in December 1964 and it was made public on 27 February 1965. The report pointed out, in the following excerpt, an important difference between its views, which seemed to reflect those of the government of Ontario, and those of the Royal Commission on Health Services released in June 1964.

The Royal Commission recommended establishment of programs operated by governments, whereas the Ontario program, as approved by the Committee, is based on continued activity of private insurance carriers issuing standard contracts under regulations adopted by a government appointed body subject to a degree of supervision by that body.

In this statement, the Hagey Committee indicated its support for the major recommendations in Bill 163. Although some relatively minor changes in the Bill were proposed, these were largely of a more permissive type, such as a recommendation that physicians be paid 100 per cent of the OMA tariff for their services. (PSI was paying only 90 per cent of the tariff; the remaining 10 per cent was accumulated in a "reserve" fund.)

Based in large part on the Hagey Report, the government presented a revised Bill 163 to the legislature at its spring session in 1965. Again there was strong dissent by the opposition parties. Public hostility became apparent in regard to the use of private insurance companies as public carriers, following published reports on the substantial profits these carriers were expected to receive under the proposed government plan. The high premium rate proposed for those in the "poor risk" categories also invited criticism. The most direct and frequent comments were that the government was trying to find a compromise, having given its unwilling agreement to a compulsory, nationwide scheme as recommended by the Royal Commission on Health Services.

As might have been expected, Dr. Hannah did not waste much time in giving his response to the Hagey Committee report. Before doing so, however, he talked with the Minister of Health, Dr. M.B. Dymond, and urged him to withdraw the revised Bill 163, but without success. In the April 1965 issue of the *Ontario Medical Review*, there appeared an article over the signature of Dr. Hannah, with the title "A Mess of Pottage", very critical of the Bill and its recommendations.

On 24 April 1965, Dr. Hannah wrote an "open letter" of fourteen pages to Premier Robarts and to the members of the provincial legislature, strongly critical of the Hagey Report. He emphasized that the report had done little to ease the concerns of AMS, which he had expressed about Bill 163 at the time it had been presented to the legislature a year previously. He noted that the recommendations contained in the report were not much different from those made in the original Bill 163. He predicted that if the recommendations adopted included the increases in medical fees that OMA was pressing for implementation in 1965, the cost of medical services in Ontario would increase by twenty to thirty per cent. In his view the increase would be about twice what had been calculated in the Hagey Report and had been used in determining the premium payment for the basic plan proposed in the report. The letter also predicted that if the proposed

"Medical Carriers Incorporated" were established to pool the "bad risks", the result would be that the prepayment plans sponsored or supported by OMA (AMS, PSI, and WMS) would be forced into competition with the private insurance companies and would inevitably disappear.

Dr. Hannah's letter was well received by the Liberals and New Democrats, both parties having stated their support for a national plan of medical care insurance. The Hagey Report, in their opinion, was a Conservative party endeavour to find some compromise in providing medical insurance to residents of Ontario without recognizing that a nationwide plan was inevitable.

While there was no direct reply to Dr. Hannah's letter to the premier, it was apparent that the Conservative party in Ontario was considering its options, the Hagey Report being one. The reaction of OMA, as the spokesman for PSI, and that of WMS were not as vehement as that of AMS. Their attitude seemed to be more to "wait and see" what happened at CMA in its consideration of the report of the Royal Commission. The Ontario press did respond in several editorial comments to Dr. Hannah's letter, some supportive and some critical; but the general opinion seemed to be that the most important aspect of the whole subject was what action the federal government was planning to take in response to the report of the Royal Commission.

In his article in the *Ontario Medical Review*, Dr. Hannah had substantially reiterated the arguments in his brief to the Royal Commission and his "open letter" to the premier. He went on to say:

Further, AMS is prepared to put their experience at the disposal of the Ontario government and demonstrate that the cost of medical care, given reasonable support, freedom and time, can eventually be made a self-sustaining entity rather than a threat to both good medical care and the economy of the Province as a whole.

As a final comment in the article, the members of both the public and the medical profession were asked to contact the Ontario government and request "that the non-profit prepayment plans which have done so much for medical economics since 1937 be exempt from legislation which will force them out of the non-profit prepayment concept to become a part of the commercial insurance industry – thus destroying the pioneering leadership which has done so much for the advancement of coverage for 78% of the population now covered in Ontario."

There is no written evidence that the government of Ontario accepted or even considered the offer by AMS to provide advisory and consultant services. It is probable that Dr. M.B. Dymond, the Minister of Health, was more inclined to seek advice from the largest prepayment plan in Ontario, PSI, which at this time had about two million subscribers (AMS numbered less than three hundred thousand). As a politician, Dr. Dymond was certainly aware that some action seemed to be imperative if the government was to proceed with its plan to offer universal-coverage insurance of a comprehensive type. It is of passing interest to note that, as would be expected, the private insurance companies were in favour of the Hagey Report and its implementation. The comments on the report coming from OMA, as sponsors of PSI, were quite mild, and even supportive of the report, in comparison to the reactions coming from AMS. The opinion of OMA was that too much time had been given to the problem; it had no easy solution; and the time for action on the part of government was overdue.

When the recommendations contained in the Hagey Report were debated in the legislature in the early months of 1965, they were again strongly criticized by the opposition political parties, both of which were aligned in pressing for a government-operated form of medical care insurance applicable to all residents of the province. There was also opposition to the report from labour organizations and from the prepayment plans, again most vocally from AMS. It was in the midst of this debate that the federal government convened its July 1965 meeting of provincial representatives and, as described previously, endorsed the recommendation for a national plan as proposed by the Royal Commission on Health Services. With this federal initiative, Ontario now had another approach to consider – that being to enter into the proposed national plan.

It was decided, however, pending further study of the federal proposal, to proceed with examination and revision of the Hagey Report, seemingly a "rearguard" action. Progress was slow, and it was not until the early part of 1966 that a Bill dealing with the report was presented to the legislature. Most of the numerous changes and revisions to the Hagey Report included in the Bill seemed to be acceptable to AMS. Among the revisions was the decision of the government to assume the responsibility for insuring residents of the province who were unable to pay an "eligibility" premium as well as low-income and high-risk groups; this disposed of the original proposal that the prepayment plans and the insurance companies develop mechanisms for insuring these groups and sharing their costs. The "Medical Carriers Incorporated" concept was abandoned, and the prepayment plans and the insurance companies were left free to conduct their business without a central control over their operations. Other amendments provided for the payment of physicians serving patients insured by the province at 90 per cent of the OMA fee schedules, and the removal of a waiting period for maternity benefits and previously proposed limitations on certain medical services. Amidst accusations of delay and compromise, the new Act, known as the Ontario Medical Services Insurance Plan (OMSIP), was enacted effective 1 July 1966.

By the end of 1966, 585,000 residents of Ontario were enrolled in OMSIP and 6,154,000 were covered by the prepayment and insurance company plans. These numbers meant that 95.2 per cent of the population of the province had some measure of protection against the costs of medical care. It was repeatedly stressed to the provincial government, particularly by the insurance companies, that this high percentage of coverage had been achieved with a minimal amount of government assistance and there was no real need for a universal national government-sponsored plan.

The federal government had stated in July 1965 its intention of preparing and submitting for approval by Parliament an Act to establish a national medicare plan; however, it was not until about a year later that the Medical Care Insurance Act was put into final form. It was passed by the House of Commons on 8 December 1966, with Senate approval following quickly. At this time, inflation was affecting government costs and revenues, and a delay followed in implementing the Act while the federal and provincial governments struggled with the problem of determining how to find the funds to meet their additional obligations under the terms of the Act. It was not until 1 July 1968 that the provisions of the Medical Care Insurance Act could be put into effect.

In Ontario the government was having difficulty in deciding what to do about medicare. The intent of the Medical Care Insurance Act was to permit the establishment of a national medicare program with all provinces participating in a cooperative federal-provincial arrangement. But there was no requirement, as had existed when national hospital insurance was inaugurated in 1959, that a majority of the provinces must participate in the program to ensure the contribution of federal funds. The stipulation was that the federal government would pay to each province 50 per cent of a "national" per capita cost. To arrive at this figure, the per capita cost in each participating province would be determined yearly, and the results from all participating provinces would be averaged to produce the national per capita cost figure. Fifty per cent of that amount, per resident, would be paid annually in quarterly instalments to the province. The result was that a province such as Ontario with high per capita costs would receive about a quarter of its real costs, whereas a province such as New Brunswick with low per capita costs would receive as much as three-quarters of its real costs. Thus the cost-sharing formula for medicare continued the generally accepted arrangements between the federal and provincial governments whereby the less prosperous provinces receive proportionately greater federal payments than the richer provinces.

The Ontario government's examination of this formula led to the conclusion that if Ontario did not participate in the medicare program, it would be denying itself a substantial amount of federal moneys, determined as approximately $100 million for the fiscal year 1968/69. This was probably the most important factor in leading to the decision, late in 1968, to participate in the federal medicare program. An additional factor in the decision was the obvious support by Canadians for a national medicare plan: the vote on the Medical Care Insurance Act in the House of Commons had been 177 "ayes" against two "nays". In Ontario also, the very strong vocal opposition of Dr. Hannah was counter-balanced by the resigned attitude of OMA and PSI that a national medicare program was inevitable. The medical profession, as represented by OMA, believed that the national program presented no challenge to three of the basic tenets of the profession in Ontario – the free choice by the patient of his or her physician; the prerogative of the profession to determine the fee through its provincial association, to be charged by the physician to the patient; and the fee-for-service principle, which had long been cherished and protected. The retention of these three tenets presented a strong argument against those, rather few in number at the time, who contended that medicare was a preliminary step towards "socialized medicine".

Early in 1969, the provincial government arrived at an agreement with the federal government. The starting date proposed for the program was originally 1 July 1969, later changed to 1 October 1969. It was also decided that its administration and operation in Ontario would be a government responsibility carried on initially by the existing organization known as OMSIP, the Ontario Medical Services Insurance Plan. When these decisions were taken, the government met with the non-profit prepayment plans (PSI, WMS, and AMS) and the insurance companies to seek their cooperation in developing a non-profit consortium to deal with the administration of existing subscriber plans and policies until OMSIP could take them over. Both PSI and WMS refused to join the consortium and handed over their lists of subscribers by the starting date of 1 October 1969. Subsequently, PSI surrendered its charter and became a private foundation under the federal Registered Charities Act. It retained its reserves of about $15 million and has since used the income to support medical education and medical research in Ontario. Many of the staff of PSI became staff members of OMSIP in Toronto. WMS also surrendered its charter and, after some dispute with the provincial government, distributed its reserves to the physicians in Windsor and Essex County who were its initial financial supporters. Most of the staff of WMS were engaged by an OMSIP office set up in Windsor to transfer some 300,000 WMS subscribers into the provincial plan.

AMS as a Provincial Agency

AMS, after some rather prolonged debate in its Board of Directors and with officials from the Ministry of Health, decided to enter into an agreement with the provincial government to act as the latter's agent, undertaking the collection of premiums and the assessment of claims and their payment, all on a non-profit basis. Although the agreement had no termination date, AMS recognized that it would not be an indefinite arrangement; but it would give AMS time to proceed with plans to close its offices, sell its building, release its staff, and consider a future role or roles.

The private insurance carriers in the province agreed to accept an arrangement similar to that of AMS on a "non-profit/non-loss" basis. In mid-August they formed a corporation known as Healthco, which concluded agreements with twenty-nine companies to act as their representative and to deal with the transfer of some two and a half million policyholders into the government plan.

As 1 June 1937 was a momentous day in the life of AMS, so was 1 October 1969 – after thirty-two years as one of the pioneering prepaid medical care plans in Canada and a model for several plans that followed, AMS ceased to exist as a prepayment plan. The Board of Directors and its Managing Director now had to consider what its future should be.

The Ontario government decided that its medicare plan would be supported in part by the payment of a monthly premium by, or on behalf of, all residents of the province; this payment would complement the premium payment required to support the hospital insurance plan, which had started some ten years previously. At first the programs in hospital insurance and medicare were placed under separate administration. In 1972, however, the government set up, under its Ministry of Health, the Ontario Health Insurance Plan (OHIP), which assumed the responsibility for operating and administering the two programs. Thus "health insurance" was brought entirely under the authority of a government ministry. The Ontario Hospital Services Commission disappeared accordingly.

AMS Operations, 1960-72: An Overview

During the early 1960s there was a moderate degree of economic inflation; in 1965 and the following years it became more pronounced. Resultant increases in the cost of medical services were compounded by the costs of additional services being offered, especially in medical technology, both therapeutic and diagnostic; these new services were increasingly represented in the OMA schedule of fees. The fee increases in 1962 and again in 1965 – approximately ten per cent – caused the prepayment plans and the insurance companies to make several upward adjustments in fees and premiums.

Commencing in 1960, AMS had in rounded figures 201,000 subscribers to its plan, about three-quarters of these belonging to group plans.

In the 1960s, AMS continued to offer its plans, often in competition with PSI and the insurance companies, in the more heavily populated areas of Ontario centred in Toronto, Hamilton, London, Kingston, and Ottawa. Regional offices were maintained in Hamilton and Ottawa into the early 1960s, largely as information and enrolment centres, but were given up in favour of concentrating all operations at the Toronto office. Like other providers of medical care insurance, AMS had become predominantly an organization offering coverage to groups of employees.

Dr. Hannah, supported by his Board of Directors, contended that AMS should not endeavour to become "big business" in seeking a constantly enlarging enrolment. He maintained that a smaller number of subscribers, which in his mind seemed to approximate 300,000, was of sufficient size to permit utilization and research studies, and that this number would provide enough useful information about "medical economics". He continued to stress the vital importance to the medical profession of embracing and supporting the concept of medical care by prepayment as the means of keeping the practice of medicine under the profession's control. He said on numerous occasions that if the medical profession was interested only in methods, such as those developed by the insurance companies, of obtaining payment for their services, there was the danger of government intervention and control in the affairs of the profession. In any event, AMS did not make any really concerted effort to bring about any substantial increase in the number of its subscribers, which was approximately 273,835 at the end of 1969.

In the 1960s, the experience of AMS led to the modification of some of its enrolment and payment policies. The first change was to pay general practitioners' fees in full (in contrast with PSI, which paid 90 per cent of the fee). Over the years AMS gradually reduced the "waiting period" for coverage for obstetrical care, for elective surgery such as herniotomy and tonsillectomy, and for examinations of the eye by ophthalmologists. Payments for surgical care were at the OMA tariff. Limited payment for laboratory and radiological services rendered by physicians was almost entirely removed by 1960. With group plans, limitations related to pre-existing health conditions were largely removed, as were age limits. Some ten years previously, in 1950, AMS had removed home and office calls from its benefits, having concluded after some twelve years of experience that it was not possible to stay solvent if they were included. By 1960, AMS decided to reintroduce home and office calls as a benefit; this benefit was popular, and PSI had covered home and office calls from its inception in 1947. It had become evident that AMS subscribers wanted the coverage and were prepared to pay for it.

On at least two occasions in the 1960s, OMA made overtures to AMS about the possibility of an amalgamation of AMS with PSI. Several meetings between the two followed, but terms for amalgamation as proposed by AMS were not acceptable to PSI, the principal proposal being that Dr. Hannah be appointed Director of Research at PSI at a substantial salary. AMS was also insistent that it retain its reserve funds. No common grounds for amalgamation being found, the subject was not raised again by either party.

The most significant development affecting AMS in the 1960-72 period was the substantial growth in its reserve funds. These funds became of much importance when decisions about the future of the corporation were considered. Previous reference has been made to the procedure instituted by AMS in the 1950s, described as "experience rating", whereby the utilization of medical services was examined for each group of subscribers over a period of several months and compared with the expected utilization and with that of other groups. This procedure continued to be applied to practically all groups in the 1960s. The results were used to adjust subscribers' fees – either upwards or downwards – and to determine new rates related to the periodic fee increases of OMA. The experience-rating studies were developed into quite accurate predictions of the changes in benefits and adjustments in their costs, which would be reflected in the fees charged to subscribers. These adjustments enabled AMS to function without a loss. Of more importance to the future was the addition to the fee structure of an amount calculated to permit the transfer, each year, of about ten per cent of total income to the reserves of AMS.

Careful attention was given to the cash flow reaching the central office monthly, and all cash-flow surpluses were invested in short-term certificates. An investment policy was continued whereby the existing and accumulating reserves were placed in bonds and similar securities.

In 1964-65, the policy of AMS of confining investment of its reserves to government and municipal bonds and debentures was changed, and AMS began to invest, to the maximum permitted by the Department of Insurance, in preferred and common stocks of Canadian companies with the objective of achieving capital gains. An internal committee, consisting of Dr. Hannah as Managing Director, Dr. Boyd Upper as Chief Medical Officer, and Mr. K.W. Atcheson as Secretary-Treasurer, was formed to deal with the investment and reinvestment of the reserves. This committee sought the advice and assistance of investment counsellors and brokers. A strong stock market during much of the 1960s enabled AMS to steadily increase the value of its reserves and the derived income.

The result of these management decisions was to develop substantial reserves, which reached $11,278,574 at the end of 1969. This increase was the result, in large part, of careful attention to investment, but most of the funds for investment came from the addition to the reserves, each year, of about ten per cent of the income from subscribers. In 1959, the income from subscribers was shown as $5,799,593 and the reserve as

$1,657,970. In 1960, as a result of increases in subscribers' fees and continuing increases in their numbers, that income had become $6,534,858. It rose as high as $8,066,000 in 1966 and remained in the $6.5 million to $7 million range in the 1966-69 period. The reserve thus increased steadily in the range of $750,000 to $900,000 each year in the period 1960 to 1969.

Between October 1969 and July 1972, when AMS was functioning as a government agency, the reserve funds were invested and reinvested. Since only small expenditures were being made, their total had become $12,608,115 at the end of 1972.

In carrying out its role as agent during this period, AMS had to engage some additional staff to deal with the changed situation. Several thousand people had now become eligible for membership in the provincial plan; waiting periods for benefits had been removed; compulsory enrolment now permitted group arrangements for groups much smaller in numbers than had been accepted previously by AMS; and the changes in the premium rates now recognized only "single" and "family" premiums.

The operation of AMS as a government agency was a new experience for Dr. Hannah, and it was not long before some elements of friction developed in the government-AMS relationship. These culminated in July 1970, when the government gave notice to AMS and Healthco that their agent status would terminate in July 1972. This notice was acceptable to Healthco, whose members were eager to retire from any participation in the provision of medical care insurance. AMS, however, reacted strongly against the termination notice, claiming that the original agreement had contained no indication as to how long the status of agent would continue and that the termination date had been an arbitrary decision of government without any prior consultation. What followed reflected Dr. Hannah's antipathy, expressed in numerous memoranda, towards government intervention in the medical care insurance field and towards government indifference to the problems AMS faced in releasing its staff, many of whom had ten to twenty years' service. An additional complicating factor was a dispute over an amount of $37,000, which AMS claimed was owing. The numerous meetings and the voluminous exchanges of correspondence between AMS and the government resulted in the inevitable acceptance by AMS of the termination date for its agency function. The financial issue was ultimately resolved by discussion and compromise, and the government made substantial contributions to the cost of severance allowances for AMS staff.

Between January 1972 and 14 July 1972, fifty-two members of the staff of AMS were terminated and given their severance pay. A few outstanding matters remained for resolution beyond 30 June 1972, mostly cases of third-party liability whose resolution had to await court action. An audited statement was prepared that permitted conclusion of the AMS/OHIP agency agreement.

Seeking a New Role for AMS

The development of the Jason A. Hannah Institute for the History of Medicine is treated in detail by Dr. Paterson in the second part of this volume. It will only be noted here that at this juncture the Board of Directors of AMS had decided that such an institute would be established and would be located at the AMS premises at 615 Yonge Street in Toronto. The fifth and sixth floor in the building would be retained for that purpose, and real estate agents would seek tenants for the four lower floors.

In August 1972, Mr. K.W. Atcheson, Secretary-Treasurer of AMS since 1938, retired. The only AMS staff remaining in the building were Dr. Hannah, Dr. Boyd Upper, and a secretary serving both of them.

As far back as 1960 and 1961, Dr. Hannah, in his reports to the Board of Directors of AMS, had begun to indicate the need for an examination of the future role of AMS in the event of medicare. The Board of Directors thought that only as a last resort should it consider a "winding-up" of the corporation. This procedure, described in the AMS constitution and by-laws, required that the assets of AMS be distributed to "institutions" in the province promoting medical education. For planning purposes, the Board agreed that AMS should endeavour to develop a role, or several roles, that AMS could assume within the three objects in its charter, these reading as follows:

(c) To encourage medical research and preventive medicine;
(d) To cooperate with organized medicine in the advancement of the standards of medical services; and
(e) To do all such things as are incidental or conducive to the attainment of the above objects.

During the 1960s and especially after 1965, Dr. Hannah and the staff of AMS studied at least twelve projects, some of them with several components, and each was the subject of one or more lengthy reports to the Board of Directors. Among the studies were the possible acquisition of, or participation in, a drug manufacturing plan, involvement in the operation of Connaught Laboratories and its production of vaccines and sera, assistance to medical clinics in Ontario in improving their "office" functions, the provision of extended health care benefits, the possibility of developing dental and drug plans, and the sponsorship of research studies in the health care system. For a variety of reasons, none of these projects, after much study, were considered suitable for AMS participation.

Two "role" projects probably merit some separate comment. The first of these was the hospital-clinic project, which first engaged the interest of Dr. Hannah in 1953 and continued until 1965. Dr. Hannah thought that the most effective way of controlling the rising costs of hospital and medical care would be by the development of a clinic in which a number of physicians would engage in the group practice of medicine. As an adjunct to the clinic, there should be in close physical relationship a hospital of about two hundred beds with full supporting services including laboratories, X-ray, and operating rooms. Only physicians who were clinic members would be permitted to use the hospital, and there would be rigid control over the selection of patients for admission, their length of stay, and the services rendered to them. Dr. Hannah pictured AMS having a major part in establishing, building, and operating such a hospital-clinic complex and in providing, from its reserves, some "seed" money to get the project started. At various times over the years, he consulted with the Ontario Hospital Services Commission, where he received some support for this project but opposition to the idea of a "private" hospital with a closed medical staff. He considered quite seriously purchasing for $500,000 a private hospital of about fifty beds in Toronto, even taking an option on its purchase.

In 1961, a full-time physician, Dr. W. Wigle, was added to the AMS staff to give his attention to the hospital-clinic project. After a year of study and visits to several hospital-clinics in the United States, he concluded that in Ontario the hospital component could not be built without public funds, and these would not be forthcoming given the opposition of the Ontario Hospital Services Commission to any further development of private hospitals. Although Dr. Wigle resigned his appointment after about a year, it was not until four years later that Dr. Hannah abandoned his plans for a hospital-clinic development. It should be noted that by the mid-1960s there were several hospital-clinic organizations such as Dr. Hannah envisioned, examples being the Mayo Clinic and the Henry Ford Hospital-Clinic. In recent years there has been a great proliferation of them in the United States, developed along the lines proposed by Dr. Hannah. However, such developments are rare in Canada.

The second project was the development of an AMS-sponsored prepaid drug plan, which came to be known as Plan D1. This was an endeavour in the 1968-69 period to continue AMS's role in the prepayment field. Existing groups and other subscribers to AMS paid a monthly premium, and AMS paid the dispensing pharmacist the average cost of each prescription. This average cost was negotiated between drug stores and AMS. The number of participating stores reached 135, with the majority of them being in the Tamblyn chain. Plan D1 started on 1 January 1969. In the following months the number of subscribers fell considerably below expectations and continued to lag over the next two and one-half years. Eventually, when the plan had shown losses of about $250,000, Dr. Hannah decided that there was no possibility of its breaking even, and the Board of Directors accepted his recommendation that it be terminated as of 31 December 1971. At a meeting of the Board in October 1971, a motion was tabled that the termination be delayed in expectation that some substantial increases in enrolment might occur shortly, as the plan was being included in union negotiations. This motion led to a tie vote; in accordance with the by-laws Dr. Hannah cast the deciding vote and defeated the motion. Dr. Hannah interpreted the motion as a challenge to his authority as President and Managing Director – those who voted in favour of the motion were classed among his non-supporters. This attitude led in the future to some friction in the Board. The cancellation of Plan D1 was unfortunate, for it was the only project of diversification for AMS that had thus far been brought into operation. The timing of the plan, just as AMS was becoming a government agency, was also unfortunate. The short period of its operation was not really sufficient to permit its development.

Reflecting on the many non-productive experiences of Dr. Hannah and his staff in their attempts at diversification, the Board of Directors had concluded that AMS should seek some activity that would permit an application of the majority of the interest income from its reserves. By a sequence of fortuitous circumstances, which are described in the second part of this volume, Dr. Hannah came to see an important and needed role for AMS in the history of medicine. Early in 1971 he presented a lengthy review to a meeting of the directors recommending preliminary action on this project. The new project, as presented, appealed to the directors, although several of them claimed no knowledge about the history of medicine. The principal immediate attraction of the proposal was that it offered an opportunity to AMS to participate in a major activity that would require a large part of its income. At the June 1971 meeting of AMS, the Board of Directors directed Dr. Hannah to proceed with his plans.

In December 1959, the Ontario Labour Relations Board had advised AMS that its staff of about a hundred regular members had been certified as a bargaining unit in an office workers' union in Ontario. Eighty-two of the staff had voted to join the union, of whom about seventy-five were female and several were part-time. Dr. Hannah and his senior management staff were disturbed by the staff's taking this step without any previous discussions with them. Many weeks followed in discussion between the union and AMS about its "supervisory staff", most of whom AMS claimed should be excluded from union membership. Numerous related matters, with their attendant delays, were referred for rulings to the Labour Relations Board. Matters came to a head in mid-1960 when a female employee was dismissed for promoting union membership during business hours. The union appealed the dismissal, and a long series of hearings followed. Dr. Hannah published an article quite critical of the Ontario Labour Relations Board in the *Toronto Board of Trade Journal.* He claimed that the board had too much power and authority and that there was a very limited right of appeal on its decisions. The procedures of hearings, conciliation, and mediation with legal representation from both sides continued. On 9 October 1961 a judge ruled that AMS should rehire the dismissed employee. AMS appealed this ruling to the Supreme Court of Ontario, which sustained the ruling; AMS then appealed to the Supreme Court of Canada. The Supreme Court's judgement was received on 23 March 1964 and supported the appeal of AMS but with no award for legal and other costs, which came to about $30,000. By this time, interest in the union had died down among the AMS staff and decertification of the union soon followed.

The original constitution and by-laws of AMS approved by the provincial authority in 1937 have been described elsewhere. The composition of the Board in respect to its membership was continued; in the ensuing years a relatively small number of members of the corporation, both medical and non-medical, served on the Board for up to three years. From the start of AMS up to 1946, Dr. Hannah held the title of Chief Medical Officer and was a member of the Board. In 1939 he was given the title of Managing Director. Dr. J.G. Palmer, appointed Chief Medical Officer in 1946, also became a director. In 1960 the medical directors were Dr. Hannah, Dr. Palmer, Dr. H. Baker, who had joined the Board in 1937 and had been President continuously since 1938, and Dr. C. Laidlaw, who became director in 1945. The non-medical directors were Mr. K.C. Hossick, who had joined the Board in 1941 and had been Vice-President since 1945, Mr. D.B. Strudley, a director since 1945, and Mr. K.W. Atcheson, a director since 1959 and Secretary-Treasurer of AMS since 1938. In April 1964, Dr. Palmer resigned from AMS and was replaced as Chief Medical Officer by Dr. Boyd Upper, who also became a director. In early 1964 Mr. Atcheson resigned as a director but continued as Secretary-Treasurer. He was replaced by Mr. R.H. Hyndman. On 9 June 1965, Dr. Baker died in his eightieth year following a brief illness, and early in 1966 Mr. Strudley resigned from the Board. Dr. Laidlaw, in poor health, continued as a director until his death in 1968, although he was unable to attend any meetings subsequent to 1965.

At the first meeting of the Board in 1966, changes in the constitution and by-laws were approved: the office of President and Managing Director of AMS was created, and assumed by Dr. Hannah; and the office of Chairman of the Board was created, and assumed by Mr. Hossick, who also continued as Vice-President.

Late in 1966, Dr. J.B. Neilson was elected to the Board as a medical member and Mr. Eric Barr as a non-medical member. No replacement for Dr. Laidlaw was elected until 1972. These several changes meant that after 1968 there were only two directors who had been directors in 1960 – Dr. Hannah and Mr. Hossick.

Meetings of the Board of Directors were usually held in March, June, September, and December of each year; the annual meeting of members came at the time of the March meeting of the directors. Over the course of the years there had been a gradual falling off in the number of the members of the corporation to the point where the total membership, including the directors, numbered between ten and fourteen. In fact, it was unusual to have more than two members who were not directors attend the annual meeting. By custom, from the start of AMS, meetings of the directors were held at the AMS offices in Toronto on a Sunday morning. For several years in the 1960s, however, the September meeting was held on a Sunday morning in Stratford. This change of meeting location permitted directors and members and their wives to attend the Stratford Shakespearean Festival and to accept the hospitality of Mr. and Mrs. Strudley at their home in Stratford.

Other Interests of Dr. Hannah

Predominantly during the 1960s, Dr. Hannah engaged in a number of activities, most of them not a part of his position at

AMS. A description of some of these activities is given to illustrate the diversity of his interests and his participation in them.

The College of Physicians and Surgeons of Ontario. In April 1958, Dr. Hannah was elected to the Council, the governing body of the College of Physicians and Surgeons of Ontario. The elected term was four years, and he was subsequently re-elected for two more terms, so that he served on the Council a total of twelve years. The College is the licensing body for physicians practising in Ontario and is also responsible for the general surveillance of physicians in regard to their professional and personal conduct. Dr. Hannah was a member of several committees of the College, especially those having a liaison relationship with the Minister of Health, OMA, and the university schools of medicine. His active interest in the affairs of the College led to his appointment to its executive committee, to his election as Vice-President in 1961, and to his election as President in 1962. In 1961 he had also accepted the chairmanship of the Building Committee to plan and construct a new headquarters for the College at 57 Prince Arthur Avenue in Toronto. The building was completed on schedule and in time for Dr. Hannah as President to preside at its official opening in April 1963. At that time, he presented to the College a presidential chain of office. In 1964 Dr. Hannah became a member of the Discipline Committee of the College and served for a period of four years. He gained the respect of many College members for the helpful contributions he made to the deliberations of the committee, faced as it was, on many occasions, with what should be done about the disposal of complaints brought against physicians. In his diary, Dr. Hannah noted that in the 1961-63 period, he gave about twenty full days of his time each year to Council business.

Queen's University, Kingston. A graduate of Queen's University, Dr. Hannah maintained his interest in the university by becoming an active member of its Alumni Association and by making frequent donations. He kept in touch with several members of his graduating class in Medicine and helped in planning the class reunions held about every ten years. He rarely missed a football encounter between Queen's University and the University of Toronto. In 1965 he was elected for a three-year term to the Board of Trustees of the university, where his voice was heard frequently on two of his favourite subjects. His belief was that in selecting medical students more attention should be given to evidence of personal aptitudes for becoming a physician rather than, in the current practice, to standing in the high school matriculation examinations. His other topic was the loss of autonomy by the university, which he believed would follow its looking to government as the chief source of its income. In recognition of his services to the university, Dr. Hannah was granted an LL.D. in 1974.

Articles, Writings, and Speeches. Dr. Hannah was a prolific writer of reports, memoranda, articles, and speeches, as well as having a large correspondence of a personal type. The volume and diversity of his writings reached their peak during the 1960s.

During the years 1960 to 1968, an article by Dr. Hannah appeared in almost every monthly issue of the *Ontario Medical Review;* most of the articles also appeared in the monthly *Toronto Board of Trade Journal.* Initially, the articles were paid for by AMS at advertising rates. In 1964, both publications discontinued the articles completely, protesting that several of them were controversial and political. When OMA continued the articles, it was only with agreement that they be edited by OMA before publication. The articles, usually one page in length, covered a wide range of subjects, with titles such as "Pioneering Days in Saskatchewan", "The Art of Graciousness", "Education", "Employment", and "The Advantages of Growing Old", but as time went on the predominant theme was medical care insurance with increasing criticism of government activity in that field. There was often pointed comment about the failure of physicians in the province to support the principles of prepayment by medically sponsored plans as a means of ensuring that physicians' business would remain in their control. Although Dr. Hannah established himself as an interesting and at times entertaining writer, his writings on medical economics and the political aspects of medical insurance seemed to bring forth little reaction and comment from his readers, aside from some statements that he was at least consistent in opposing any form of government-sponsored medical care insurance.

Prior to 1960, Dr. Hannah had composed a few poems, but from 1960 to 1970 his venture into this field of expression resulted in a large number of "poems" prepared for almost any occasion. Poems often accompanied letters he wrote to his daughter and members of his family, and several of them appeared in the *Ontario Medical Review*. At Christmas in 1968, he had a selection of fifty-six of his poems printed and bound, bearing the title *Poetic License with Prose*. A copy of this book was sent to the directors of AMS, some senior members of the AMS staff, to members of his family, and to a number of friends. It was "Dedicated to Insomnia and Stress which this Effort Changed from Ennui to Pleasure". This dedication recalls that Dr. Hannah throughout his lifetime was an early riser, usually leaving his bed about five o'clock in the morning. From then until 7 or 7.30 in the morning he did much of the writing in his diary, as well as completing reports and memoranda and composing poetry.

Even in his early years, Dr. Hannah was a diarist. Later, during the 1950s and more especially in the 1960s, his diary entries became more frequent and lengthier; for most of the 1960s there were daily entries. In 1962 he acquired a typewriter, and most later entries were typed in single spacing and on both sides of the page. The diary material between 1960 and 1974 filled about a thousand closely typed pages. It is replete with his comments and observations on the passing scene and with frequent references to AMS and its operating problems.

Flying. In 1951, when he was fifty-two years old, Dr. Hannah achieved a lifetime ambition when he obtained a private pilot's licence. Later he became the owner of a Cessna 182. During the 1950s and into the mid-1960s, the aircraft was kept at an airport in Oshawa, and from there he made numerous flights, all without mishap, to Montreal, Ottawa, Windsor, and elsewhere in Ontario, sometimes on AMS business. On one occasion, he flew to Regina to attend a family reunion. He was never able to persuade his wife to be his passenger, although she flew often in commercial aircraft. In the early 1960s he made considerably less use of the aircraft – most of his trips were to an airstrip at Northbrook, Ontario, about five miles from his summer cottage at Cloyne. He sold the plane in early 1966.

At Home. Dr. Hannah and his wife over the years lived in three houses, each located in Toronto and reasonably accessible to the AMS offices. Each of these houses had some surrounding property in which Dr. Hannah planted flowers and vegetables. He found much pleasure and relaxation in tending the garden. He also became rather competent in dealing with the plumbing, electrical, and other maintenance problems that face the homeowner. Most years he and his wife managed to get away for periods of two to four weeks, usually in February and March, to Florida or the Caribbean Islands. They both enjoyed the theatre, being regular attendants at the O'Keefe Centre and the Royal Alexandra Theatre. Dr. Hannah was a hockey fan, usually viewing the games on television. He and his wife were both active members of Rosedale United Church.

CHAPTER VI

Transformation – 1973 to 1976

This rather short period in the history of AMS marked the transition of AMS from a non-profit corporation to a registered charity and the withdrawal of Dr. Hannah from active participation in its affairs.

Late in 1972 a small committee of the Board of Directors, consisting of Dr. Hannah, Mr. Barr, and Dr. Neilson, was appointed to consider the "future of AMS". In requesting a committee study, the Board was expressing its concern that the future goals of AMS and the several factors that would influence them should be set down in writing along with a timetable for achieving them. Although this subject had been presented to the Board in numerous memoranda and reports, and some progress was being reported by Dr. Hannah in developing the interest of AMS in the history of medicine and the proposed Hannah Institute for the History of Medicine, clearly stated objectives and their target dates were missing. The reorganization of AMS to meet its role in the history of medicine and to ensure that the assets of AMS were available to support that role had not, in the view of the Board, received the attention it deserved.

The report of the committee to the Board, initially considered at its December meeting in 1972 and at later Board meetings in 1973, contained several recommendations, many of which did not have the endorsation of Dr. Hannah. All of the recommendations need not be reviewed here, but a number of them of them called for action by Dr. Hannah and should be noted.

In 1972 the Board had considered two recommendations from Dr. Hannah about a suitable location for the Hannah Institute for the History of Medicine and its library acquisitions and had decided early in 1973 against Dr. Hannah's preference, the AMS building at 615 Yonge Street. At that time the sole occupants of the six-storey building were Dr. Hannah, Dr. Upper, and a secretary, and arrangements were being made to sell the office furniture and equipment. It was then decided by the Board, on the recommendation of Dr. Hannah and with the agreement of the committee, that the appointment of Dr. Upper as Chief Medical Officer should be terminated, and Dr. Upper ceased to be a member of the staff of AMS in March 1973. On the insistence of the Board, the AMS building was offered for sale.

In September 1973, following a period of negotiations, an agreement was reached with the National Trust Company whereby that company would accept into its custody all corporate records of AMS and all its investments and securities. National Trust also agreed to act as the manager of all AMS investments and to be its financial agent, making payments of expenditures as authorized by Dr. Hannah. Additionally, it agreed to provide corporate secretarial services to AMS, and Mr. P.J. Sewell, a staff member of National Trust, became corporate secretary of AMS in September 1973. He served AMS in a capable and satisfactory manner until AMS decided in 1981 to have a corporate secretary as a member of its staff.

The "operational" records of AMS, which filled some hundred and twenty file boxes dating back to 1937, were brought together and were moved into the archival storage area of the Fisher Rare Book Library, which is a part of the John P. Robarts Library building of the University of Toronto. These records were subsequently inventoried.

The sale of the building at 615 Yonge Street required considerably more time than was anticipated by the Board of Directors because Dr. Hannah insisted that he could receive a sale price in excess of its valuation at approximately $500,000. In September 1973 the building was sold for about $600,000. Required to vacate the building, Dr. Hannah proposed the leasing of office space on Eglinton Avenue, space that the Board considered to be in excess of requirements; the Board withdrew from the lease. Late in 1973, the Board accepted a recommendation that AMS continue to function under the direction of Dr. Hannah from space in his home at 5 Douglas Drive in Toronto, with agreement that a sum of $200 be paid to him each month for the space.

In the years 1974 to 1976, the Board had to deal with several important matters relating to AMS organization and operation. The most pressing of these was its future administration, now that Dr. Hannah's health was declining. His health problems are described in considerable detail in several memoranda he presented to the Board and in frequent diary references. A summary of these problems will give some indication of the difficulties they caused for the Board.

In February 1964, Dr. Hannah developed symptoms of prostatic obstruction, which were relieved by surgical removal of portions of the prostate gland. A follow-up examination in July 1965 found malignant changes in the prostate gland, and he was placed on hormone medication, which was continued for the duration of his life and fortunately prevented any further growth of the prostatic malignancy. At the same time, an X-ray examination showed a small cyst of the right kidney. The cyst was removed by surgery in September 1965, and there was no evidence of malignancy in the cystic material. However, post-operative complications developed – pneumonia and acute intestinal diverticulitis – and were life-threatening for several days. Some ten weeks of convalescence was necessary. In August 1967, he had a sudden onset of blood in the urine and was again admitted to hospital. The cause of the bleeding was found to be a malignant tumour, a hypernephroma of the left kidney, and both kidney and tumour were removed by surgery.

In his diary entries and at Board meetings, Dr. Hannah referred to the physically debilitating results of this succession of illnesses. Yet although he later claimed that he had thought about retirement even prior to 1973, it is evident in the records that he never seriously considered retiring. During the 1969-72 period, while AMS functioned as a government agency, the Board had accepted Dr. Hannah's assertion that he was essential to AMS. He refused, however, to consider stepping down from his position at the end of this period. By 1969 there had been some return of Dr. Hannah's physical and mental vigour, but not to the point where the Board believed that he could continue indefinitely as

Managing Director. Some improvement in Dr. Hannah's health enabled him to resume some physical activities at his home and cottage, and in his diary he wrote about the possibility of acquiring a bulldozer, which he planned to operate in improving the landscaping of the cottage area.

But the time of feeling better and eager to be about his business was short-lived. About mid-year in 1970, Dr. Hannah began to record in his diary increasing physical and mental lassitude that restricted his physical activity and made many days at his office long and trying. The cause of his symptoms was found to be a moderately severe but persistent anaemia of the iron-deficiency type. Initially it was possible to maintain satisfactory blood levels of haemoglobin with iron therapy, but by early 1971 it had become necessary to treat the anaemia by frequent blood transfusions. In 1971 or 1972 Dr. Hannah was getting transfusions every seven to ten days of two units of whole blood. In 1972 he had something like forty transfusions. About this time he was away from the office for almost four months in Florida.

Extensive investigations showed that the anaemia was due to blood loss from the stomach and possibly the upper small intestine. By gastroscopic examination, the cause of the bleeding was found to be the presence in the stomach of several benign small tumours composed of blood vessels that tended to bleed into the stomach. By then Dr. Hannah's chronic anaemia was physically evident in his pallor and his restricted tolerance for exercise and any prolonged period of mental activity. Appearances at his office became less frequent and of shorter duration; holidays were longer, usually in Florida in the winter and at his cottage in the summer. In early 1975, the bleeding became more frequent and severe, requiring transfusions at least once or twice weekly. As a life-saving measure, it was decided to surgically remove the portion of the stomach that contained the vascular tumours. This major surgical procedure was accomplished without any complications, and a satisfactory recovery followed.

For several weeks following the operation there was no evidence of any further bleeding, but hopes for relief were dashed by the reappearance of bleeding, fortunately not as frequently or in as great quantity as previously. The weekly blood transfusion procedure was again initiated. From 1976 until his death in May 1977, Dr. Hannah became progressively disabled by chronic disease and spent most of his time at his home.

As the possibility of Dr. Hannah's being restored to a better state of health became increasingly remote, the Board of Directors began to press him to propose an administrative organization for AMS that would include a suitable person as his successor. In 1974, Dr. Hannah was carrying on the business of AMS from his home as its sole remaining staff member. His limited energies were devoted almost entirely to developing and promoting the interests of AMS in the history of medicine. He kept up a steady production of memoranda, drafts of agreements with universities, and estimates of the costs to AMS of this new activity.

In Board meetings, Dr. Hannah was reluctant to discuss the future of AMS, and it became more and more apparent that he was determined to retain the control and management in his own hands. In June 1974, however, in response to pressure by the Board, Dr. Hannah announced, and received approval of, his intention to engage as his assistant Dr. G.R. Paterson, who was prepared to join Dr. Hannah on 1 October on a half-time basis until 30 June 1975. Dr. Paterson was a senior professor in the Faculty of Pharmacy at the University of Toronto who had a demonstrated interest in and knowledge of the history of medicine. His primary responsibility was to proceed with the development of the history of medicine concept in its several applications to universities in Ontario. Later, Dr. Hannah announced that he had engaged the full-time services of Miss Mary Wildridge as a secretary effective 2 January 1975, and that, as an interim measure, she had been provided with office space at his home. Later, in January 1975, the offices of AMS were moved into 50 Prince Arthur Avenue, and Dr. Hannah, Dr. Paterson, and Miss Wildridge were located there.

In the Board of Directors, discussions continued in 1975 about the future of AMS and its administration. It was recalled that in 1965 Dr. Hannah had told the Board that he would retire when he reached the age of seventy in 1969. At that time the Board had agreed to pay $200,000 to the Confederation Life Insurance Company for a lifetime annuity that would pay $20,000 a year starting at his seventieth birthday. Subsequently, in 1969, the Board had signed a contract with Dr. Hannah to continue his appointment as President and Managing Director for a five-year period dating from 1 January 1970 to 31 December 1974, at a salary of approximately $46,000 per year. When this five-year period concluded, the Board had some reservations about its renewal. Dr. Hannah had requested an extension for a period of one year, during which, he assured the Board, the administrative structure of AMS would be developed and his successor would be found. With the assurance of Dr. Hannah that he was capable of continuing as President and Managing Director, a contract for the period 1 January 1975 to 31 December 1975 was approved, but with a clear understanding that the administration and management of AMS for the future would be clearly defined.

Early in 1975, the Board of Directors received a report from Dr. Hannah that the performance of Dr. Paterson was equal to his expectations and he was prepared to recommend that Dr. Paterson become his successor at the end of 1975 as Managing Director. To consider this recommendation and the role or position of Dr. Paterson in the AMS administrative structure, the Board appointed a small committee from its members to examine the relationship between the proposed Hannah Institute for the History of Medicine and AMS, and the role of Dr. Paterson in this relationship. The recommendation of the committee to the Board was that, giving recognition to his obvious interests in the history of medicine and his demonstrated abilities in furthering the interests of AMS in the history of medicine, Dr. Paterson should be appointed Executive Director of the Hannah Institute effective 1 July 1975. This recommendation was approved by the Board. Dr. Paterson having arranged a two-year, full-time leave of absence from the Faculty of Pharmacy at the University of Toronto, his appointment was to continue until 30 June 1977.

Later in 1975, another small committee of the Board of Directors was struck to recommend the appointment of a "Chairman" or "Chief Executive Officer" or "Managing Director" of AMS to succeed Dr. Hannah at the end of the year. It was agreed that Dr. Paterson should not be considered for that position, in spite of Dr. Hannah's belief that a suitable period under his own guidance would be sufficient preparation. Further, the committee, in analysing the requirements of the position and in relating them to the full-time appointment of Dr. Paterson, concluded that only a part-time appointee giving two to three days each week should be sought. Several possible choices were considered. A person with considerable business experience having declined the position, in March 1976 Dr. J.B. Neilson, who had been a member of the Board of Directors since 1966, was appointed Acting Managing Director to replace Dr. Hannah as of 1 January 1976. At the subsequent annual meeting in May 1976, Dr. Hannah resigned as a director of AMS and Dr. Neilson was elected President on a part-time arrangement. The "Managing Director" title was deleted. At the same meeting, Dr. Hannah was named an Honorary President of AMS in recognition of his services: its founder in 1937, its Chief Medical Officer from 1937 to 1946, its Managing Director from 1939 to 1975, and its President and Managing Director from 1965 to 1976. Shortly afterwards, a testimonial luncheon was held in honour of Dr. Hannah with all present and former members of its Board of Directors in attendance.

Of rather pressing importance to the Board of Directors in 1974 was the question of the corporate status of AMS. The purposes and objects of AMS in its original provincial charter granted on 9 April 1937 were as follows:

(a) To arrange for the provision to others of any or all services required in the prevention, diagnosis or treatment of illness as recognized by legally qualified medical practitioners in the Province of Ontario on a non-profit, prepayment and voluntary basis;
(b) For the purposes aforesaid to establish reserves and administer the same;
(c) To encourage medical research and preventive medicine;
(d) To cooperate with organized medicine in the advancement of the standard of medical services; and
(e) To do all such things as are incidental or conducive to the attainment of the above objects.

To give some added emphasis to clause (a), later in the charter appears the statement:

And it is hereby ordained and declared that the said Corporation shall be carried on without the purpose of gain for its members, and that any profits or other accretions to the Corporation shall be used in promoting its objects.

The Board of Directors had approved in June 1971 a recommendation from Dr. Hannah that the major continuing activity of AMS should be in the history of medicine. However, the progress in planning and initiating this activity had been considerably slower than the Board had expected. It was not until some three years later, in mid-1974, when some substantive progress was evident and the appointment of Dr. Paterson gave needed impetus.

An additional concern of the Board was the non-profit status of the corporation. There was general agreement that AMS had functioned until 30 June 1972 in accordance with object (a) in its charter, and that to that date, at least, AMS should be entitled to non-profit status. The opinion of Dr. Hannah, expressed in memoranda to the Board, was that the original charter with its stated objects under items (c) and (d) in particular would permit AMS to continue to operate as a non-profit corporation and that no change in these objects was either indicated or necessary. This opinion of Dr. Hannah prevailed until December 1974, when Dr. John Deutsch, Principal of Queen's University, became a member of the Board. Dr. Deutsch expressed views that differed from those of Dr. Hannah: he believed its current operations rendered AMS liable for the payment of income tax on its investment earnings, which, at the time, were about $900,000 annually. At the request of Dr. Deutsch and the Board, an opinion on the tax liability status of AMS was sought in October 1975 from the Ministry of Consumer and Commercial Relations. In a letter dated 24 October 1975 from the Chief Examiner of the Ministry, the pertinent comment was:

It would appear to us that AMS *as it is presently operating would not qualify for exemption of these [quoted] provisions of the Income Tax Act . . .*

We would therefore recommend that you seek independent legal advice in this matter in order to avoid a potential tax liability which could reduce significantly the funds available for your worthwhile research projects in the field of medical history.

At the December 1975 meeting of the Board, it was decided to form a committee of the Board consisting of Dr. Hannah, Dr. Deutsch, and Dr. Neilson as chairman. The committee was directed to select legal counsel and in meetings with counsel to investigate and determine the arrangements that would be necessary to continue AMS's exemption from federal income tax. The committee was also directed to consider and recommend any necessary revisions needed to the charter and to the Board structure to give effect to any changes that counsel considered to be advisable or necessary.

Mr. John Hodgson, Q.C., was engaged, and two meetings of the committee followed, with Mr. Hodgson and Mr. P.J. Sewell, Secretary of AMS, in attendance. Mr. Hodgson believed the existing charter of AMS could be amended acceptably to continue its tax-exempt status. He also believed that its tax-exempt status as a medical care by prepayment plan ceased in September 1972, but he was confident that the Department of National Revenue would grant exemption dating from 1972 on being made aware of the present plans of AMS in the history of medicine. If AMS were to operate under the exempting section 149 of the Income Tax Act, the most appropriate designation for it would be that of a registered charity and further classified as a "charitable organization".

When Mr. Hodgson later met with officers of the Department of National Revenue in Ottawa, no problems were foreseen in having AMS registered as a charitable organization. At a special meeting of members of AMS on 26 April 1976, approval was given to a recommendation that AMS make formal application for such registration. At the same time, the necessary changes in the AMS charter were proposed to be included in supplementary letters patent for submission to the Provincial Secretary. The principal changes were in the objects of the corporation, which were now listed as:

a) To receive and maintain a fund or funds and to apply from time to time all or part thereof and the income therefrom for charitable purposes;
b) Under the name of the "Hannah Institute for the History of Medicine" to establish, maintain and advance studies in the history of medical and related sciences by every available means;
c) To encourage medical research and preventive medicine;
d) To cooperate with organized medicine in the advancement of the standards of medical services.

The by-laws of AMS were also revised to reflect changes in the composition and functions of the Board in its new role as a charitable organization. When approval by the Provincial Secretary had been obtained, the application to the Department of National Revenue was duly submitted in May 1976. That too being approved, AMS became a charitable organization as of 1 July 1976. Thus, after almost four years of indecision, the new organization had been achieved and the security of its reserve funds was in the hands of the Board of Directors.

The third subject of concern to the Board of Directors of AMS in the 1973-1976 period was its reserves. Previous reference has been made to the rapid increase in these reserves in the 1960-1972 period, to the point where the reserves were shown in an audited statement at 31 December 1972 as $12,608,000. By 31 December 1975 they were approximately $15,000,000.

In September 1973, as noted previously, the financial assets of AMS (its reserves plus what was realized from the sale of the AMS building) were placed in the custody of the National Trust Company in Toronto, and thereafter Dr. Hannah, as the sole staff member of AMS, became, in conjunction with National Trust, the custodian of these assets in the form of invested securities. In the following three years the Board received rather meagre current information about the assets and their administration, aside from the annual report of the auditor, which was given to the directors and subsequently to the annual meeting of members of the corporation. Dr. Hannah rejected a suggestion that the auditor be asked to attend the annual meeting to present and discuss his report. Several directors were not satisfied with Dr. Hannah's presentation of the financial position. Dr. Hannah contended that he acted on the advice of National Trust, which he considered to be reliable. On questioning in Board of Directors' meetings, Dr. Hannah seemed unable to define an "investment policy"; nor did he have a satisfactory explanation of "decline in market value of investments" in the auditor's reports of both 1973 and 1974, in the amount of $1 million for each year. The Board concluded that the attention given to AMS investments was not adequate, because of Dr. Hannah's continuing illnesses and his inability to deal quickly with investment recommendations sent to him by National Trust as the only designated decision source. Moreover, Dr. Hannah in 1974 authorized, without Board approval, the purchase of the Lambo collection of rare books at a cost of $125,000.

The period 1974 to 1976 was a crucial one for AMS. Since 1937 Dr. Hannah had had a Board of Directors who rarely challenged his recommended policies. He had exercised over the years a free hand in writing about, and speaking on, several subjects on health insurance that were controversial. His articles in the *Ontario Medical Review* and the *Board of Trade Journal* did not have any previous endorsation by the Board of Directors, so that his interpretation of AMS policy prevailed and resulted in some conflict with OMA and PSI. Those who knew Dr. Hannah recognized that he was an outspoken person who did not mince words. As time went on, however, it became apparent that his views on medical care insurance and his strong opposition to government involvement were out of touch with the political times.

At its annual meeting in April 1974, Dr. Hannah and his supporters opposed the proposed re-election of Dr. Boyd Upper as a member of the Board and defeated the proposal in a close vote. In reaction to what some Board members interpreted as the intention of Dr. Hannah to gain control of the Board, Mr. Eric Barr, a Board member since 1966, and Mr. R.H. Hyndman, a Board member since 1964, tendered their resignations. In the following year Dr. Ian Macdonald, a Board member since 1972, resigned and was replaced by Dr. W.B. Spaulding. Judge Robert

J. Cudney was elected as a member of the Board in 1975, but health problems left his position on the Board vacant in 1976. To complete the complement of members, and on the recommendation of Dr. Hannah, Dr. John Deutsch, Principal of Queen's University, and Judge Walter Little joined the Board in 1975.

Thus, in this rather crucial period, when primary concerns were the future of AMS and the protection and use of its assets, the Board of Directors had an instability of membership, an ailing president, and a lack of clear-cut objectives. To this scene came the energy, perception, and organizational abilities of Dr. Deutsch. He chaired the committee of three members whose efforts established continuity of the administrative organization, through the appointment of Dr. Paterson as Executive Director of the Hannah Institute and Dr. Neilson as Acting Managing Director. He initiated the course of action necessary to establish AMS as a registered charity and thus prevent its assets from being subject to income tax. A rapidly progressing cancer resulted in his death in April 1976, but his endeavours on behalf of AMS built a firm foundation for its future activities.

At the time of the annual meeting in 1976, it was apparent that Mr. K.C. Hossick was suffering from serious heart disease, which, as he came to his eightieth year, rendered him able to carry on only limited activity and led to his death a few months later. Elected to the Board in 1941, Mr. Hossick was a long-time contributor to the success of AMS as its Vice-President since 1945 and Chairman of the Board since 1965. He resigned from the Board in 1976. To complete the Board membership, Dr. Boyd Upper and Dr. John W. Scott were elected as directors. It was decided that in addition to the President there should be a First Vice-President (Dr. Spaulding from 1976 to 1979) and a Second Vice-President (Dr. Scott from 1976 to 1984). Dr. Upper became First Vice-President in 1979. The President and the two Vice-Presidents constituted an Executive Committee, which met at least four times each year and made subsequent reports to the Board. Judge Little continued as a Board member until 1977, when the demands of his professional duties resulted in his resignation.

CHAPTER VII

Operation as a Charitable Organization – 1977 to 1987

From 1977 to the present, the principal activity of AMS has been the development and expansion of its interest in the history of medicine.

As noted previously, AMS became a registered charity in 1976. As a registered charity AMS is required to file an annual report on its charitable activities to the Department of National Revenue on a prescribed form, accompanied by a financial statement. Its designation as a "charitable organization" rather than a "charitable foundation" provided exemption from the requirement applicable to charitable foundations to expend 90 per cent of income on charitable activities not later than in the year after the receipt of the income. As a charitable organization, AMS is permitted to accumulate its income and to spend the income on a continuing basis over long periods of time. Using its estimates of income, it thus is able to determine what funds will be available and to give some assurance to those involved in a project of the duration of the assistance that may be expected, thus permitting them to plan prospectively. The income has varied in the past fourteen years between $1.7 million and $2.1 million per year, and has permitted AMS to fund its charitable activities to the extent of $1 million to $1.4 million a year.

In its charter, the primary object of AMS is to promote interest in, and knowledge of, the history of medicine. Two additional objects in the charter are:

(c) To encourage medical research and preventive medicine;
(d) To cooperate with organized medicine in the advancement of the standards of health services.

Both of these objects are interpreted as permitting AMS wider scope in supporting almost any activity in the field of medicine.

The Board of Directors agreed that the major portion of income should be expended on the history of medicine. Reviews of income and expenses for the ten-year period show that after meeting the costs of programs in the history of medicine and the administrative expenses, an amount estimated at about $250,000 to $300,000 annually remains. The Board decided to apply this amount to support proposals for assistance coming under objects (c) and (d).

With regard to object (c), it was decided that medical education should be a part of this object. The directors were hesitant about engaging in the support of medical research because of its cost and the tendency for many medical research projects to continue over several years. Thus the criteria for support of a medical research proposal are that it can be completed within a specified period and holds the expectation of achieving some tangible results. Few medical research proposals have received AMS support. The whole subject of preventive medicine was considered to be difficult to assess, in terms of how it might be encouraged and in its research applications. In the ten-year period, no project in preventive medicine has been directly supported.

In 1979, the Board had discussions with representatives of the Council of Faculties of Medicine in Ontario about some of the current problems in medical education and how AMS might offer assistance. These discussions resulted in a one-day seminar in Toronto in May 1980, co-sponsored by AMS and the Council of Faculties of Medicine. The expenses of the seminar, approximately $1,200, were met by AMS. A summary report on the seminar, which was well attended, indicated agreement by those attending that medical education should try to provide medical students, as part of their education, with information about medical economics, law as applied to the practice of medicine, and the ethical matters facing physicians in their professional and societal relationships. It should also stress the necessity of good communications between physician and patient. This seminar has had some desirable results. In the next two to three years, most of the medical schools in Ontario, in conjunction with their affiliated teaching hospitals, developed teaching programs that give medical students information about these subjects.

In June 1980, as an expression of its interest in geriatric medicine, AMS offered financial assistance to the University of Toronto and the University of Western Ontario to meet the cost of the salary and benefits payable to a medical student training in geriatric medicine. Between 1980 and 1982 the costs thus paid by AMS were $60,000. Support was then provided for geriatric and gerontology programs in all the Ontario universities with medical faculties and a total of $275,000 was spent on these programs in 1981 and 1982. AMS tried to interest other charities and the provincial government in providing grants to training programs in geriatric medicine, but without success. AMS then withdrew its support from further funding of geriatric programs.

In 1982 the Board made a grant of $340,000 to University Hospital in London as the major cost of a computerized digital angiographic unit. This unit, installed in the Department of Radiology, has had extensive research and experimental use, and with some modifications is now a service component in Radiology. It provides a more accurate and safer method of examining the flow of blood in the arteries serving the heart and brain and has an essential function in the diagnosis of disease of arteries.

With regard to object (d), the Board has approved a few projects considered as qualifying under this object. AMS has made inquiries as to how it might exercise some influence in support of this object. With comprehensive hospital and medical care insurance plans in effect in the province, any projects designed to "advance" health services could involve AMS in political issues. Care has therefore had to be exercised in terms of this object.

In discussion of object (d), the directors of AMS became interested in the problems of an ageing population in the province and in their impact on the social, economic, and health resources. This interest was stimulated by a proposal from the University of Toronto in 1978 that AMS provide financial assistance for a study program in gerontology. The proposal had been developed as a cooperative effort by several departments in the university that had some interest in gerontology. It was designed to determine what role the university might assume in dealing with the problems presented by an ageing population. Impressed with the proposal, AMS agreed, starting in July 1978, to commit an amount of $100,000 each year for four years to support the program and to publish the reports, conclusions, and recommendations emanating from it.

During the four-year period, AMS was provided with information from the study, and some members of the Board served on committees set up as part of the program. The final payment of $100,000 was made in 1982. Late in 1982 an assessment of the study was made by an outside consultant. In June 1983 the university advised AMS that the comments of the consultant had been most favourable and that the university was proceeding to act on the recommendation that it establish a Department of Gerontology.

In 1983 a grant of $25,000 was made to the Royal Botanical Gardens in Hamilton to assist in developing its Medicinal Herb Garden. The garden was officially opened in 1985.

By the end of 1978, all vacancies had been filled on the Board of Directors. At the annual meeting of the Board in April 1981 Miss Mary Wildridge was appointed Corporate Secretary. At the same time, management consultants were selected to study the organization and operation of AMS.

The report of the consultants was received by the Board early in 1982. Of particular interest to the Board were the following recommendations:

— That the Board of Directors consist of nine members including the President (this being an increase of two in the number of directors), and that it be representative of the medical profession, the teaching profession, and the public interest.

— That directors be elected for a three-year term such as to allow for a rotation of membership. (The term had previously been one year but renewable each year.)

— That an age limit for directors be established so that no person could be elected a director after the age of seventy, nor be re-elected after the age of seventy-five. (There had been no previous age limit.)

— That the existing Investment and Finance Committee, consisting of the President and the First and Second Vice-Presidents, be called the Executive Committee.
— That the President of AMS should be a physician with a knowledge of the health care system, government health agencies, and hospitals.

These recommendations were approved by the Board of Directors and were subsequently made part of the regulations respecting the by-laws of AMS. At the same time, the by-laws themselves were revised, and from that time on there were no members of the corporation other than the directors.

The report of the consultants made several references to the present and future role of AMS in the history of medicine. The consultants had also reviewed the financial status of AMS and confirmed that with careful attention to the reserves and their investment, AMS would be able to continue to meet its commitments in the history of medicine.

By 1982 it was evident that the office space at 50 Prince Arthur Avenue was not adequate to meet current needs – a point also remarked upon by the consultants. The deficiency was remedied by a move in October to new accommodation at 14 Prince Arthur Avenue.

Early in 1982, Dr. J.B. Neilson announced his intention to resign from the position of President. Later that year Dr. D.R. Wilson was chosen by the Board to replace Dr. Neilson.

Since 1983, AMS has continued its interest in the history of medicine to the point where it has become known internationally. In the coming years AMS is committed to supporting the Hannah Chairs in the History of Medicine in Ontario and is considering the possibility of giving some financial support to departments of the history of medicine in other universities in Canada. But AMS continues to be interested in its other objects.

In accordance with proposed new federal legislation, Revenue Canada stated they would inform all registered charities of their reviewed designations – private or public foundations, or charitable organizations. Early in 1985 AMS received notice of its designation as a public foundation. This designation was appealed on the grounds that AMS had been operating continuously as a charitable organization since July 1976. The appeal was accepted; AMS continues to function as a charitable organization, defined as "an organization – all of the resources of which are devoted to charitable activities carried on by the organization itself and no part of the income of which is available for the personal benefit of any proprietor, member, shareholder, trustee or settlor thereof". Unless further changes are made in federal legislation affecting registered charities, AMS will be able to continue functioning as it has since 1976.

With the completion of the first ten years of active participation by AMS in the history of medicine, the Board decided to appoint a committee chaired by Dr. W.B. Spaulding to evaluate the program. The committee presented its report to the Board in December 1985. The principal recommendation of the report was that AMS continue to support the Hannah Chairs in the History of Medicine at the Ontario medical schools, and continue also – within its financial resources – most of its other activities in support of the history of medicine. The committee also recommended considering support to history of medicine outside Ontario. Study of the report was proceeding in 1986.

A special meeting of the Board convened in September 1986, with the question to be debated: "What other activities, aside from those in the history of medicine, should attract AMS's support, to what amount, and for how long?" A report on this meeting will give the Board more opportunity for thought and action in 1987.

CHAPTER VIII

Some Retrospective Comments on Associated Medical Services

In April 1937, Dr. Hannah resigned from the position of Provincial Neuropathologist, which he had held since October 1930. While his memoirs record several reasons for the growing disenchantment with his position, the principal reason for his resignation must have been his discovery of a new venture which had more appeal to him than a career in neuropathology.

His studies of medical economics over a period of some six years had convinced Dr. Hannah that he had an idea which, under his guidance and direction, could become a useful and remunerative enterprise. Although he sought advice and assistance from several sources, notably the Civil Service Association and government officials, the decision to form AMS was his and he was able to move quickly to produce his plan for providing medical care by the mechanism of prepayment.

The timing of AMS was certainly favourable, there being an obvious need in Ontario for a practical method for people to meet the costs of medical care on some budgeted basis. A considerable number of civil servants could be expected to become subscribers to AMS, and government authorities had shown their willingness to support its ideas and proposals. Of major importance was the full-time personal involvement of Dr. Hannah in developing and promoting the concepts of AMS, with the principal concept being that of "prepayment". All of these factors placed the chances of success of the prepayment plan on the side of AMS, and even more so when the entrepreneurial skills of Dr. Hannah became evident in the development of this new venture.

Much of Dr. Hannah's knowledge about methods of meeting the costs of medical care on a "budgeted" or "prepayment" basis had come from study of reports on prepayment plans operating in Europe, the United States, and a few locations in Canada. Dr. Hannah claimed that the AMS prepayment plan was the result of "extensive research" and that it had several exclusive features; however, the AMS plan was very similar to other plans in operation elsewhere, and his research had resulted in the selection of the most desirable features of the other plans.

In his writings Dr. Hannah gave emphasis to the importance of the concept of "prepayment" as distinct from "insurance", although admitting that the prepayment concept did include some of the principles of insurance. His explanations of the differences between prepayment and insurance were confusing and not very convincing, and the differences were of no real interest to a potential subscriber.

The AMS prepaid medical care plan as presented for sale to the public in 1937 required proof of good health by the subscriber, excluded benefits to subscribers for pre-existing health conditions, and limited enrolment to subscribers under fifty-five years of age. With these conditions AMS was making use of the insurance principle of selecting its risks. The requirement that a subscriber name his own family physician and that the named physician become a participant in the plan seemed to be quite restrictive. But in the 1930s in the midst of severe economic depression, most physicians seized any opportunity that offered payment for their services. The plan was popular with physicians from its beginning, although as time went on some of them began to complain about the administrative controls on their claims for payment.

In its first ten years, AMS had a steady increase in the number of its subscribers – not remarkable in view of the number of potential subscribers in the province. Some early financial worries had been dispelled by the accumulation of about $600,000 in reserve funds. And there had been a clear demonstration that AMS was able to provide medical care by prepayment to its subscribers while satisfying most of its participating physicians and remaining financially solvent.

By 1939 AMS had repaid its loan of $3,800 from the Ontario Medical Association and then asserted its independence from any sponsorship or control by OMA. Efforts by OMA to have AMS and Windsor Medical Services amalgamate to produce the nucleus of a province-wide plan of prepaid medical care were unproductive, as were similar approaches to the Ontario Blue Cross plan. Finally, OMA, not totally convinced that it should become involved in prepaid medical care, nevertheless decided in 1947 to establish Physicians Services Incorporated (PSI) as its sponsored plan.

In the 1950s AMS, along with other providers of medical care insurance, particularly PSI and the private insurance companies, had its greatest growth period. Dr. Hannah had become the foremost and most vocal of the supporters and proponents of prepaid medical care. The success of AMS was cited as an example of what could be done without the assistance of government. Between 1946 and 1954, eleven prepayment plans, predominantly under the sponsorship of provincial medical associations, had developed across Canada and had by 1954 an enrolment of some two million subscribers. Dr. Hannah pointed to these plans as being patterned after AMS and as further evidence of the value of prepayment. By 1953 these plans had joined together to form Trans Canada Medical Plans (TCMP) to promote their common objective of offering medical care by prepayment. Although offered membership in TCMP, the directors of AMS decided not to join. This decision was interpreted again as the desire of AMS to go its own way and to maintain its independence, and did not enhance the profile of AMS across Canada. It seemed incomprehensible to members of TCMP that AMS, the oldest prepayment plan in Canada, should continue to preach the virtues of prepayment and yet remain aloof from joining an organization whose primary objective was to expand prepaid plans across Canada. Although AMS was not publicly critical of the medical sponsorship of the plans joined together in TCMP, it was well known that in Ontario, for reasons not too evident, AMS had refused to cooperate with OMA in developing a medically sponsored plan. Considering the independent nature of Dr. Hannah, it is not difficult to understand why he maintained the independent status of AMS, which was his creation, but there may have been some deeper motives which began to appear in later years.

In January 1959, Ontario decided to participate in the

federally sponsored national hospital insurance scheme. In spite of the unanimous approval of the scheme by Parliament and the support of the scheme by all political parties in Ontario, Dr. Hannah, in a letter to the premier of the province, criticized the action of the Ontario government. Aside from stating his basic objection to a government role in any form of health insurance, his main argument seemed to be that the costs of the scheme would soon get out of hand because of the inability of government to say "no". He had no alternative to the scheme to offer except to claim that the government missed its opportunity to support the Blue Cross plan for hospital care and its prepayment approach. He received no response to his letter that is on record, it probably being acknowledged in government circles that this was the reaction that could be expected from Dr. Hannah. A couple of years later in the *Ontario Medical Review* he dwelt at some length on the recently published costs of the hospital insurance plan in Ontario, pointing out that they had increased as he had predicted. He made no attempt, however, to analyse the reasons for the cost increases, and there was again no response to his article.

The 1960s brought the birth of medicare and the demise of the prepaid plans. The 1964 report of the Royal Comission on Health Services was followed a year later by the federal government announcement that it was accepting the major recommendation in the report that it initiate and financially support a national plan of medical care insurance in cooperation with the provincial governments. These two events resulted in two articles by Dr. Hannah in the *Ontario Medical Review* and the *Toronto Board of Trade Journal* that were very critical of the report and of the federal government's reaction to it. His criticism reiterated his view that government was planning to take on responsibilities in respect to health insurance that should rest with the citizens of Canada. He predicted that the costs of medicare would soon far exceed its estimates and that both the federal and provincial governments would be unable, because of political pressures, to exercise any real control over the costs. His criticism was also directed at the medical profession for not being more aggressive in promoting his prepayment concepts and for accepting what he believed would ultimately lead to government control of the profession. These articles led to a refusal by the Board of Trade to accept any more articles for publication, claiming that it did not wish to have its publication used by Dr. Hannah for expression of his political views. The *Ontario Medical Review* also indicated to Dr. Hannah that any future articles he wished to have published would be subjected to careful editing. As might have been expected, Dr. Hannah protested these attempts to limit "free speech" but to no avail.

These criticisms by Dr. Hannah were hardly unexpected because they were consistent with the beliefs and opinions he had held and expressed for many years. What was missing was some constructive criticism about what might be done to produce a medical care insurance plan applicable to all Canadians and not operated by government. If prepayment as pictured by Dr. Hannah and reflected in its spread across Canada was the answer, there had not been enough convincing evidence to persuade the political parties in Canada to a prepayment concept, and the political opinion, supported by all the political parties, was expressed in support of the "medicare" plan.

The critic could point to the fact that in some thirty years of operation, AMS had achieved in Ontario a membership of some 300,000 subscribers, which represented only about five per cent of the population of the province. Further, if the success of a prepayment plan required the sponsorship and cooperation of associations of physicians, the obvious question was why AMS had decided to pursue an independent course from cooperation with OMA and, later, had refused membership in Trans Canada Medical Plans.

Later, Dr. Hannah objected to the proposal of Ontario to form the Ontario Medical Services Insurance Plan (OMSIP) as an alternative to a government-sponsored medical care insurance plan. He also objected to the proposal that private insurance companies be included in OMSIP, which offered an arrangement to all of the providers of medical care insurance, including AMS, to "pool" the costs of insuring the "high risk" members of the population entitled to enrolment in OMSIP.

The described events of the 1960s and Dr. Hannah's reaction

to them must have persuaded those who read, or listened to, what he said that he was not in touch with the reality of the times. Medicare was going to come to Canada and Ontario in spite of Dr. Hannah's views and opinions. The medical profession had at least accepted the realities and was trying to ensure that medicare preserved some of the basic tenets of the profession such as the fee-for-service principle, the setting of its fees by the profession, and the right of the patient to have a free selection of physician. The efforts of Dr. Hannah to preserve his prepayment principles, or some portion of them, had been unavailing and his credibility had become submerged in the progress of political decisions and actions.

A Personal Recollection

In the 1961-65 period, I had had several meetings with Dr. Hannah as well as telephone conversations while I was Director of the Hospital Services Branch of the Ontario Hospital Services Commission. He was seeking advice about his proposal to develop a hospital-clinic project and the possibility of acquiring such a project in Ontario. He hoped that AMS could sponsor such a concept in one hospital-clinic unit, largely for experimental purposes. He believed that the concept, which pictured a tightly controlled hospital with a closed medical staff, could save hospital and medical care costs. Although his concept had some merit, it could not be developed because of the Commission policy, which did not permit any further issue of private hospital licences or the transfer to a new owner of an existing licence. Dr. Hannah seemed to accept this policy with reluctance; he was a forceful advocate of his project and obviously did not relish a "no" answer.

I was, therefore, somewhat surprised when, in mid-1966, Dr. Hannah invited me to join the Board of Directors of AMS. Early in 1966 I had moved to London to become associated with the design and building of a new teaching hospital on property of the University of Western Ontario. A few months later Dr. Hannah asked me to join him for lunch on one of my periodic visits to Toronto. Probably out of curiosity I met him, and after he had given me a rather lengthy description of AMS, past and present, and some comments about its future, he invited me to become a member of the Board. He thought that my experience in hospital and health administration and in government service could be helpful to AMS. I accepted the invitation largely out of interest, having developed a favourable impression of Dr. Hannah through our previous meetings. I was also being offered a chance to keep abreast of developments in Ontario in health care insurance, which were of interest in my new position. In December 1966 I attended my first meeting of the Board of Directors and remained as a director until April 1984.

The principal discussion item on the agenda of this first meeting and in most of the meetings in the following five years was the future of AMS following what was considered to be inevitable at an early date – a national scheme of medical care insurance in which Ontario was expected to participate. In reviewing the past minutes of the Board of Directors back to 1960-61, I found that Dr. Hannah's approach to the future of AMS was to diversify its operations by seeking enterprises in which it might become engaged, all of these having some reference to the health care field. As pictured by Dr. Hannah, when national medicare came to Ontario, there would be no future role for the prepaid medical care plans.

This "diversification" process in the following years resulted in the examination by Dr. Hannah and the staff of AMS of at least a dozen possibilities, all of which were the source of lengthy reports to the directors. All of these possibilities were rejected, usually for valid reasons, but one was accepted and promoted in a two-year period from 1969 to 1971. This was a prepaid drug plan, which, although innovative in its approach, failed to meet the condition of being self-supporting and was abandoned. As time went on I, along with other Board members, came to think that diversification, as pictured by Dr. Hannah, would never be the future of AMS.

After a long time of examining alternatives – which included the "winding up" of the corporation – Dr. Hannah in 1971 presented his recommendation that AMS become interested in supporting the history of medicine. The idea of the history of medicine was not original to him, but had rather been suggested to him. In any event, the Board of Directors, long exposed to many hours of "diversification" in which a waning of interest on the part of Dr. Hannah was apparent, grasped the history of medicine idea even though none of the directors knew very much about the history of medicine. But at long last something had been found that held a future for AMS and tied that future to one project, a much more manageable activity than "diversification". It was, however, almost three years later before the history of medicine received the direction it required with the appointment of Dr. G.R. Paterson in September 1974.

The quarterly reports presented to the directors gave much detailed information about the operations of AMS, financial and otherwise. The most significant item in the reports was the remarkable increase in the reserves – in the 1960-69 period about $1 million a year, of which the greater part was the difference between income and expenses, the remainder being income from investments. The explanation offered for this very favourable financial picture was the rate increases instituted in the 1960s and the careful attention to the utilization of benefits by subscribers. The directors' concern about this increase in reserves of a non-profit corporation was alleviated by Dr. Hannah's statement that the Superintendent of Insurance had made no comments about the amount of reserves or the rapidity of their accumulation, nor had there been any direction about how much in the way of reserves would be required or permitted.

A director did not attend many meetings before he recognized the control Dr. Hannah exercised over the Board. All elections of new directors were at his instigation. The Board composition was seven members. Of these, one was the Chairman, who had been on the Board for about twenty-five years and was completely subservient to Dr. Hannah; a second was Dr. Hannah; and a third was the Chief Medical Officer, an employee of AMS reporting directly to Dr. Hannah. Since all of Dr. Hannah's submissions and recommendations met with the approval of the other two, the four remaining members, all selected by Dr. Hannah, were unlikely to vote together to defeat some motion coming before the Board. Although the Board members were kept informed by numerous reports prepared by Dr. Hannah and his staff, these were rarely discussed in any detail in the Board. The only committees of the Board were ad hoc, created to deal with some specific subject. Dr. Hannah routinely "edited" the minutes of the Board before they were sent in final form to the members. As time went on, with many delays in getting things done and with the failure of Dr. Hannah, partly because of health problems, to respond to some suggestions of the Board, members of the Board became restive.

The 1969 agreement with the provincial government to act as an agent for the provincial insurance plan did not contain a date for termination, it being decided to leave the date open for future consideration. About a year after the agency operation started, the Ministry of Health advised AMS that it would be terminating the agreement in September 1972, almost two years later. This "unilateral", "arbitrary", and "inconsiderate" action of the Ministry stimulated Dr. Hannah to begin numerous exchanges of correspondence, his being usually provocative and critical, and the Ministry replies being firm yet conciliatory. A series of meetings was held between Ministry officials and Dr. Hannah and Dr. Upper as representatives of AMS. In reporting to the Board, Dr. Hannah even suggested bringing legal action against the Ministry on some vague grounds of breach of contract. This suggestion did not meet with Board approval. In the midst of this controversy Dr. Hannah decided to depart on a winter vacation, and in his absence Dr. Upper continued meeting with Ministry officials. The whole problem was soon resolved, and the acceptance of the termination date and the later dissolution of the staff of AMS, with their fair treatment in terms of severance allowances, was concluded without further difficulty.

In the view of the Board this episode was magnified beyond reasonable proportions and was evidence that the deterioration in Dr. Hannah's health was bringing into question his abilities to direct the affairs of AMS in the important period of transition.

Another episode occurred in 1971 after the Board had decided on the advice of Dr. Hannah that the AMS prepaid drug plan should be finished at the end of 1971. Dr. Upper, who had developed the drug plan, believed that it might become self-supporting if some large unions in Ontario should accept it as a negotiated benefit. He suggested to Dr. Hannah that it remain open until union negotiations were completed, there being a reasonable expectation that it might be accepted. When Dr. Hannah rejected the suggestion, Dr. Upper approached me and another director with the suggestion that at a forthcoming Board meeting the matter of keeping the plan open for a short time beyond the end of 1971 be presented for discussion. Dr. Upper's suggestion seemed reasonable to me, and I raised the matter at the Board meeting, asking that the termination date of the plan be extended. Another director, Mr. Barr, supported me in a motion I made to that effect. Dr. Hannah's reaction was almost violent; he claimed that Dr. Upper had no right to approach me on the matter and that the motion was in defiance of his position and authority. I tried to persuade Dr. Hannah that I did not believe there was anything wrong in having a "second look" at a previous decision, especially when there was good reason to do so. I also defended the action of Dr. Upper in approaching me when his suggestion had been completely rejected by Dr. Hannah. When the vote was held, one director was absent and the vote was three in favour and three opposed. In accordance with the by-laws, Dr. Hannah was permitted a second or casting vote, and the motion was defeated. This episode lingered in Dr. Hannah's memory and, as later events would prove, turned him against Dr. Upper and me.

In at least one meeting of the Board in the years 1969 to 1972, Dr. Hannah offered his resignation, citing reasons of health, but at no time did he present a written resignation. Up until 1972 his retention in the position of President and General Manager seemed essential as long as AMS was functioning as an agency of government, and he was given no encouragement to resign. On each occasion he took the renewal of his appointment as an indication, expressed verbally or in writing, that the Board had his confidence and that he could expect their support. By the end of 1972, however, there was more deterioriation of Dr. Hannah's health with the need for blood transfusions, and in spite of gentle pressure from the Board to develop a detailed description of the role of AMS in the history of medicine and to seek an assistant who could preferably become his successor, there was no real evidence of progress in either of these matters. The conclusion of the Board was that Dr. Hannah had no real intention of resigning his position in AMS – perhaps could not bring himself to the act of resignation.

By 1973 Dr. Hannah's health had shown some improvement and a two-year contract, including salary terms, was signed with him for the years 1973 and 1974. Some progress was being made in developing the programs in the history of medicine, and the AMS building at 615 Yonge Street was sold. Early in 1973 I raised in the Board my concern about the substantial reserves of AMS, then in excess of $12 million, because AMS was no longer operating as a non-profit corporation and was, in effect, adding interest to interest with the reserves. I suggested that whatever steps were necessary should be taken to ensure the retention of the reserves by AMS and to avoid the possibility of being required to pay taxes on investment income. It had become obvious to me, and I believe to most Board members, that the future of AMS was dependent on the financial resources it had to support its activities in the history of medicine and in whatever other activities it might become engaged. Dr. Hannah dismissed my suggestion with the observation that if I understood the charter of AMS, I would appreciate that I should have no cause for concern. This, to me, was far from being a satisfactory explanation, and I subsequently put my concerns into a letter to Dr. Hannah, which he acknowledged with the general observation that I had become unduly concerned about a matter that he believed did not merit the concern I expressed. It was at that time that the differences between Dr. Hannah and myself began. I was not prepared to accept his assurances that "all was well" with AMS and that I should have more faith in its President and Managing Director to look after its affairs. Later, there were several episodes that failed to rally me to Dr. Hannah's support.

Unfortunately, Dr. Hannah had become unduly sensitive to any questions by Board members about his management of AMS, and he interpreted any questions, generally designed to be helpful, as challenges to his authority and his ability to continue in his position. At the 1974 annual meeting, the re-election of Dr. Boyd Upper to the Board of Directors was brought forward. Although it was anticipated that Dr. Hannah would oppose the re-election, the other Board members were believed favourable. When a vote was called, however, Dr. Hannah was supported by another Board member in opposing Dr. Upper's re-election; within the voting requirements of the AMS by-laws, this opposition was sufficient. I was particularly disturbed about this action, because I believed it to be a vindictive move on the part of Dr. Hannah with origins back in 1971 and the difficulties associated with the termination of the drug plan. In my opinion, Dr. Upper had been a conscientious member of the staff of AMS and a strong and loyal supporter of his superior, Dr. Hannah; that Dr. Hannah should react against him by removing him from the Board of Directors was incomprehensible to me. The repercussions of this meeting were important to AMS at this time of finding its future in that, as a reaction to the removal of Dr. Upper, two other members of the Board tendered their resignations in protest. My inclination at the time was to tender my resignation also; but, if I did so, I would be endorsing the "supremacy" of Dr. Hannah in the Board, and I decided that Dr. Hannah would not be able to arrange my removal from the Board as he had Dr. Upper's.

From that point on I suppose I could describe my relationship with Dr. Hannah as adversarial. I had become convinced that his deteriorating health and his desire to hang on to AMS were not compatible, and that the future of AMS had to be placed in other hands.

During my time on the Board, as a physician I recognized more than some other Board members that Dr. Hannah was suffering from an incurable illness and that his life was being sustained only by the repeated blood transfusions. This illness had serious effects on his physical and mental health, and should have led him to decide to give up his position in AMS, but this he was unable to do. It therefore devolved upon the Board to determine what should be done primarily in the interest of AMS.

When Dr. Hannah's contract with the Board of Directors expired at 31 December 1974, it was renewed for one year only. During this time AMS was being established as a registered charity and its role in the history of medicine defined. Dr. Hannah was a participant in these changes, and I recall numerous visits to his home to discuss the future of AMS, as well as to his bedside at the Toronto General Hospital while he received his life-preserving transfusions of blood. When his contract expired at the end of 1975, Dr. Hannah, with the evident intention of continuing as President and Managing Director of AMS, sought its renewal. Chiefly because of his serious health condition, the Board refused. With obvious reluctance, Dr. Hannah resigned from his position and as member of the Board prior to the annual meeting in April 1976.

In these later years the Board had come to recognize that, with a fatal illness facing him, his thoughts had been directed towards recognition of his accomplishments. One of his confreres acknowledged having had few acquaintances who were as concerned with "recognition" as Dr. Hannah. The Board believed that AMS as a monument to Dr. Hannah was hardly a suitable form of recognition; however, the future of AMS predominantly in the history of medicine could be. Recognition that must have been pleasing to him is found in the Hannah Chairs in the history of medicine at the five medical faculties in Ontario, the Hannah Institute for the History of Medicine, and the Hannah Collection in history of medicine in the Fisher Rare Book Library at the University of Toronto, as well as in various grants bearing the Hannah name as approved over the succeeding years by AMS and its committees.

Although Dr. Hannah and I were never friends, I believe we had some respect for each other and that, before his death, he came to appreciate that I had inherited some of his beliefs about AMS and its future.

APPENDIX I

AMS Board Members and Officers

Atcheson, Kenneth W.	1959-64
Secretary-Treasurer	1938-64
Baker, Herbert W.	1937-65
President	1938-65
Barr, G. Eric	1966-74
Secretary-Treasurer	1973-74
Beardall, Frederick G.[1]	1937-45
Vice-President	
Bocking, Douglas	1976-77
(ex officio)	
Broughton, Ernest A.	1938-45
Caldwell, William S.[1]	1937
Cudney, Robert J.	1975-76
Deutsch, John J.	1975-76
D'Iorio, Antoine	1984-
Eames, Leonard C.	1943-45

[1] Charter member and provisional director from the date of incorporation to the first general meeting, September 8, 1937.

Fleming, Shirley A.	1976-84
Godfrey, E. Ray	1983-
Hannah, Jason A.[1]	1937-76
Chief Medical Officer	1937-46
Managing Director	1939-75
President	1965-76
Hon. President	1976-77
Higgins, Douglas G.	1938-56
Hossick, Kenneth C.	1941-76
Vice-President	1945-76
Hunter, H.A.	
Secretary-Treasurer	1938
Hyndman, Robert H.	1964-74
Jackson, Alan B.[1]	1937-38
President	1937-38
Jackson, Harold M.[1]	1937
Johnson, J. Ragnar	1938-42
Kelly, John M.	1978-84
Kuehner, W.C.	1943
Laidlaw, Campbell C.	1945-68
Little, Walter	1975-77
Lynch, Abbyann D.	1984-
Macbeth, Robert A.	1984-

MacCarthy, George S.	1941-46
Macdonald, R. Ian	1972-75
Mackenzie, Thomas P.	1941-42
McCutcheon, John W.	1941-43
McGuire, John A.	1943
Neilson, John B.	1966-84
Acting Managing Director	1976
(position terminated 1976)	
President	1976-83
Palmer, J.G.	1959-64
Chief Medical Officer	1946-64
Playfair, Lawrence L.	1941-43
Pollock, Allan D.	1944-45
Reid, Leslie F.	1978-81
Scott, John W.	1976-
Vice-President	1976-84
Seidelman, William E.	1985-
Sewell, Preston J.	
Secretary	1973-81
Spaulding, William B.	1975-85
Vice-President	1976-79
Strudley, Donald B.	1944-66

Sword, John H.	1983-
Vice-President	1984-
Upper, S. Boyd	1964-74
	1976-
Chief Medical Officer	1964-73
Vice-President	1979-
Waddell, R.C.	1946-55
Wales, Henry C.	1938-41
Waugh, Douglas O.W. (ex officio)	1975
White, C.C.	1942-45
Wildridge, L. Mary	
Secretary	1981-
Wilson, Donald R.	1983-
President	1983-

PHOTO SECTION

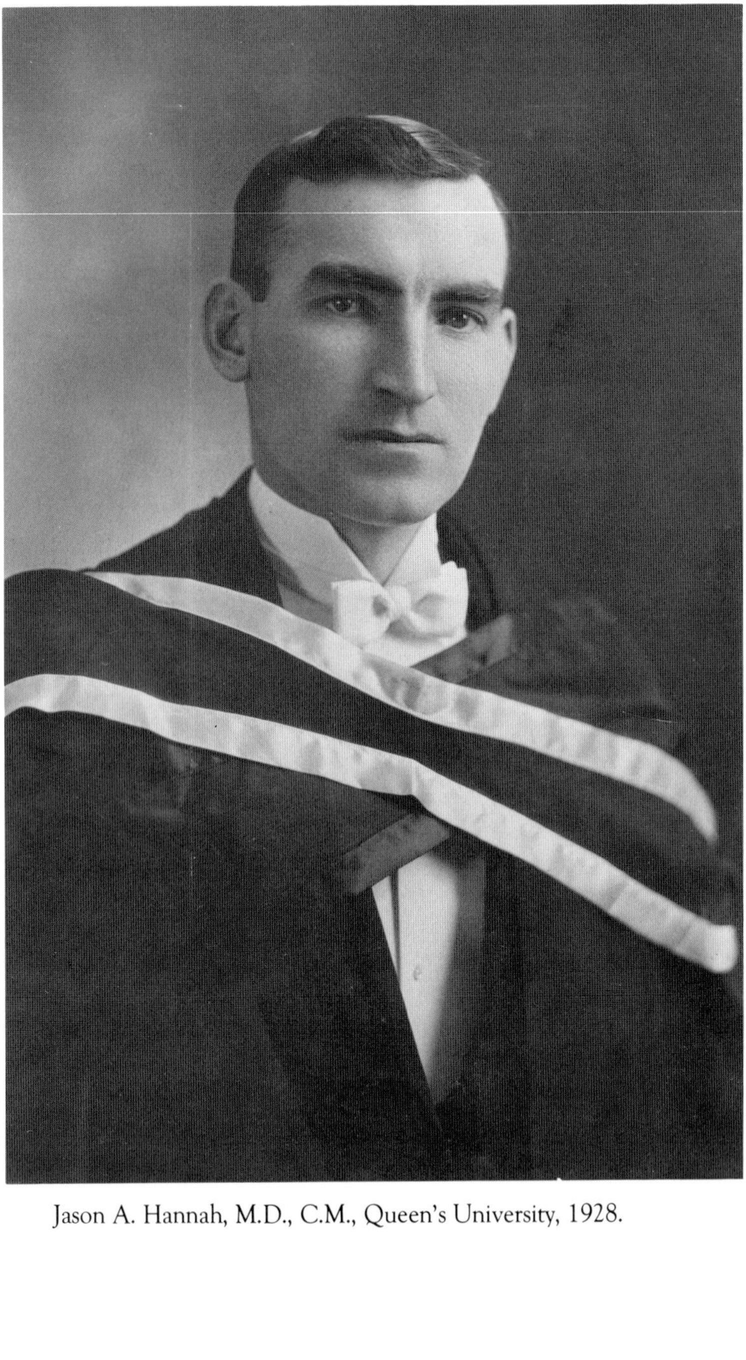

Jason A. Hannah, M.D., C.M., Queen's University, 1928.

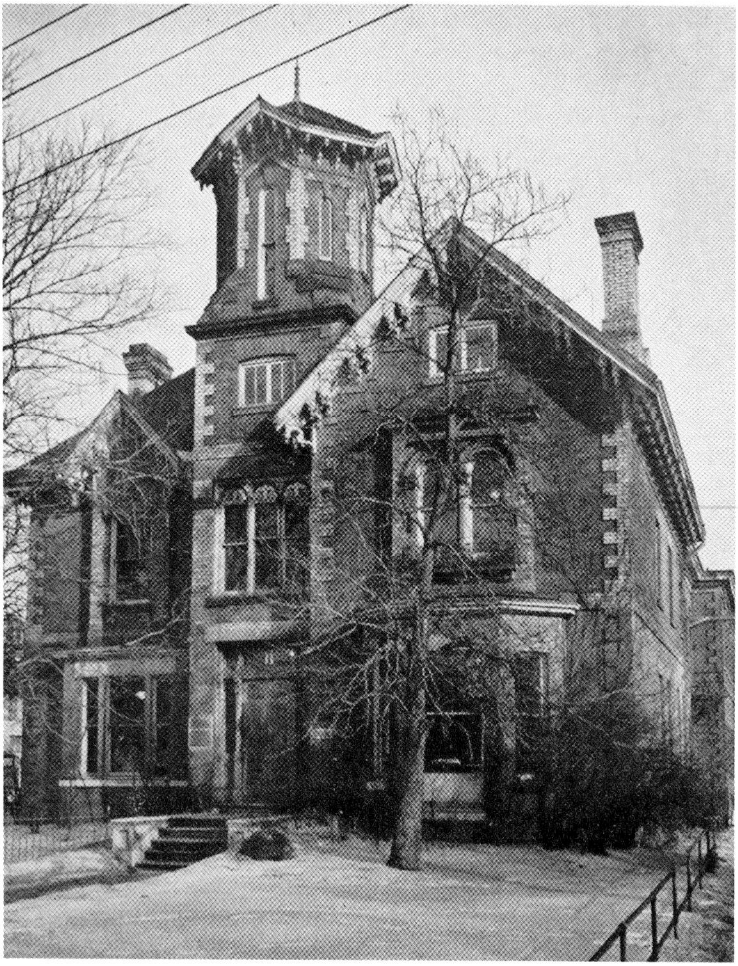

First offices of AMS, 11 Queen's Park, Toronto.

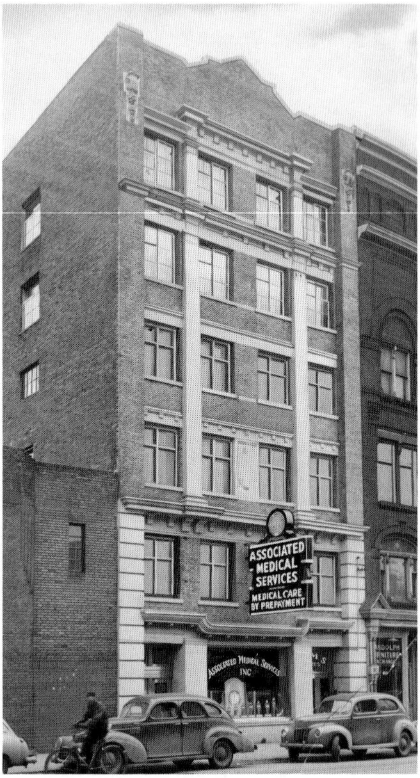

Headquarter offices of AMS,
615 Yonge Street, Toronto.

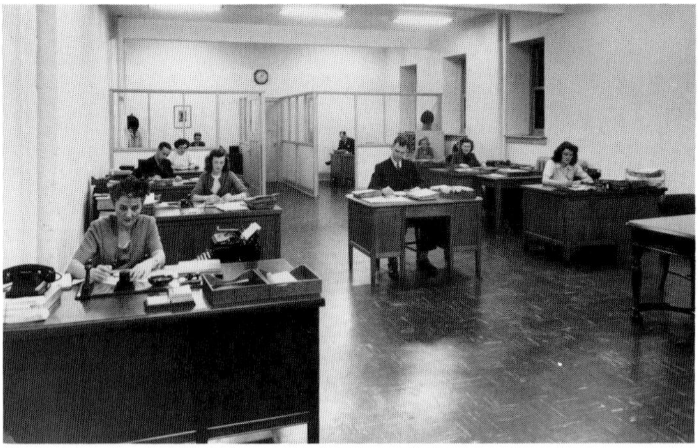

Main floor (Reception) AMS offices.

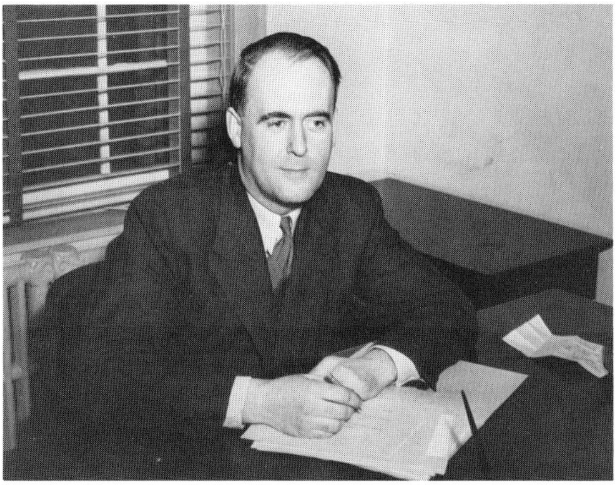

Dr. J.G. Palmer,
Chief Medical
Officer 1946-64.

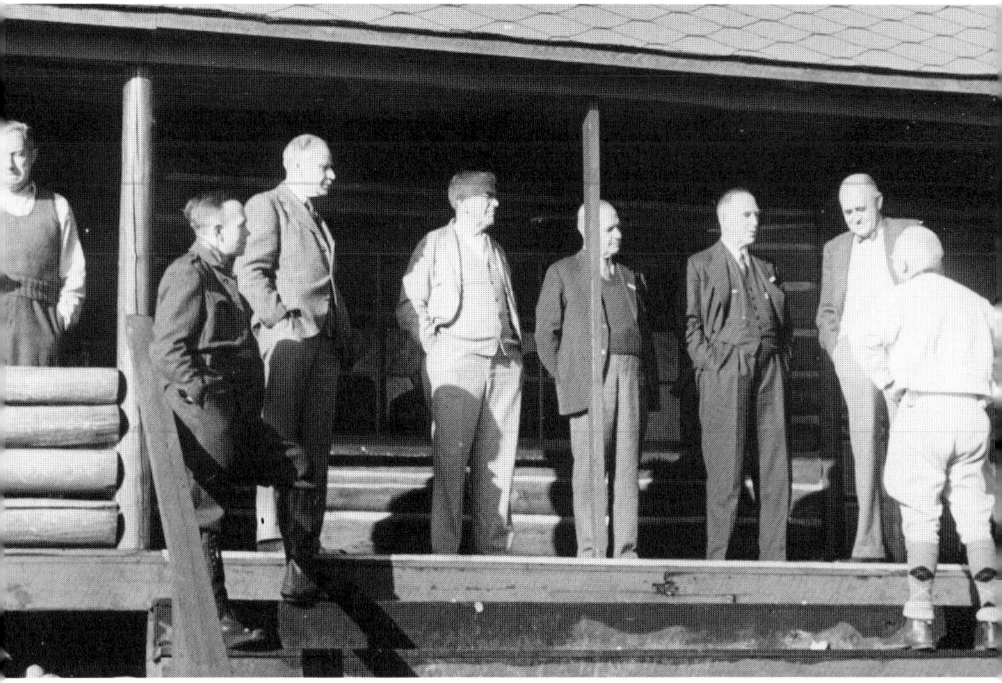

Guests at Mazinaw conference on health economics, October 1946.
L to R: J. Ragnar Johnson, Dr. A.D. Kelly, Dr. H.S. Dunham, Dr. R.L. Gardner, Dr. D. Smith, Dr. C. Laidlaw, Dr. T.C. Routley, Dr. W. Wilson, Dr. H. Agnew.

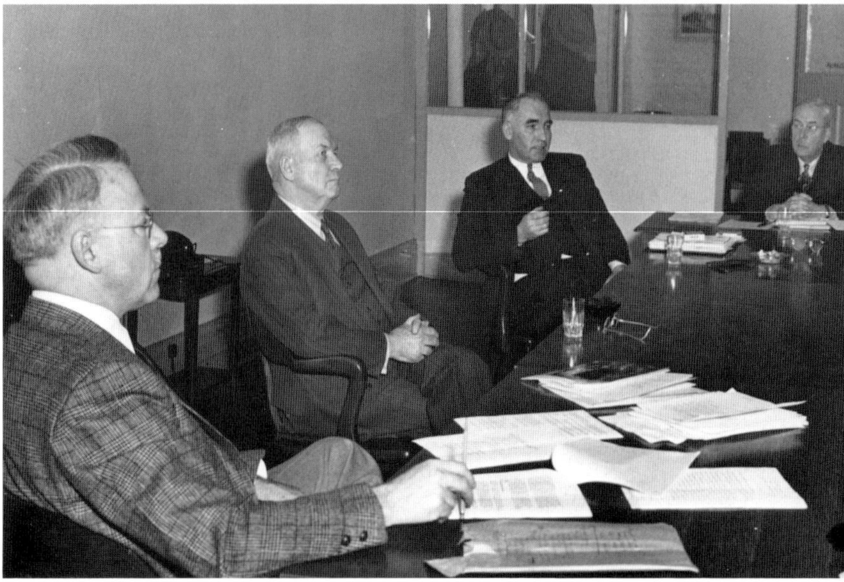

Board of Directors, c. 1946
L to R: D.G. Higgins, Dr. C.C. Laidlaw, Dr. J.A. Hannah, Dr. H.W. Baker (President).

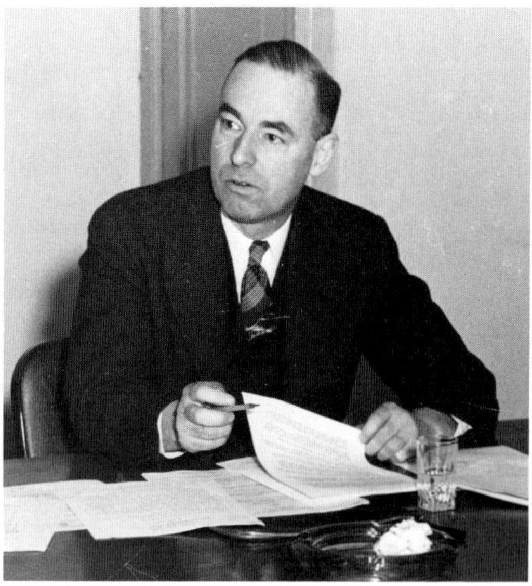

Dr. D.B. Strudley
(Director 1944-66).

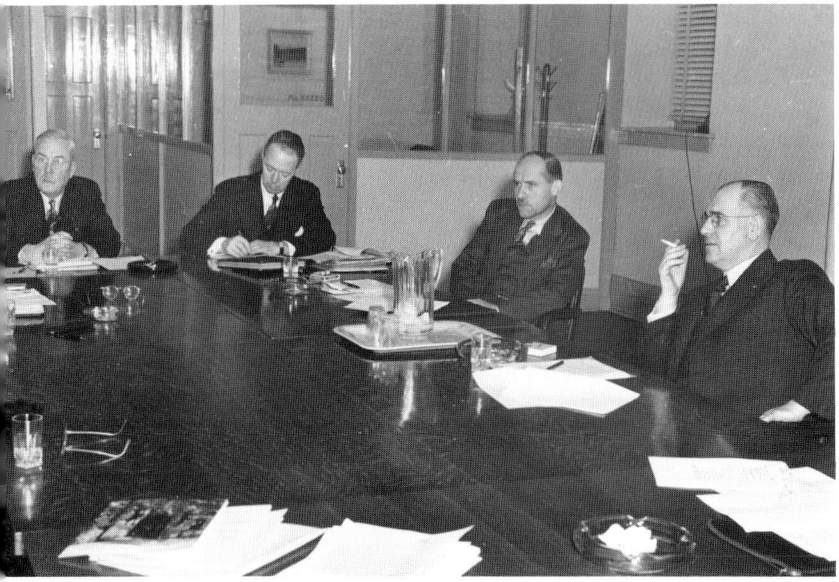

Board of Directors, c. 1946. L to R: Dr. H.W. Baker, K.W. Atcheson (Secretary), Dr. R.R. Waddell, K.C. Hossick.

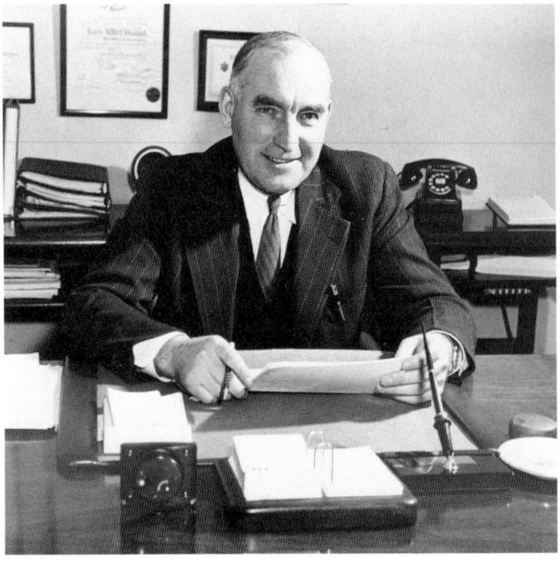

Dr. Jason A. Hannah in his office at AMS headquarters, 615 Yonge Street, Toronto (c. 1946).

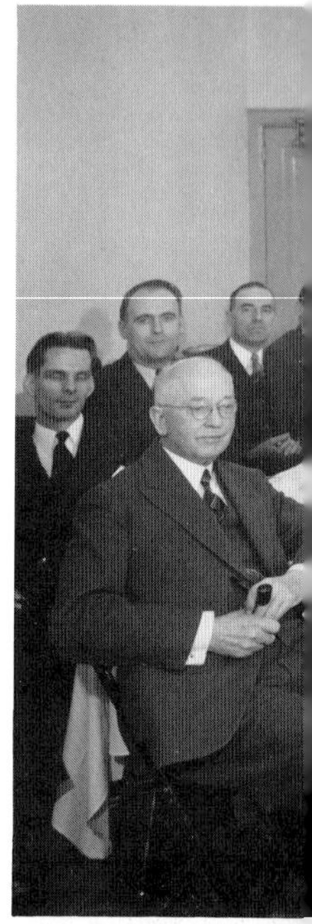

AMS 10th Annual
Meeting Dinner, 1948.

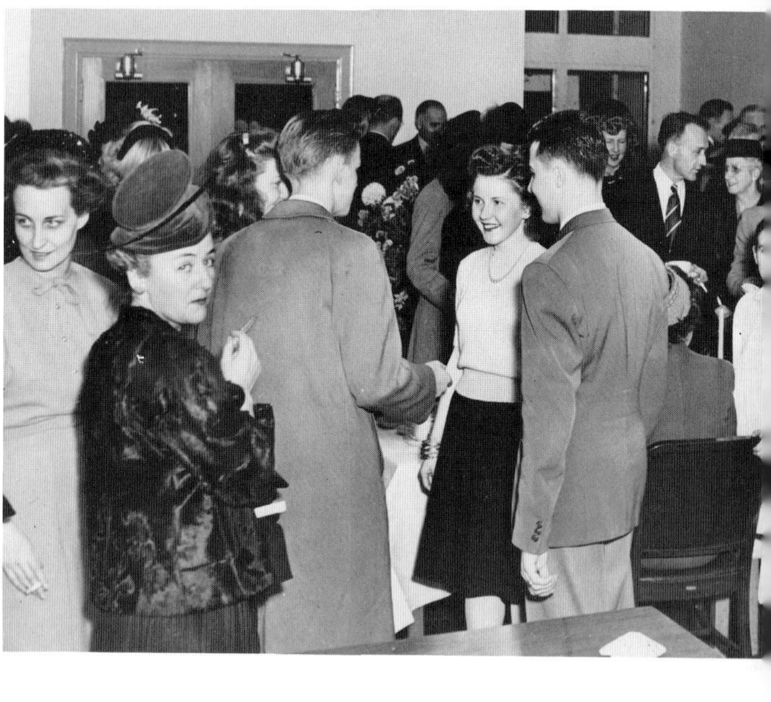

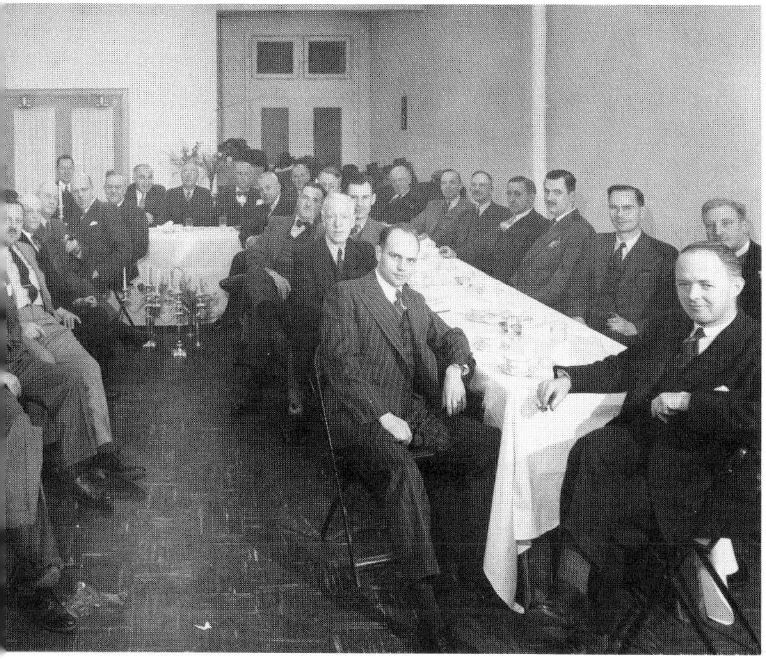

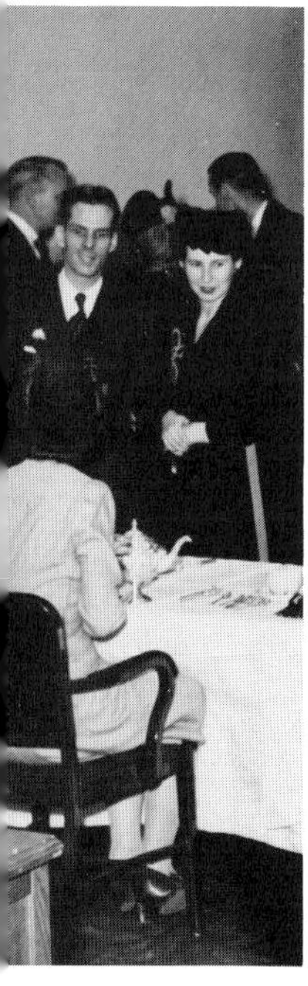

Open House, AMS offices, 1960.

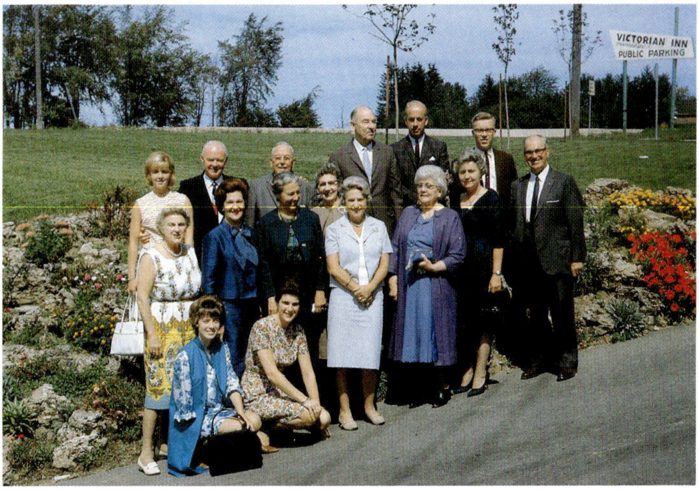

AMS Board members and their wives, Stratford 1964.

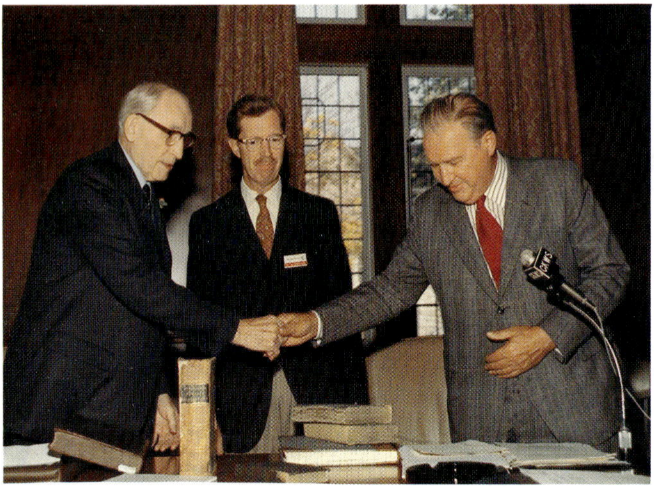

Presentation of rare books to Queen's University Library by Dr. Hannah, October 1973. L to R: Dr. Hannah, D.A. Redmond (Chief Librarian), Dr. J.J. Deutsch (Principal).

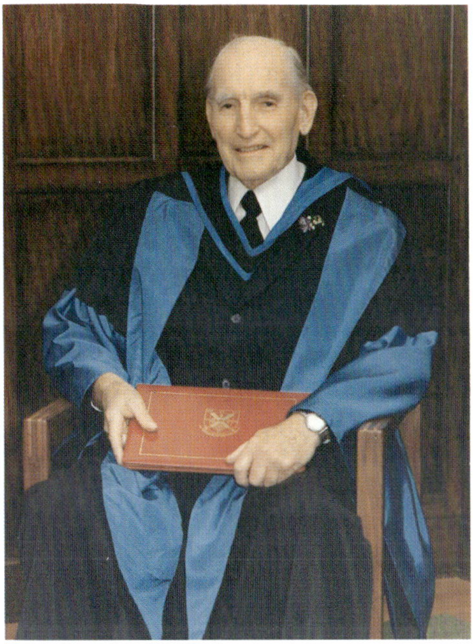

Dr. Hannah presented with Honorary LL.D., Queen's University, May 25, 1974.

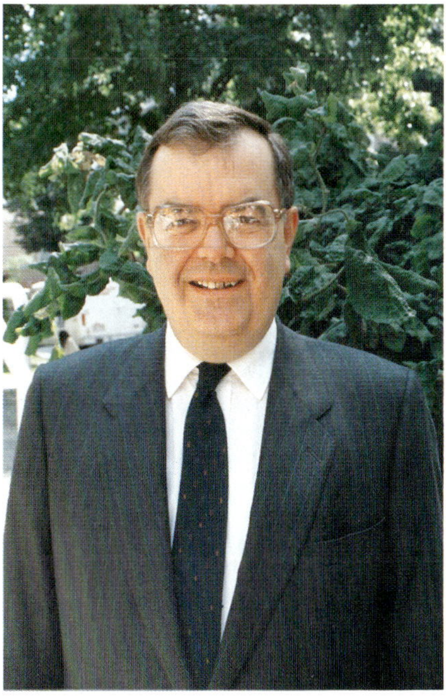

Dr. S.B. Upper, Chief Medical Officer of AMS 1964-73, Vice-President 1979- .

Dr. Hannah receiving gift from
the board, daughter Katherine
in foreground.

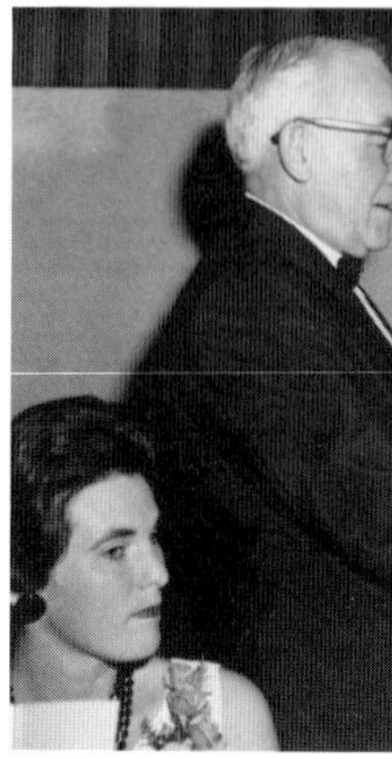

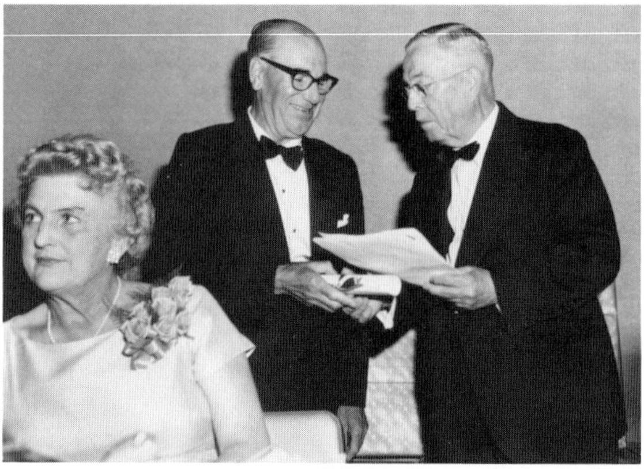

K.C. Hossick (Vice-President) being presented with AMS life membership by Dr. H.W. Baker (President). Mrs. Hannah in foreground.

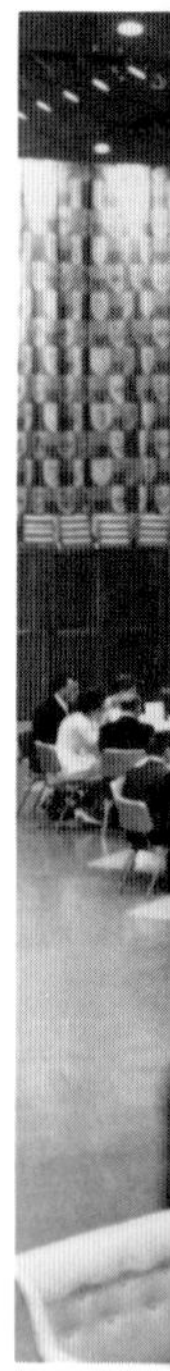

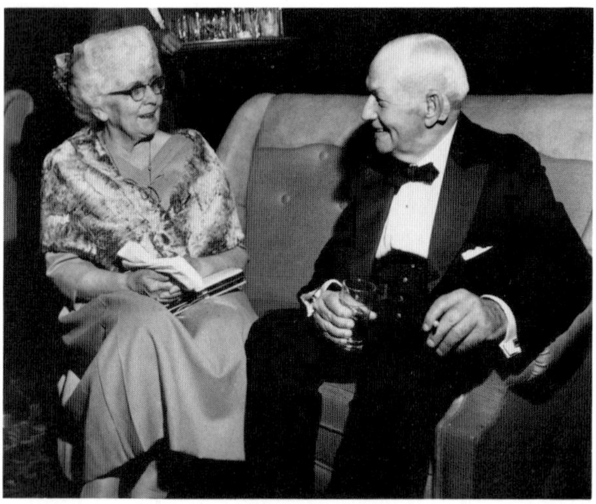

Mrs. H.W. Baker, Dr. C.C. Laidlaw (Director 1945-68).

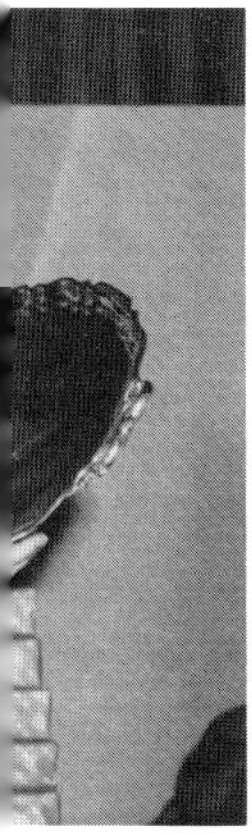

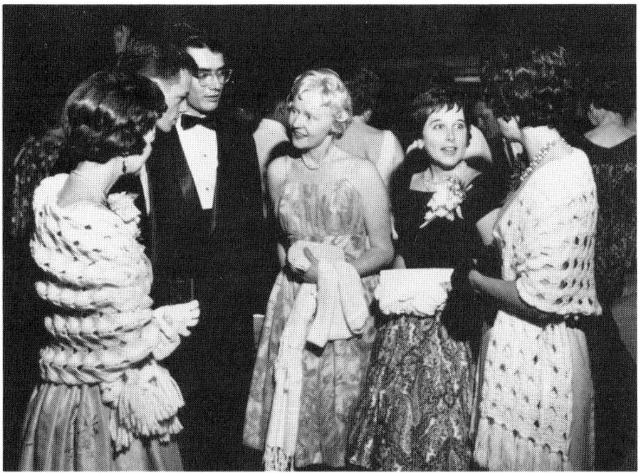

AMS staff members.

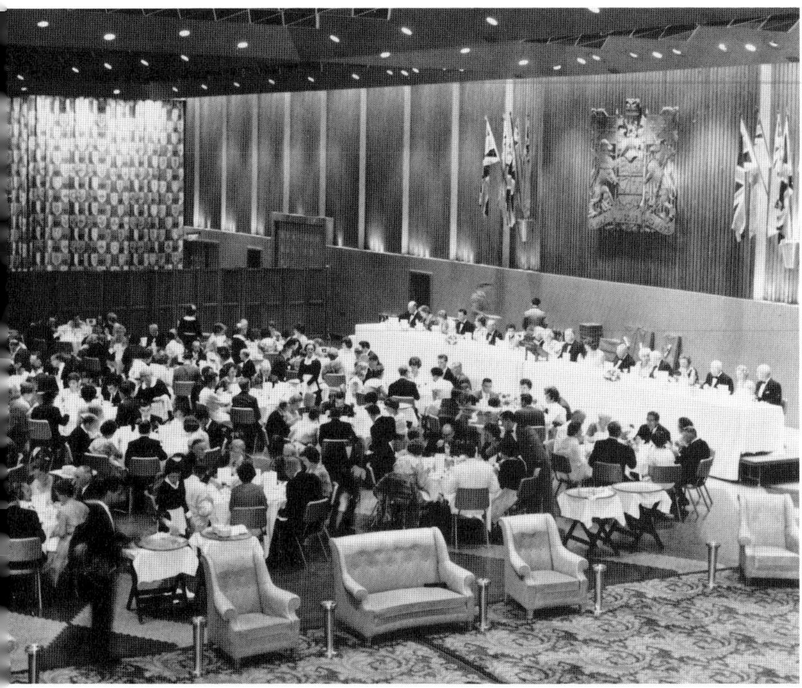

AMS 25th Anniversary Dinner, June 1, 1962, Royal York Hotel.

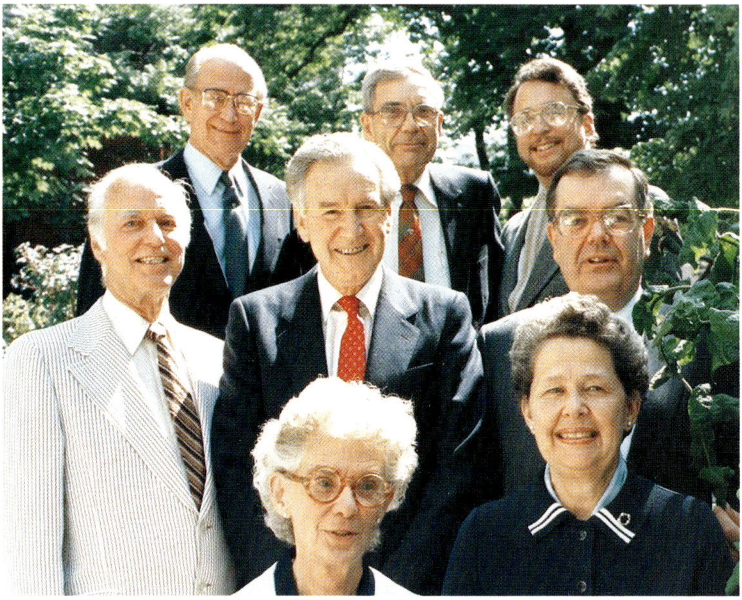

AMS Board of Directors 1986. L to R from rear: Dr. R.A. Macbeth, Dr. J.W. Scott, Dr. W.E. Seidelman, Dr. J.H. Sword, Dr. D.R. Wilson, Dr. S.B. Upper, Prof. E.R. Godfrey, Dr. A.D. Lynch. Absent: Dr. A. D'Iorio.

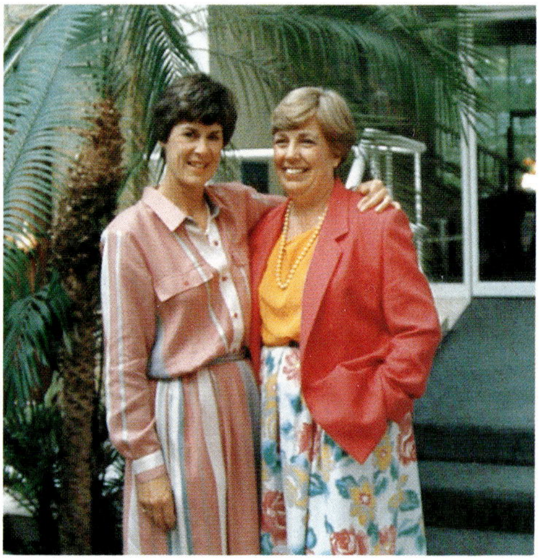

AMS and Hannah Institute office staff 1986: Mary Wildridge (Secretary, AMS), Sheila Snelgrove (Administrative Assistant, Hannah Institute).

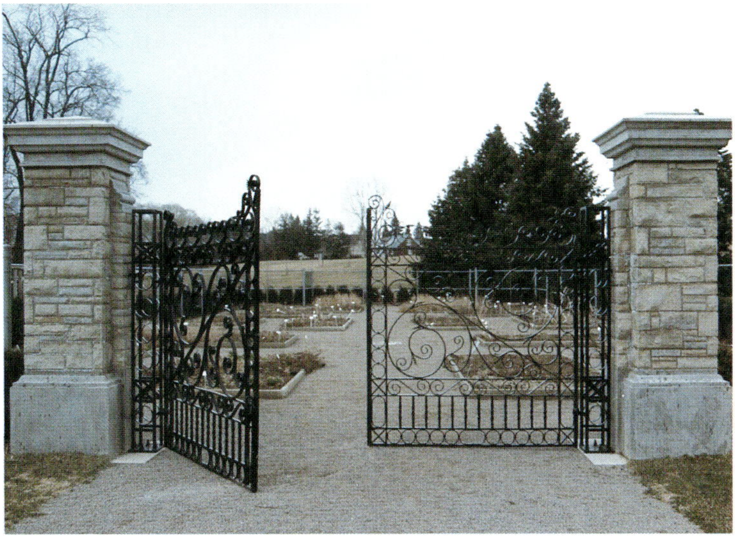

AMS Medicinal Garden, Royal Botanical Gardens, Hamilton. The garden was developed with a grant from AMS.

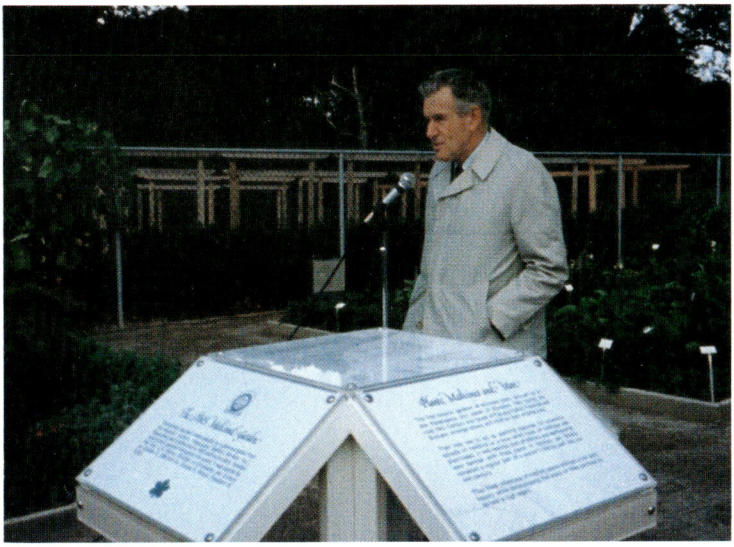

Opening of garden by Dr. D.R. Wilson, President of AMS, October 1985.

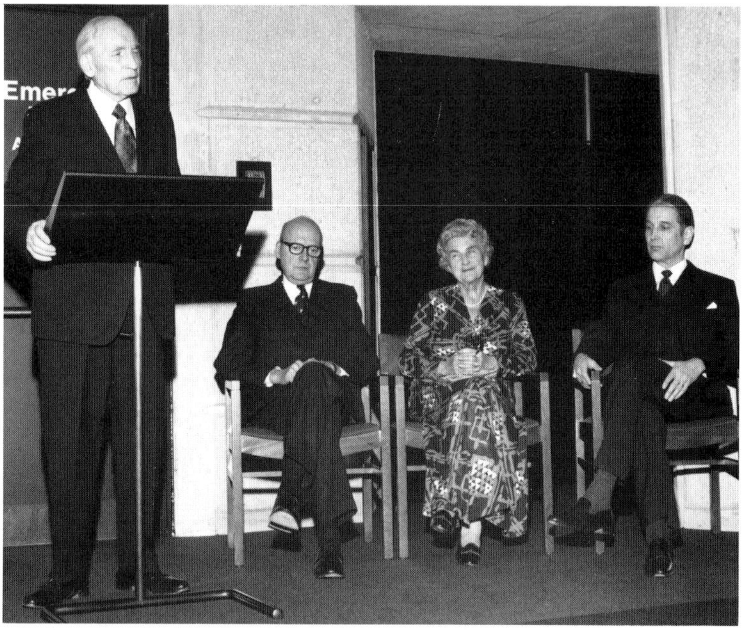

Reception for Dr. Hannah in Thomas Fisher Rare Book Library, University of Toronto, March 1974, in conjunction with an exhibit of early history of medicine books from the Hannah Collection.

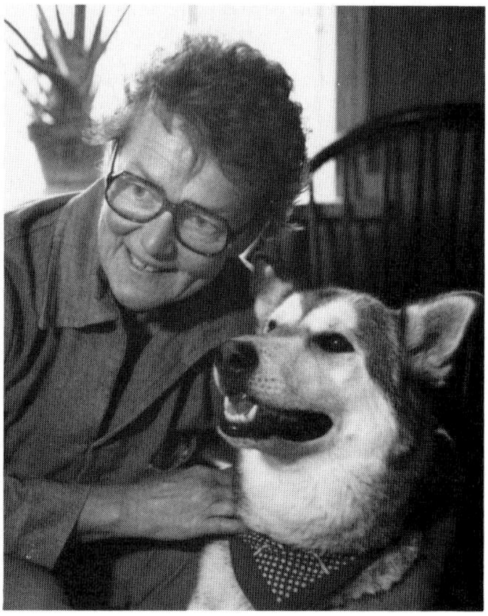

Frances Gage, sculptor, designer of a bronze portrait head of Dr. Hannah and of bronze medals for the Royal Society of Canada Hannah Medal awards. (with Mindy)
– Photography by Doris Huber

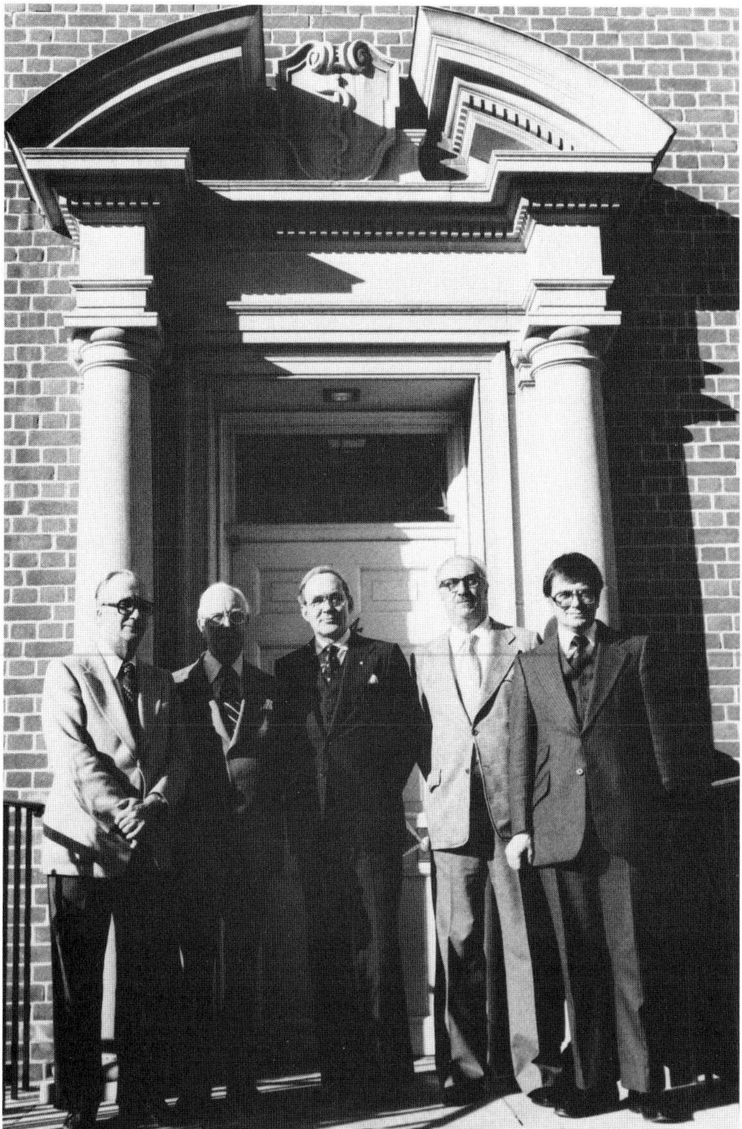

Participants in the first Hannah Symposium held as part of the International Congress of the History of Medicine, Quebec, August 1976. L to R: Dr. G.R. Paterson, Dr.W.E. Swinton, Dr. R.B. Salter, Dr. M.L. Barr, Dr. G.D. Hart. (Photo taken in front of College of Physicians and Surgeons building, Prince Arthur Avenue, Toronto)

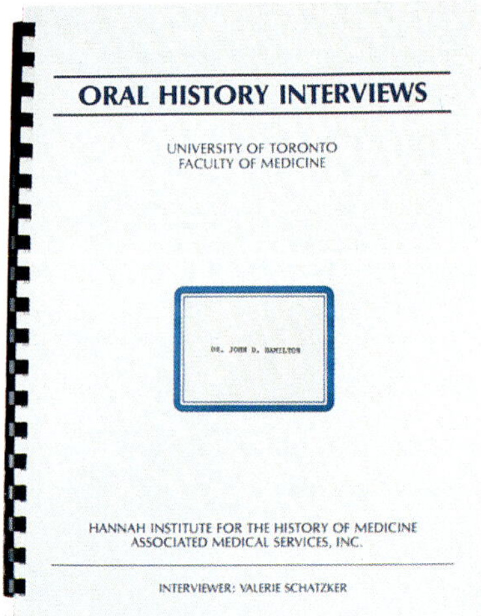

Oral History program – transcript, interview of Dr. J.D. Hamilton by Mrs. V. Schatzker.

– Photograph by Birgitte Nielsen

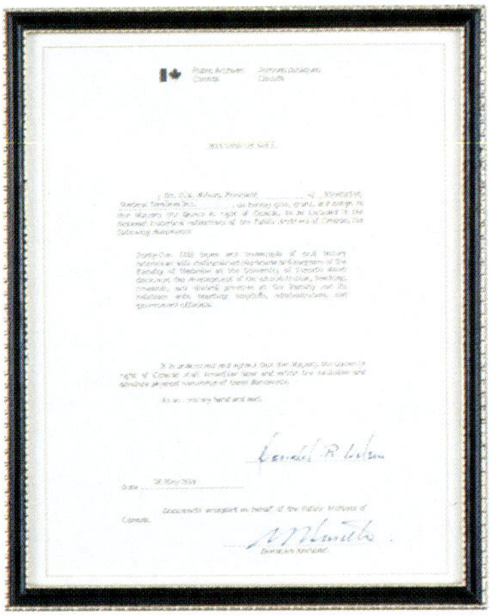

Oral History program – acknowledgement of gift of tapes and transcripts to Public Archives of Canada, May 1984.

– Photograph by Birgitte Nielsen

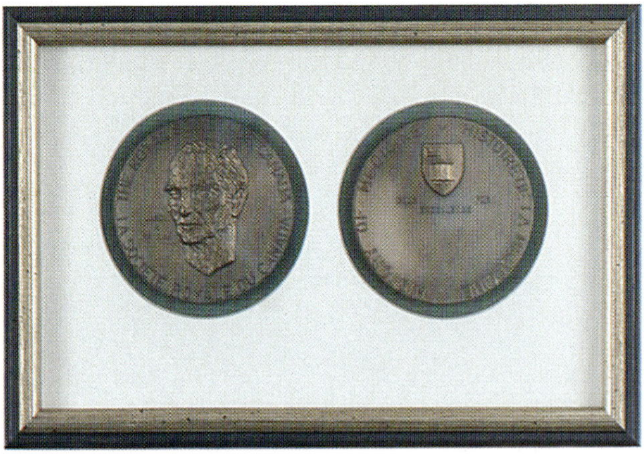

The Hannah Medal of the Royal Society of Canada, established in 1976 and awarded annually for Canadian publications in history of medicine.

– Photograph by Birgitte Nielsen

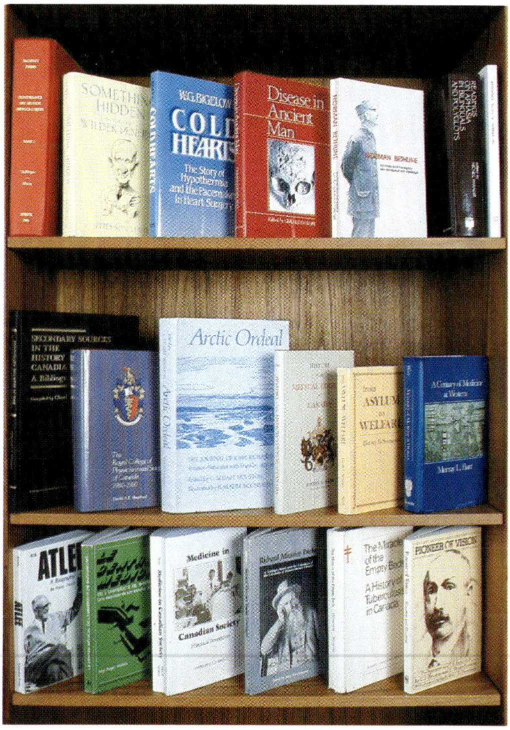

Books published with financial assistance from AMS and the Hannah Institute.
– Photograph by Birgitte Nielsen

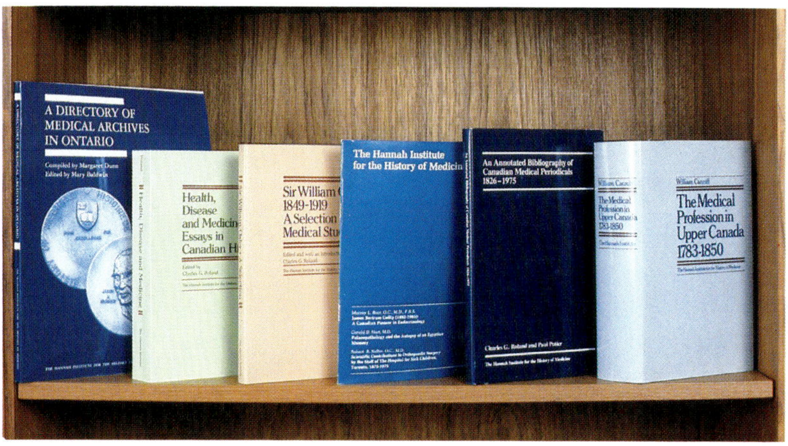

Books published by AMS and the Hannah Institute.
– Photograph by Birgitte Nielsen

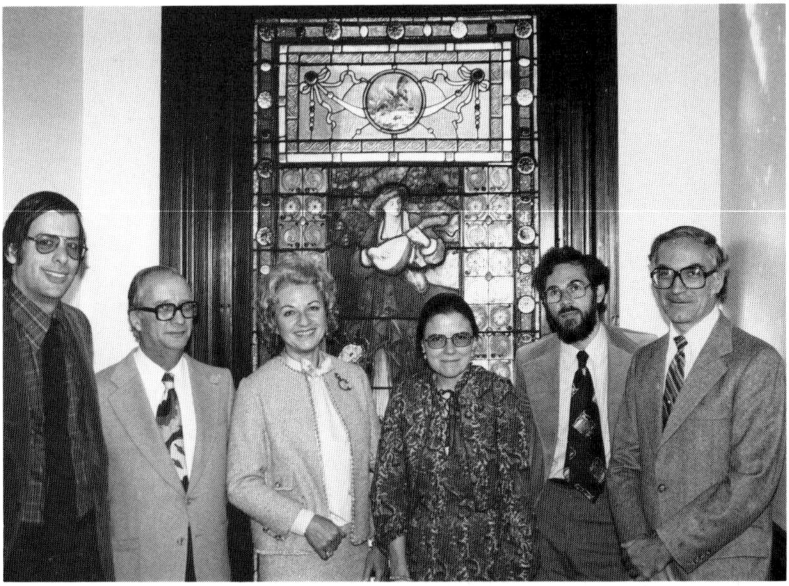

First meeting of Hannah Professors, Academy of Medicine, Toronto, November 1977. L to R: Dr. Toby Gelfand, Dr. G.R. Paterson, Dr. Ruth Hodgkinson, Dr. Pauline Mazumdar, Dr. Paul Potter, Dr. Charles G. Roland.

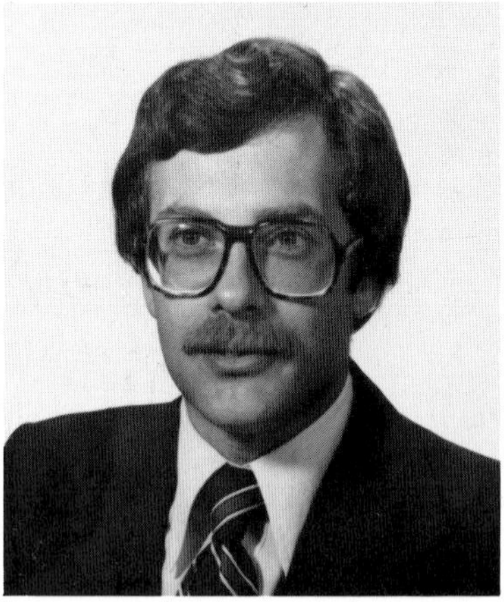

Dr. Samuel E.D. Shortt, Hannah Professor, Queen's University 1979-84.

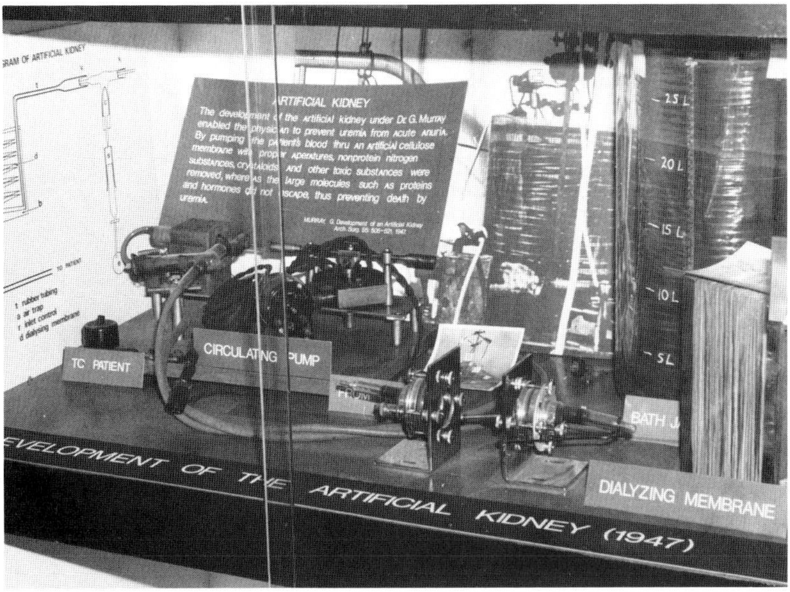

Cardiovascular Surgical Teaching Museum, Toronto General Hospital, May 1978, developed with a grant from AMS.

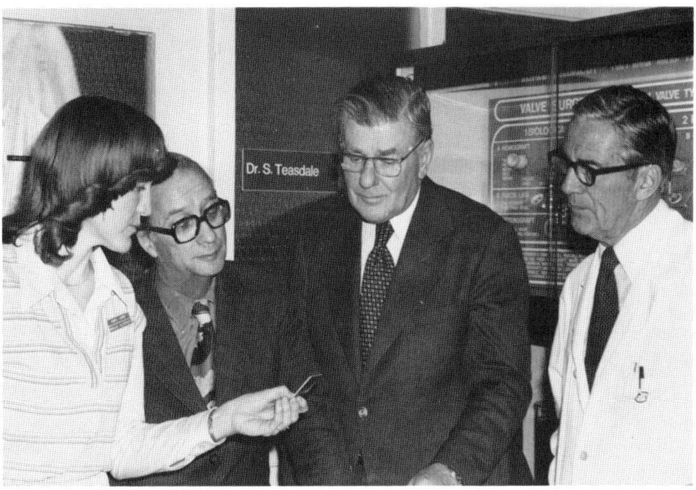

Cardiovascular Surgical Teaching Museum. L to R: Mrs. Karen Young, Dr. G.R. Paterson, Dr. J.B. Neilson, Dr. W.G. Bigelow.

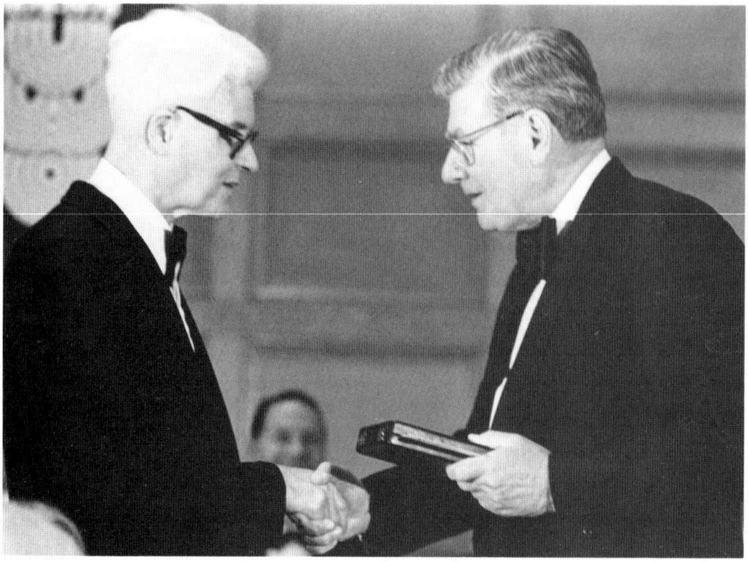

Dr. Henri Ellenberger of Montreal being presented with the first Hannah Medal of the Royal Society of Canada, London, Ontario June 1978.

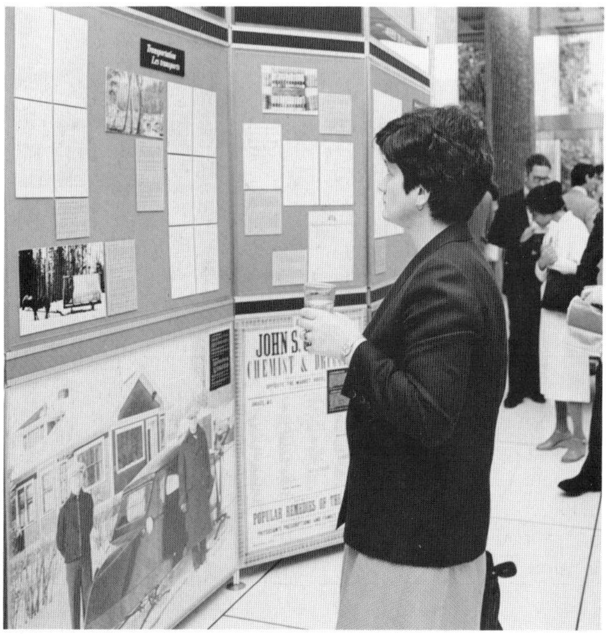

Canadian Medical Archives exhibit, sponsored by AMS and the Hannah Institute with the Public Archives of Canada. Opening reception, Royal College of Physicians and Surgeons of Canada Annual Meeting, Ottawa, June 3, 1980.

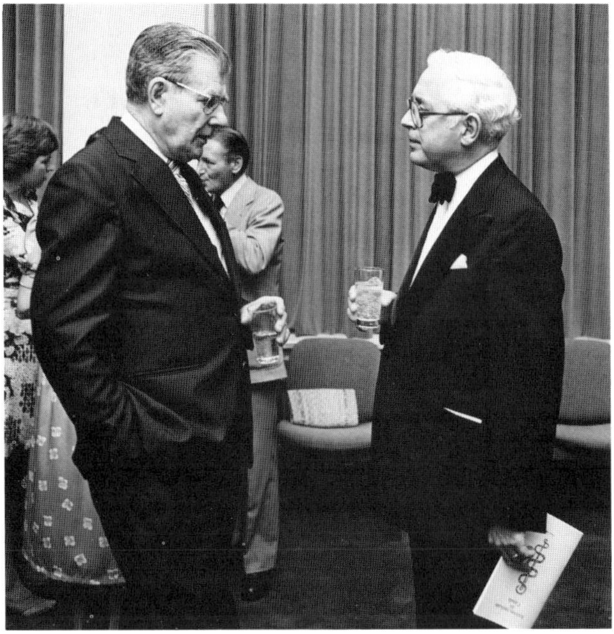

L to R: Dean G.D. Hurteau, University of Ottawa; Dr. J.B. Neilson. Background left: Miss M. Dunn, AMS Archives project coordinator.

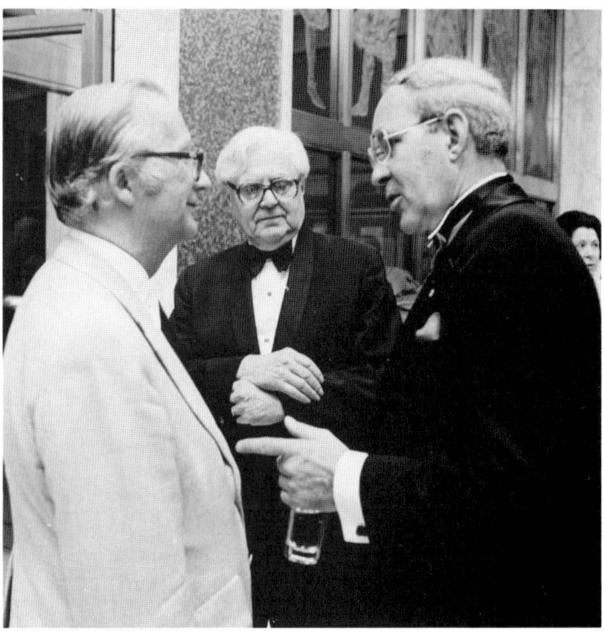

L to R: Dr. G.R. Paterson; Dr. R.B. Kerr, Vancouver; Dr. R.B. Salter, Toronto

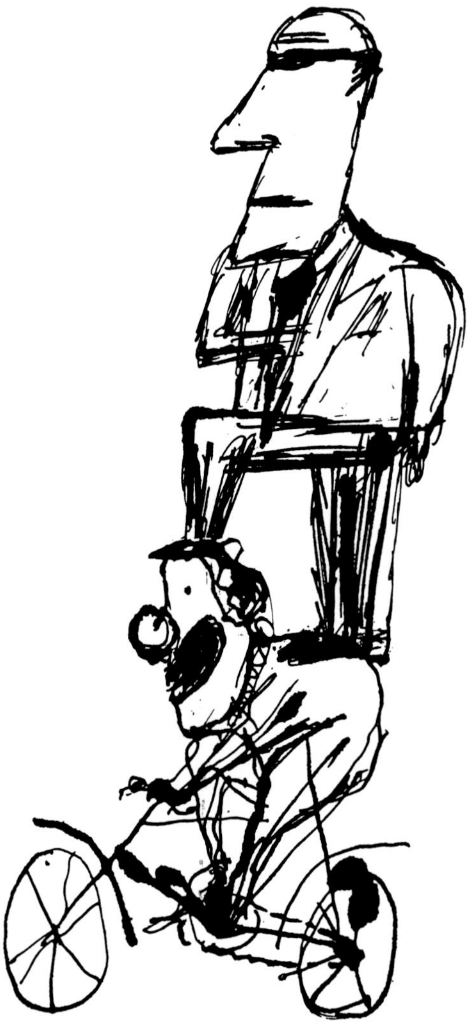

We should know on whose shoulders we stand.

Philosophy of **Jason A. Hannah**, Toronto neuropathologist, who established the Hannah Institute for the History of Medical and Related Subjects, which endowed chairs in medical history in five Ontario universities. Quoted by Joan Hollobon in the Globe and Mail, January 20, 1977.

PART TWO

No Better Float Through Posterity
The Hannah Institute for the History of Medicine

by

G.R. Paterson

"There is no better float through posterity than to be the author of a good bibliography. Scores know Conrad Gesner by the 'Bibliotheca' who never saw the 'Historia Animalium'. A hundred consult Haller's bibliographies for one that looks at his other works; and years after the iniquity of oblivion has covered Dr. Billings' work in the army, as an organizer in connection with hospitals, and even his relation to this great Library, the great Index will remain an enduring monument to his fame."

Sir William Osler, speech delivered to a memorial meeting for John S. Billings, 21 April 1913

PREFACE

Jason Albert Hannah (11 November 1899 – 2 May 1977) was a remarkably determined man. Most members of the human species go through life with few ideas, original, good, or otherwise. Some produce one good idea or exploit an unusual or exceptional talent or circumstance. Dr. Hannah, in a long and busy life, produced two considerable developments. One, in all likelihood, at least in Dr. Hannah's opinion, was the first of its kind in Canada, although it is certain others had proposed and probably developed private prepaid medical care plans elsewhere, perhaps even in Canada. The second idea did utilize the organization, expertise, and resources he had created, in order to leave behind a memorial. It proved to be not a memorial he planned, so much as a somewhat eccentric one on which he happened, during the course of investigating ways of retaining control of the capital accumulated while developing the first idea.

The first came early in his productive adult life and led to the establishment of Associated Medical Services, Incorporated, in 1937 for the purpose of providing prepaid medical care. My colleague Dr. John B. Neilson has dealt with the implementation of the first idea in Part One of this history of the corporation.

The purpose of Part Two is to deal with the beginnings and development of the second idea. It cannot be said that the economic times were ripe any more than for the first idea. Nor can it be said that personal background was to any great extent responsible for the involvement of a man near the end of his productive span, victim of a decade of serious illness, in the elaboration of a plan for promoting history of medicine. Certainly, developments in the first field to which he contributed, and the passage of time which brought increasing interest in the second field, will be seen to be definite factors for change in the activities of Dr. Hannah and the corporation. At no time, however, did increasing provincial and federal government involvement in health care delivery dictate the nature of the changes that were to take place in the corporation and in its use of its financial and other resources.

AMS interest in and promotion of history of medicine was the result of a long period of thinking, discussion, and exploration. The original charter, wisely drawn up, made this long gestation and birth possible. The purpose of this second part, then, is to examine in detail how the history of medicine became the chief activity of the corporation and to look for the significant developments that have resulted from that activity, the acceptance of the discipline by five medical schools and by many individuals.

The success of AMS and its plan for prepaid medical care, overwhelmingly due to the imaginative hard work of Dr. Hannah himself, led to several happenings and consequences. The first was the interest on the part of others in the idea. Governmental interest increased too, owing to many political factors. These happenings meant the corporation would eventually lose its role in a field in which it had been a pioneer. A second consequence, however, possible because of both a far-sighted charter and the accumulation of reserves as required by law, was the freedom to make choices of new plans for the betterment of the profession of medicine. One option available under law, returning the accumulated funds to the general revenues of the province in the procedure called winding-up, obviously was not considered to be in the best interests of medicine.

The search for what would be best for medicine in the opinion of Dr. Hannah and his Board members brought forward many suggestions, usually referred to in the minutes under the heading "diversification". Selective and most frequently unproductive discussion consumed a considerable amount of time, at the end of which the Board decided in favour of the history of medicine by the founding of an institute of the history of medicine and by the establishment of chairs in the subject at the five Ontario universities possessed of faculties of medicine. The institute, quite unlike any of the other medical historical institutes in existence, was intended to coordinate the universities' activities and to extend history of medicine beyond the five campuses. A third consequence of the corporation's success was that money was available to make a substantial contribution or endowment to a medical field, compatible with the 1937 charter.

This being so, Dr. Hannah's idea of supporting history of medicine began to take shape, although he did not live to see all five chairs filled. Nor did he see the development of the institute as it has evolved. However, tribute must be paid him for his determination, which contributed greatly to what has developed. It is, of course, not possible to say that he would have been pleased by all that has come about in history of medicine in the name of Hannah. It is, however, possible to hope that he would think the balance of accomplishments positive.

In a spirit of admiration and gratitude, then, this account and the accompanying analysis of the growth of his second idea are dedicated to the memory of Dr. Jason A. Hannah.

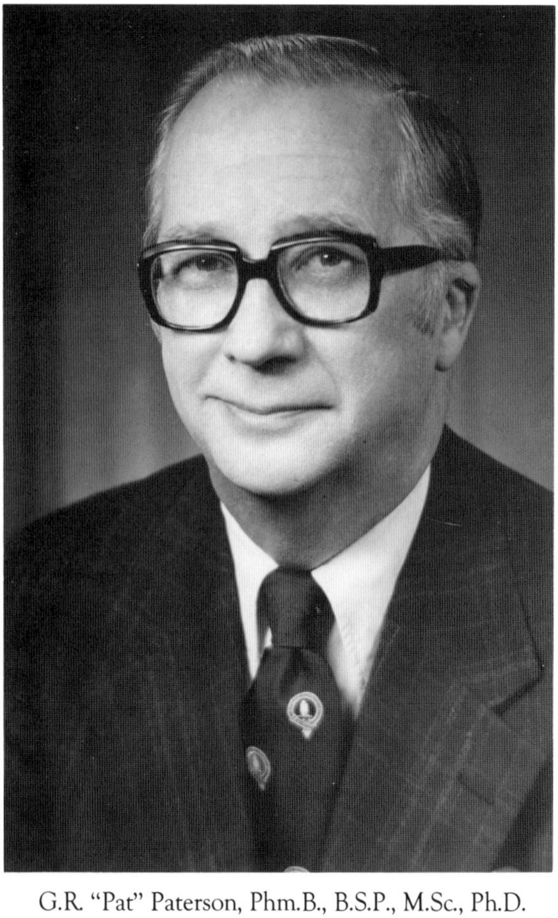

G.R. "Pat" Paterson, Phm.B., B.S.P., M.Sc., Ph.D.
Executive Director, Hannah Institute 1975-87.

– Photograph by Milne, Toronto

ACKNOWLEDGEMENTS

I have received much help in locating, identifying, and gaining access to relevant archival material from the following: George Connell (President), Kirk Haworth (Director of Archives) and his assistant, Harold Averill, and Richard Landon (Head, Fisher Rare Book Library), all of the University of Toronto; Dean D.L. Wilson, Faculty of Medicine, Queen's University; Dean Gilles D. Hurteau and Mlle Andrea Courtemanche, Faculty of Health Sciences, University of Ottawa. I am particularly grateful to Queen's and Ottawa for having retained essential files of the Council of the Faculties of Medicine. I am most thankful to all mentioned for their courtesy.

Three interested and deeply involved individuals have made their files available to me. To Dr. John W. Scott, Professor Emeritus of Physiology, University of Toronto, and Dr. A.A. Travill, Professor of Anatomy, Queen's University, both members of the *ad hoc* COFM Committee, and to Dr. W.C. Gibson, now Chancellor of the University of Victoria, one of Dr. Hannah's two principal historical advisers, I say that I could not have managed without the material they made available to me so graciously.

Interviews were granted me not only by Drs. Scott and Travill, but also by two other members of the COFM Committee: Dr. C. Barber Mueller, Professor of Surgery, McMaster University, and Dr. Frederic L. Holmes, who represented the University of Western Ontario on that Committee. The late Dean Jacques J. Lussier of the University of Ottawa chaired that Committee; some of his notes about the meetings were found in the archives of the Faculty of Health Sciences, University of Ottawa. Both of Dr. Hannah's advisers, Dr. Gibson and Dr. W.E. Swinton, talked to me at some length – profitably. All of the following talked freely of their memories of Dr. Hannah and his second great idea: Dr. Robertson Davies, Master Emeritus of Massey College; Dr. E. Harry Botterell, Dean Emeritus of Medicine, Queen's University;

the late R.B. Hyndman, Dr. S. Boyd Upper, and Dr. John B. Neilson (who talked to me as former members of the Board of Directors of AMS); Mrs. Kathy Davis, daughter of Dr. Hannah; and Dr. Holmes, now of the Section of the History of Medicine, Yale University. To all, I express sincere thanks. Dr. A. Rupert Hall made available a proof copy of his forthcoming book, *Physic and Philanthropy,* for my reading. This is a history of the Wellcome Trust, and reading it proved most helpful.

Dr. Upper read the chapter "Diversification" critically and offered most useful information and many helpful hints. Dr. Scott, a member of the Executive of the Academy of Medicine at the time when Dr. Hannah was negotiating with that body, read that chapter critically. I am very grateful to both Drs. Upper and Scott.

Four colleagues read the complete manuscript critically at my request. They are Mr. Eric J. Freeman, Librarian and Deputy Director of the Wellcome Institute for the History of Medicine; Dr. Paul M.J. Potter, Hannah Professor of the History of Medicine, University of Western Ontario; Dr.Holmes; and Dr. John M. Norris, Director, Division of the History of Medicine, Faculty of Medicine, University of British Columbia. To all four, I am most grateful for positive criticism. To Dr. Norris especially, I am indebted for much editorial and structural advice, which, I feel sure, has improved the earlier draft I sent to my readers. That it still has shortcomings will be obvious to my readers; I accept responsibility for them.

I should also like to thank my Administrative Assistant, Mrs. Sheila Snelgrove, for guiding me in the use of the word processor with which this book has been written. Too, I thank the officers of AMS, beginning with Dr. Hannah, for the opportunity to undertake a fascinating second career. Doing so would not have been possible without the loving and thoughtful support and devotion of my wife, to whom I am forever thankful.

G.R. Paterson

CHAPTER I

Diversification

Associated Medical Services, Incorporated, was founded as a corporation without share capital 9 April 1937 by authority of the Honourable Harry Corwin Nixon, Provincial Secretary in the Government of Ontario.

Clauses (a) and (b) in the statement of purposes and objects in the letters patent granted the five applicants for a charter were concerned with Dr. Hannah's first idea, how it would be realized and maintained. Clauses (c), (d), and (e) were designed to permit other activities than those associated with prepaid medical care. They were stated as follows:[1]

> (c) To encourage medical research and preventive medicine.
> (d) To co-operate with organized medicine in the advancement of the standard of medical service, and
> (e) To do all such other things as are incidental or conducive to the attainment of the above objects.

In the early 1960s, three factors began to come into play that would cause the officers and Board of Directors of the corporation to consider alternative activities – what the Board would term "diversification". As noted in the preface, one of these factors was the increasing government interest in its assumption of responsibility for provision of health care facilities and services for the electorate. A second factor was the approaching twenty-fifth anniversary of the corporation and its celebration in 1962. A third factor was the beginning of Dr. Hannah's ill health. The second and third were to combine, in Dr. Hannah's mind, to make more urgent some form of permanent memorial to his first great idea and accomplishment. It is certainly not apparent in the early years of the decade that he saw the memorial itself in the history of medicine.

In late 1960 and again in 1961, Dr. Hannah discussed with his Board and, in company with the Medical Director of AMS (then Dr. William Wigle), with provincial government officials the subject of supplementary letters. Factors dictating the need to do this probably included the Lesage government's adoption of provincial health insurance in Quebec, as well as growing interest at Queen's Park in health services provision.[2]

At the same time, the Board began to discuss, or at least hear Dr. Hannah talk of, more specific options, such as closed panel clinics,[3] a medical centre research reserve (the Board made $250,000 available for such a fund),[4] and the actual operation of a hospital by AMS.[5] Dr. Hannah reported too on discussions he had with many hospital experts.

History Enters the Picture

There was other evidence in the same sets of minutes of concern about the corporation's future. Dr. Hannah and Board members were of the opinion they should deal with the subject of winding-up by means of supplementary letters patent, which would provide for employee separation, a specific endowment to Queen's University (Dr. Hannah's alma mater), and the disposal of surpluses in principle but not in detail.[6] The endowment reference concerned a medical historical museum, whose cost was estimated at $100,000. This is the first reference found in all available sources to the subject of medical history.

Anniversary Plans and Other Discussions

Initial discussion of anniversary plans centred on recognition of charter subscribers or those who had been enrolled for at least twenty years. There is no indication of the number who would be honoured if a formula were devised and applied. There was a distinct slowing down of discussion of specific suggestions for diversification at this time, undoubtedly due, at least in part, to the work and influence of the Royal Commission on Health Services (the Hall Commission).[7]

When anniversary plans were next discussed in early 1962, they did take a different form, an anniversary acknowledgement of the Managing Director's (i.e., Dr. Hannah's) accomplishments. A motion was passed at the 6 May 1962 Board meeting unanimously:

> In order to create a suitable memorial to J.A. Hannah, B.A., M.D., C.M., the Founder and Developer of Prepaid Medical Care Plans, it was agreed that the Board of Directors should offer to donate $250,000 to Queen's University at Kingston, Ontario to be paid over a two year period for the provision of facilities to encourage and facilitate medical research at the University or for such other uses as may come within the scope of the purposes and objects as set out in the A.M.S. Charter.

The minutes went on to record that the gift would be for the establishment and endowment of a suitable display of historical objects of medical interest. Such a display was to be housed as a predominant part of the reading or study area of a medical library. Authorized correspondence between Dr. Hannah and Dr. J.A. Corry, Principal of Queen's University, then ensued, as a result of which the motion was amended in the next month to read:[8]

> That in reference to the Resolution passed at the meeting of the Directors on May 6, 1962, and the amendments to this resolution made at the meeting held on June 1, 1962, the Board of Directors of Associated Medical Services, Incorporated, hereby authorizes a donation of $250,000 as a contribution to assist the medical research programme at Queen's University at Kingston, Ontario through the establishment of a Medical Library to bear the name of Dr. J.A. Hannah and in which continuing provision would be made for a suitable display and endowment of objects of historical medical interest.

The Board specified that one-half the grant would be paid if and when construction began no later than 1 July 1964, and the second half would be given during the succeeding calendar year. Dr. Corry responded in July saying, "It may not be possible to build a medical library as a separate and self-contained building for several reasons but the decision in this matter would be for the Trustees of the University to make."[9] Later, the principal said he would await a study of the situation by the new Dean of Medicine, Dr. E. Harry Botterell. Dr. Hannah made it clear he would not favour having a library (especially one named for him) as part of another building on campus. Such a situation would fail to fulfil the purposes of such a gift, he said. Later, a request from Dean Botterell for help in acquiring a medical sciences librarian, even though authorized by the directors, was not acted upon by the Managing Director.[10]

Little (perhaps no) progress was made towards implementing clinic and hospital diversification. At this time, the reader may well be wondering what the relationship of Dr. Hannah to his fellow directors was (his title was still Managing Director), and how serious he was about various diversification thoughts recorded in Board minutes. The best source of firsthand knowledge and thoughtful opinion about these subjects has been conversation and other personal communication with Dr. S. Boyd Upper, AMS Medical Officer from 1964 until 1973. His personal opinion was expressed in these words: "In ten years, no diversification had occurred. Why? In hindsight, it is clear that Dr. Hannah was personally unwilling to invest money in any business other than prepaid medical care. He was uncomfortable outside his chosen field."[11] These views must be taken seriously, for Dr. Upper was observing in an uncomfortable dual role in AMS, as an employee and as a member of the Board of Directors. He also believes Dr. Hannah dominated his Board by "a personality of great power", as another observer has expressed it. In an oral history interview in 1982, Dr. John B. Neilson, a director from 1968, and Dr. Hannah's successor as President of AMS (he served as President from 1976 until 1983), said: "And it got to be obvious to me that his attitude on the Board was that he was all-powerful, he was president and general manager, and you did things at his pleasure and according to the way he thought they should be done, or else. There was history for this; you were got rid of from the Board. You were one of the 'yes' boys or else you didn't belong."[12]

It is quite probably true that Dr. Hannah had always had a somewhat difficult personality. However, it must also be always borne in mind that the period of diversification and the coming of history of medicine as AMS's principal activity coincided with his many severe illnesses.

In late 1962, still no progress could be reported by Dr. Hannah to the Board.[13] This time, the reason was the meeting called by Dr. Matthew B. Dymond, Minister of Health for Ontario, on 12 November 1962, "to investigate the possibilities of offering coverage in Ontario through existing carriers". One of the attending groups was AMS. This governmental move could have been expected to exert more pressure for AMS to diversify, but there were probably other reasons, some within government and government agencies, that negated developments in the field. More or continuing delays were recorded for the 1 September 1963 Board meeting held at Stratford.[14] (The Board was accustomed to holding one meeting each year at Stratford in order to combine some culture with Board work.) At the end of the year, Dr. Hannah expressed disillusionment that anything would develop in the areas he had investigated.[15]

At the 3 May 1964 meeting, concern about winding-up bylaws reappeared. The Board agreed on the high desirability of facing up to the problem before it might present itself suddenly. For the first time, there was a suggestion that surplus assets might be distributed to medical schools in Ontario, which would constitute a solution to the problem of disposal of reserves to other than the government coffers.[16] In September, the Board reaffirmed that a gift to Queen's should bear the Hannah name. Additionally, the view was expressed that an impartial yardstick concerning distribution of assets to the medical schools would be necessary. The motion, introduced for study, read as follows:[17]

> Should AMS for any reason be wound up, all its remaining assets "after payment of all debts and liabilities" shall, prior to dissolution be distributed or disposed of to promote medical education in the Province of Ontario;

distribution of such remaining assets shall be made in such manner and amounts to such medical schools in Ontario and in such ratio to each of them, as the Board of Directors of AMS may in its sole discretion deem advisable, prior to such distribution being made.

At the 9 May 1965 meeting, the clause was passed as part of the Amendments to the Constitution and By-Laws.[18] The Managing Director reported having received a letter from Dean Botterell at Queen's noting progress in the development of the university's objectives for basic medical and clinical sciences. The letter also requested a contribution from AMS to develop these plans. Dr. Upper remembers that the dean's letter made no mention of naming a medical library or any other building after Dr. Hannah; it was to be a straight gift.[19] This was unacceptable to Dr. Hannah and probably explains Dr. Botterell's inability to remember any response or action.[20]

On 18 December 1964, the Government of Ontario released the Hagey Report, which followed on Dr. Dymond's investigations of the possible introduction of government health insurance, initially to use existing carriers. This document was, of course, studied by AMS personnel with respect to its effects on the corporation. It was thought that legislation based on the Hagey Report could not be proclaimed before 1 June 1966. The Board decided AMS did not wish to be a carrier (because of the insurance concept of the Report) except possibly for a brief period of time that would enable AMS to complete plans to channel its funds and energies into other activities permitted by the charter.

The Future of AMS

In 1965 occurred the death of Dr. Herbert W. Baker, AMS President for 26 years. Dr. Hannah assumed, in succession, the dual role of President and Managing Director, which titles he maintained until 1976, the year before his own death. At the 29 August meeting of the Board, the new President offered for consideration four courses that AMS might follow, under the existent charter, after the institution of the government's plan. They were:[21]

> Formation of a mutual insurance company to sell group life and weekly indemnity and other such items as might be deemed advisable.
>
> Development of a clinic-hospital concept as discussed on previous occasions.
>
> Utilize reserves in developing a programme and teaching in medical schools.
>
> Distribute assets to charitable or other purposes which are beneficial to the community.

Dr. Upper recalls that the first of these was barely discussed, and that the third was unrealistic – unrealistic for AMS to think it could influence university curricula – and therefore was never really discussed.[22] The fourth was a last resort only. Consequently, the new President's four courses produced no developments.

Bill 136, which coincided with the recommendations of the Hagey Report, was introduced in the Legislature in May and passed in June 1965 "after bitter debate and public opposition". Two sections only were proclaimed in November: those placing administration under the control of the Minister of Health and authorizing the government to spend money. On 21 July, the Pearson government in Ottawa offered to pay to eligible provinces, on and after 1 July 1967, one-half of the average cost (national) of medical care coverage. On 1 December, the Ontario Department of Health acquired quarters in Toronto and began to advertise for staff for the Ontario plan.[23] It was at this time that AMS began to think its limit of time in which it could operate as a carrier was four to five years at most.

The Board at its next meeting, 15 May 1966, concerned itself briefly with uncertainties caused AMS by these government actions, and then proceeded to change the winding-up clause by substituting the word "institutions" for "medical schools".[24] One might wonder if the alteration presaged the eventual establishment of the Hannah Institute. While there seems to be no clear path from 1966 to the events of 1971, Dr. Upper says the change was deliberate.[25] Dr. Hannah had lost faith that the universities would give him the personal recognition he desired. Consequently, the change, which was given the required notification of by-law changes in the *Ontario Gazette*,[26] freed him to develop a memorial to himself elsewhere, if the opportunity should arise.

At subsequent meetings of the Board, other equally inconclusive ideas of diversification were raised, including (if truth be told) other organizations seeking investment capital. Two Board changes, however, proved important in different ways. One of the strong non-medical members resigned because of what he considered lack of adaptability in investment policies, which he regarded as being of increasing importance in an altered situation.[27] The other was the election to the Board of Dr. John B. Neilson in December 1966.[28] He was to become Dr. Hannah's successor as President of AMS in 1976.

A period of more than fifteen months was to elapse between Board meetings in 1966-67 because of extremely serious surgery Dr. Hannah was compelled to undergo and the ensuing prolonged convalescence. In September 1967, when the Board met again, Dr. Upper, in the absence of the President, reported briefly on the subject of diversification and on investment limitations imposed by the Corporations Act of Ontario.[29] In reporting on Dr. Hannah's health, he told his fellow directors that, while convalescing in Florida, Dr. Hannah was anxious "to write a history of AMS and a history of prepayment for the cost of medical care in Ontario over the past thirty years". There is no indication these hopes were fulfilled. They do, however, tell us the area of Dr. Hannah's medical historical interest.

By December 1967, Dr. Hannah was back in harness.[30] The same non-productive diversification topics were again placed before the Board for discussion, as well as the need for a drug plan. A new member of Board asked the President "what Management might expect from the Directors to assist in these areas of possible diversification". To which the President replied, "(1) to be constructively critical both before and after the event, and (2) to give to Management the benefit of their individual experience in business as well as in the hospital and medical field".

The First Library Is Considered for Purchase

In the light of subsequent developments, the most important disclosure of Management to Board members at this time was the attempt to purchase the rare book library of the Royal Society of Medicine at the University of Edinburgh. The Board was informed that the Scots valued the library at £150,000, but Dr. Hannah proposed to offer £125,000, saying he thought this to be in order. He always liked to bargain and assumed others did too. There was no appraisal made; indeed, no complete list of the books had been secured. In discussion, the Board agreed that the $250,000 earmarked for medical research at Queen's earlier would have to be increased to $350,000 to allow the President to negotiate for the library. A motion to do that was carried.

In preparation for the next Board meeting (8 September 1968), Dr. Hannah sent out the President and Managing Director's Report.[31] In it, he had to tell members of the Board that his offer of £120,000 to the Edinburgh society for the library had been refused. Even then, he expressed the view that his failure was because Sotheby's already had part of the library for disposal. He also thought that the owners of the library might have liked to place the library at Queen's. There is no evidence for this view; nor at the time of making his offer had he received a catalogue in order to know something of the contents of the library.

At the 8 September Board meeting, diversification was again considered. Some old subjects – clinics, hospitals – were discussed, as were several new ones – a drug plan and nursing homes.[32] The drug plan was to come into being, but Dr. Upper remembers the nursing home discussion as being concerned with certain entrepreneurs seeking investment capital for their own purposes.[33] The minutes do read as if this were a serious consideration for diversification. Family care units and a student medical care plan were also on the agenda.

The Past, Present, and Future of AMS

The President and Managing Director's Report for the next

Board meeting, 15 December 1968, was a lengthy document. It dealt at great length with the past, the present, and the future of AMS: it gives much historical information and public opinion as well as considerable insight into the philosophy of this determined man.[34] His views, whether justified or not, about diversification deserve verbatim quotation:

> As indicated previously to the Board of Directors, your Management has declined to become inactive or passive, and you as a Board have approved that we seek any and all advisable and proper programs of diversification. To this extent, the future of AMS has been decided. As is usually the case, however, it is much easier to decide what not to do, than to be positive and decide what to do, and to make sure that such decisions will eventuate in further progress of AMS in discharging its obligations in regard to the objects as contained in our charter. There remain many areas in regard to which a decision has yet to be made as to our course of action, and although "the crossroads have been met" and the broad outlines of our future decided, it remains for your administration to work out the details of the various plans involved in the diversification into which it has been decided we will proceed.

The next Board meeting was to consider the *curricula vitae* of four young men to effect certain aspects of diversification,[35] although no decisions had been made concerning how to diversify, so that hiring of supervisory staff seemed, at the very least, premature. Nevertheless, the subject persisted on future agenda. Indeed new subjects of diversification were also introduced. (In hindsight what the minutes describe as a possible purchase of a drug manufacturing plant was more likely a search for equity capital from AMS on the part of a promoter.)

Still, one must examine the philosophy expressed by Dr. Hannah. Did Dr. Hannah have any real plans for diversification? Or rather was he more concerned to maintain control of the funds that had been accumulated by AMS? Dr. Upper has questioned strongly whether Dr. Hannah would have been comfortable with any new role for AMS that did not relate closely to prepaid medical care. It seems to the writer, in the light of opinions obtained from those who were there when these discussions were proceeding, and also in the light of his own experience with Dr. Hannah in the last few years of the latter's presidency, that any plan of diversification adopted would have to fulfil two conditions. First, it would have to constitute a memorial to Dr. Hannah, and, second, it would have to be run according to the principles and methods expounded and developed to make AMS the successful prepaid medical care carrier it had become. It seems in retrospect that a lot of straw figures were erected – and shot down – in order to gain time to identify the desired memorial. Confirmation of this thinking will be obtained in studying details of the establishment of the AMS role in history of medicine, once that had been accepted as the memorial long sought. Also, conditions attached to any diversification schemes put forward for adoption seemed to make it impossible for them to be successful.

A Central Library

The minutes of the 8 September 1968 meeting record another interesting idea, in these words: "Dr. Hannah indicated another approach to the Medical Library question has come up for consideration. The need for a good Central Library in Canada is becoming increasingly apparent with good communication facilities with other libraries. The establishing and managing of a Foundation for managing a central library may be a better approach than making contributions to a library at Queen's, Western or Ottawa Universities."

Dr. Hannah was left to canvass the idea further. It is apparent there is no direct connection between this idea and the ultimate choice for diversification – that is, history of medicine – but the idea does seem to have played a part in the decision that was to come in 1971. The word "central" seems to have been used as if it were synonymous with "clinical". This idea of a central library will be returned to because of its greater importance than the other ideas for diversification proved to have.

Medicare and Its Effects

The only diversification scheme related to prepaid medical care that was implemented was the drug plan, which will not be discussed here. However, key initial steps leading to the implementation of the government plan were taken in the summer of 1969. These and miscellaneous, and perhaps unrealizable, ideas for diversification seemed to consume most of the time of AMS personnel and of agenda.

Some of the young men whose *curricula vitae* were earlier mentioned had been hired. They and Drs. Hannah and Upper, according to the minutes and reports of the Managing Director, must have consumed much time in consideration of vague, perhaps even somewhat unorganized, ideas for the continued utilization by AMS of its accumulated funds. Family practice units referred to as the Satellite Programme, computerized ECG analysis, and such earlier ideas as had survived thus far were considered.

Perhaps the most detailed plan, difficult to understand in all its implications, was advanced by the Managing Director in his report intended for the 7 September Board meeting.[36] He proposed that the Board set aside a suitable amount of money, say $1,000,000, from the reserves, for diversification policies to be put into effect. For each project approved, he proposed there be established a budget for a start-up period and a reasonable period thereafter based on expectations. If the original budget were exceeded, the project would be wound up. If the project were successful and showed a surplus of 20% or more, the 20% only should be fed back to the project as it was continued. That surplus in excess of 20% would be added to the capital reserves of the corporation. He did add, "Special consideration may be given by AMS to funds to expand any successful program." However, no quick decisions were made concerning this plan, since the next meeting took the form of a retreat at the Hannahs' summer home at Cloyne, Ontario, 18-19 October.[37] Most of the time was spent discussing the effects of the government's moves. In addition, there was the first mention of the Academy of Medicine, Toronto, which wished to establish an archives wing in the new building being planned. The Board saw a relationship between this and honouring Dr. Hannah.

By the time the Board met again on 14 December,[38] little had been accomplished. The Academy of Medicine did receive a promise of $25,000 towards the cost of its archives wing. The drug plan was experiencing difficulties. Under the agenda item "central library", the President did report the possible availability of another library similar to the one he had failed to obtain from Edinburgh. This statement shows a failure to appreciate the difference between a clinical and a historical library. The most important development at this meeting was the warning issued by a member of the Board, Dr. Neilson, that he believed AMS, because of its reserves, to be in a vulnerable position. He said he sincerely hoped some disposition could be made soon from the reserves for worthy projects. He thought the central library might be one such. He added that he thought other organizations, if asked, might be able to help AMS to identify suitable projects. Dr. Hannah replied that he was aware of AMS vulnerability, but then declared he would not be pressured into action by politicians as long as the corporation continued to act within its charter.

Dr. Hannah's Evaluation of AMS

Before Board met next on 12 April 1970, the President prepared a long report.[39] This extensive document was divided into five sections – Introduction, The AMS Charter, Personnel, The Future of AMS, Recommendations – and consisted of eighty pages of material. It was highly political (bitter against the introduction of medicare), very rhetorical, shrewdly argued, and very often self-congratulatory.

In the minutes of the April Board meeting,[40] Dr. Hannah is reported as having reminded the Board of a response he had made in December 1969:

> . . . the line of our future developments have [sic] begun to crystallize. Also, because of the political involvement arising in regard to our reserves, there is some urgency to the necessity to concentrate our efforts on certain specific projects, rather than casting a wide net. Time is becoming of the essence. In my opinion, our future "casting" must

be limited and minimized . . . . I am somewhat concerned that we do not continue to "cast" as an occupation rather than concentrate on developing those "catches" which may have been netted. I am convinced that "the period of analysis" for diversification for AMS as a result of the introduction of Medicare and OHSIP in Ontario must be closed and the time for action has arrived.

This sounds like a specific call to arms, yet his newly revised recommendations do not reflect this sense of urgency. Rather do they support Dr. Upper's view. The earlier sum of $1,000,000 for establishing "diversification projects" was reduced by 75%, and approved projects were to be placed under the control of the Chief Medical Officer, who would be answerable to the Board for their administration. The same formulas for establishing budgets and for winding up projects were to be applied. Dr. Upper says all diversification ideas described previously would have required millions, and "the sum of $250,000 was designed to end diversification efforts, not extend them". He goes on to record the view that such a formula will kill a growing business. He says, "Growth requires capital to be put in and *profits* to be reinvested. No new business could survive on this basis and Dr. Hannah knew it at the time."[41]

A second Hannah recommendation was that AMS not continue under the restrictions of the Prepaid Hospital and Medical Services Act and rather develop other lines of diversification under the Corporations Act. He thought that such projects would have a more secure future.

In connection with this recommendation, he ruminated about the different foundations he had investigated – Markle, Bickell, Wellcome – and the relationship of original capital to moneys distributed over a period of time. It is rather strange, in the light of subsequent happenings, that at this stage of examining the Wellcome Trust, he drew his conclusions from the medical research side of Wellcome operations rather than from the medical historical side.

His third recommendation was that AMS should separate carrier functions from other activities because of the political controversy surrounding medicare. He concluded his report by insisting that decisions be made in whole or in part on his recommendations. He gave notice of a motion he would introduce at the next Board meeting, 12 April 1970:

> THAT the Board of Directors hereby approves of the recommendations as set forth by the Managing Director in connection with his report to the Board, An Evaluation of AMS, Its Personnel and Future as of 31 December, 1969, and:
>
> THAT the Board of Directors hereby instructs the Managing Director to proceed with the development and implementation of these recommendations.

A busy agenda in April precluded discussion of these motions, which were therefore put over to another Cloyne retreat on 7-8 August. In the meantime, however, the President reported having had further discussions with the Academy of Medicine on the subject of a central library. From this 9 April meeting and the Board meeting 12 April, there emerged the suggestion and its approval that AMS give the Academy $7,000 "to assist the work of cataloguing". It would seem this was the only decision made, despite a seemingly long meeting. Needless to say, it can hardly be termed "diversification"; rather was it a grant.

The sole purpose of the Cloyne meeting was to discuss diversification. The minutes quote Dr. Hannah as having said, "The problem of diversification requires careful study in light of AMS philosophy, its charter, existing legislation, and the management of AMS reserves."[42]

Yet the first day at Cloyne was consumed by discussion of old and discarded ideas and, in addition, the loss of some of the new senior staff to better opportunities, the consideration of whether AMS should become a foundation, the announcement of a recent grant to the Ontario Geriatric Research Society, and the President's desire that his pre-AMS pathological research be completed at Queen's. One interesting sidelight was disclosure of a talk with Dr. O.M. Solandt, a director of Connaught Laboratories and a member of the Science Council of Canada, about sources of research funds, particularly those termed seed-money.

On the second day only did Board members come to discuss the Hannah recommendations. The President said there were three things to be decided: What to do with AMS reserves, that is, how and where would they be used? How could personnel be used and developed? In what fields should AMS limit its activities?

His recommendations did not fare too badly, but he did not get everything he had asked for. Perhaps this marks the first time Board members really saw the need to take issue with him in the light of problems they could see would confront AMS within a year or two, and for which planning was now needed. Despite the number of deletions and changes voted, Dr. Hannah expressed himself as confident that Board action had given him the necessary power to proceed to take advantage of any situation that fell within the charter. A memorial?

Revisions as asked for by Board members were made before the next meeting on 13 September 1970. The minutes state:

> It was the unanimous feeling of the meeting that a motion to approve Dr. Hannah's Recommendations was not necessary, as the Board would be only restating its responsibility for adoption of policies and programs that come within the Corporation's Charter – a position which has always been carefully observed by both Management and the Board of Directors.

Dr. Neilson, who had been absent from the Cloyne meeting, again warned "that the size of AMS unencumbered reserves might expose AMS to political criticism". Dr. Hannah made his position clear: he did not want to relinquish control over any part of AMS reserves. He added that he was interested in what Dr. Solandt had said, and that he would be happy "to feel there is a source of funds in AMS for worthy research projects in the field of medical care".

Medical care. Not diversification to a number of small fields. No history of medicine yet mentioned.

AMS and Other Carriers to Be Phased Out

In his report for the meeting of the Board, scheduled for 13 December 1970, the Managing Director reported that Premier John P. Robarts had announced in the Legislature 10 October that the carriers (among them AMS) would be phased out of OHSIP on or before 1 July 1972.[43] AMS had certainly wished for such an announcement, since time was needed to deal with severance of remaining employees.

The gift of funds to the Academy for the archives wing, a suggested further gift ($100,000-$200,000) to aid members with their planned new building, and the idea of a personal gift of a Hippocratic plane tree for a roof garden at the new building, all testify to the increasing importance of a link with the Academy of Medicine, Toronto. The plane tree is also evidence of a growing relationship with Dr. William C. Gibson, Professor of the History of Medicine at the University of British Columbia, for Professor Gibson was actively engaged in raising funds for Cos, the Greek island associated with Hippocrates, by the sale of plane seedlings.

The Board, on 13 December 1970, authorized Dr. Hannah to give the Academy the promised $25,000, and to indicate to Academy officials

> that the Board of Directors of AMS is prepared to give support to the establishment of a museum and archives in the new proposed building to the extent of approximately 2,000 usable square feet of space and in addition to provide assistance for a period of up to five years in the maintenance of exhibits which may be contained in this area.[44]

The Advent of Library Developments

Before the next Board meeting in April 1971, the initial steps had been taken for the purchase of a portion of the library of the Medical Society of London. This proved to be the catalyst that would bring about major AMS activity in history of medicine in the province of Ontario.

However, because Dr. Hannah never seemed to distinguish between a central library and a specialist historical library of rare books, it is necessary to trace the birth and collapse of the idea that several medical bodies in Ontario should unite organizationally and financially to create a first-class library resource in Ontario.

CHAPTER II

Libraries

The Board's final decision that its involvement in history of medicine would constitute its major activity, after prolonged discussion and consideration of diversification projects, is beyond doubt due to the catalytic force given such a decision by Dr. Hannah's interest in libraries, both clinical and historical.

The first library decision was taken in 1962, the silver anniversary year of AMS, and the library was intended as a permanent memorial to the founder of AMS, Dr. J.A. Hannah. It was to be established at Queen's University with an approved funding of $250,000. At various times, it was described as an endowment for suitable display of historical objects of medical interest and as a medical research library. The reaction at the university was that the sum involved was not likely to result in a separate and self-contained library, which comment was not at all in agreement with Dr. Hannah's wishes and undoubtedly contributed to a delay in plan development.

Medical educational aims continued to find expression when the Board dealt with the subject of diversification. This was most evident at the time the winding-up by-law was changed in 1965 and 1966.

The Library of the Royal Society of Medicine, Edinburgh

In 1968 came the attempt to buy all or part of the library of historical works being sold off by the Royal Society of Medicine in Edinburgh. This must be examined more closely. Not all the relevant correspondence has survived, but sufficient has to give the general outline of the incident. Early in the spring of 1968, presumably through Professor William C. Gibson of the University of British Columbia, who had become the first of two principal historical advisers, Dr. Hannah learned of the intention of the Royal Society of Medicine, housed at the Medical School of the University of Edinburgh, to dispose of a major part of its library. This library was a historic one. Dr. Malcolm D.W. Low, treasurer of the society, was the contact in Edinburgh for Drs. Gibson and Hannah. The Principal and Vice-Chancellor, Dr. J.A. Corry, was the contact at Queen's University in Kingston where Dr. Hannah hoped to install the collection. Dr. Hannah was, of course, an alumnus of Queen's and very conscious of the Scottish Connection between Edinburgh and Queen's.

In a surviving response to Dr. Low,[1] dated 19 April, Dr. Hannah referred to Dr. Gibson's contacts with Dr. Low on behalf of AMS, indicated he was copying the letter to Dr. Corry, and identified himself as the principal behind Queen's interest in the library. He went on to say:

> It is my sincere hope that your Committee will see fit to reconsider the situation in this matter in order that the Library may be preserved within the British Commonwealth and become a part of Queen's University's valuable facilities to promote medical education in Canada and particularly in Queen's University. I am of the opinion that if this library could be secured for Queen's, there would be an appreciable accretion to it from various other sources.

He mentioned interest on the part of some members of the Board in the library being located at Queen's.

What was the situation Dr. Hannah wished to have reconsidered? Undoubtedly this was the placement of the library for sale at Sotheby's. He quoted liberally from two letters, one written to him by Dr. Gibson on 8 April, with which the latter enclosed a letter of 4 April he had received from Dr. Low. Neither of these letters can be found but the quotations survive in a letter written 19 April also to Dr. Gibson by Dr. Hannah.[2]

Dr. Low refers to the library thus: "the disposal of this, the Society's greatest asset, will require considerable justification to the generations of future members". Yet he writes of the library in the same letter as a "decreasingly used asset". Later in the same letter, Dr. Hannah quoted Dr. Low as having written:

> For the Society it means substitution of its historic and decreasingly used asset of old and rare books for means of rebuilding a new home and creating a permanent endowment.

In his letter to Principal Corry,[3] dated three days later, Dr. Hannah again quoted Dr. Low as having stated:

> Rightly or wrongly, the Committee by a narrow majority decided that a public sale by auction offered libraries and collectors in Scotland, the United Kingdom and abroad an equal opportunity of acquiring at least some books in fair competition.

At the same time, however, Dr. Hannah refers to Dr. Low as having told Dr. Gibson in a telephone conversation that the University of Edinburgh required "an understanding that there would be no disbursement of the collection on the part of the purchaser". One must agree with Dr. Hannah that this seemed inconsistent on the part of the society. The discussions with the principal of Queen's, by telephone and by letter, concerned the willingness and ability of Queen's to accept and to house properly the library if Dr. Hannah were able to acquire it.

In his letter to Dr. Corry, Dr. Hannah showed clearly his desire for a memorial when he wrote, "I gather it is Queen's intention to establish this as the nucleus of an historical library of the nature agreed upon some few years ago and called The Jason A. Hannah Medical History Library." He was surely thinking less clearly (possibly because of his illness) when he added:

> I believe this would be a very important acquisition for the medical school at Queen's and am most anxious to

see it come there. I believe it will be useful to Canada as a whole and might well be the beginning of making Queen's medical school the leader in Canada, if indeed not on the Continent, over a period of years.

Principal Corry did not play a passive role in this proposed acquisition of the library. On 22 April, he both telephoned and wrote to Dr. Hannah, as indicated in a letter from Dr. Hannah to AMS directors.[4] He "had another source prepared to advance the money for the purchase of the Royal Medical Society Edinburgh Library". He said that Queen's would appreciate knowing as soon as possible whether or not AMS was going to provide the purchase sum. Dr. Hannah told the principal that, while the Board might be prepared to bid £130,000, he himself felt he was being "squeezed a bit" and was not prepared to go to £150,000. The principal was prepared to send Dr. Hannah and Dr.Steele (an Edinburgh man, once library curator) to Edinburgh.

Dr. Hannah reported another call from the principal on 24 April. He had called Dr. Low, offered £130,000, and been told, "in order to have a look in, we would have to go to £150,000". Consultations among Drs. Corry, Hannah, and Gibson ensued and it was agreed to await the sales at Sotheby's. Dr. Hannah did fear it might prove too expensive that way. He closed the memorandum with the comment, "A 'horsetrader' never regards a deal as being finalized until he has got his 'horse'."

Dr. Gibson had succeeded in obtaining only a partial listing of the library's contents. Dr. Hannah had very much wanted a complete catalogue from the beginning. After he had seen the partial listing, he had commented to Dr. Gibson in the 19 April letter:

> There is the further fact that however valuable the existing volumes may be, the listing I have seen indicates an hiatus covering the last fifty to one hundred years and in order to have a complete library, it would be necessary to fill this gap. This would be a delightful project if one had the ability, the time, and finances available. At the moment, all three appear to be at least limited, if not completely absent.

In that letter Dr. Hannah had also shown considerable, but perhaps exaggerated, concern about the costs that could be associated with repair and rebinding and shelving, as well as a more realistic concern about a structure in which the library might be housed under safe and proper conditions. Time was also a factor, since it seemed Sotheby's was seeking the right by 24 April to acquire the collection for auction. Dr. Hannah did not feel he could commit AMS to the purchase price asked (£150,000) before that date – indeed not before the next meeting of the Board on 5 May.

Nevertheless, despite his having said this and the Board not yet having met, and despite not having received the complete catalogue he wanted so very much, in a letter to Dr. Low, dated 26 April, Dr. Hannah wrote, "If you can provide me with a complete listing of the Library, indicating those items which you wish to retain in respect of the history of the Society, I will be prepared to cancel my future commitments to such an extent as to make it possible for me to go to Edinburgh with a certified cheque for the equivalent of £125,000 conditional upon the collection being intact as it was prior to it being offered for sale and a portion of it having been shipped to Sotheby's in London."[5] He went on to write,

> I sincerely hope that you and your Committee will give this matter your most serious and sympathetic consideration. My personal feeling is that it is almost sacrilegious to see the collection broken up, or to see the whole or any part of it allowed to go outside the Commonwealth. I sincerely regret that my financial circumstances will not permit me to go any further than £125,000. Frankly, beyond that amount I am of the opinion that I could attend the auction in London and pick up those volumes which might be suitable and allow the remainder where it will and I believe it could be done at less expense than the amount of money being offered presently.

Sacrilegious or not, the society placed its collection with Sotheby's for sale. The plan appeared to be that the sale would take place in a number of lots at different auctions. On 3 May, Dr. Hannah asked Dr. Gibson's help in selecting books from Sotheby's sales of the society collection,[6] but three days later he declined the latter's offer to represent him at Sotheby's, saying he himself intended to be present at the auctions.[7] In the interval, the Board discussed the proposed purchase. On the basis of Dr. Hannah's stated belief that, although Edinburgh wanted £150,000, an offer of £125,000 would suffice, the Board passed a motion:[8]

> That the amount of $250,000 approved for Queen's University at the Directors' meeting held on June 1, 1962, be increased to $350,000 in order to allow Dr. Hannah to negotiate for the purchase of the Royal Medical Society, Edinburgh library if, as and when negotiations proceed to the point where a firm offer can be made.

It is really necessary here to comment on the most unbusiness-like way in which this possible purchase of a historic library was handled by the prospective buyer. At no time, it seems, did a representative of AMS see the library in Edinburgh or even a catalogue of it. Certainly Dr. Hannah did not. The services of a library appraiser were not engaged. Sometime during the summer of 1968, Dr. Hannah revised his earlier offer (not acknowledged to the Board) to £120,000, an offer that was refused by Dr. Low. In the President and Managing Director's Report, prepared for the Board meeting of 8 September, he wrote:[9]

> In brief, it eventuated that I could not obtain a listing of the books in this collection, despite which an offer of £120,000 did not prove sufficiently attractive. I am of the opinion the Edinburgh Medical School might have liked to accept our offer of £120,000 to put it at Queen's, but part of it was already in Sotheby's in London, and we came on the scene too late. We are asking for a catalogue and to be kept informed in regard to the date(s) of sale, and it may be that we can get what we want from the auction sale without some of the unnecessary or duplicate items at a lesser cost.

Unnecessary or duplicate to what? From where would come the knowledge of how to participate in an auction, how to bid, what to bid for, when not to bid? In most cases, buying from a library by bidding on individual offerings is a much more expensive proposition than buying a collection and disposing of unwanted material by sale or trade. Books do have individual characters. Did Dr. Hannah never come to appreciate this? Rare books, in particular, are not just pieces of merchandise. The costs associated with obtaining expert advice when acquiring valuable collections, such as rare books, are most frequently recovered several times over.

When he did request the catalogues from Sotheby's, Dr. Hannah added: "I would appreciate being placed on your list in respect of any important medical books of vintage prior to 1928." The significance of the date is difficult to understand. In November, Dr. Upper, Chief Medical Officer of AMS, reported by letter after a visit to Sotheby's while on holiday that the auctioneers had not yet prepared a catalogue.

A Central (Clinical) Library

A telephone conversation with Dr. Gibson on 16 November apparently caused reinstatement of the idea that Ontario badly needed a central (clinical) medical library for use throughout the province.[10] In his memorandum of the same conversation, Dr. Hannah wrote:

> Dr. Gibson feels that perhaps in view of the failure to secure this Library [i.e., the Edinburgh library] that my concept of trying to build up a suitable Library for the medical profession as a whole in the Province of Ontario, through the College of Physicians and Surgeons, probably making the Academy of Medicine Library the nucleus and securing a fee added to the C.P. & S.O. registration fee, is the best approach. He indicated to me that this is the arrangement they have in British Columbia, where they charge a fee of $25 per annum to each doctor for the maintenance of this central library. In return, the doctors

> are entitled to a stated number of Xerox copies of any articles [they] may desire for further study. The books are never sent out through the mail and consequently do not become misused, lost, etc., etc. Dr. Gibson is to forward me particulars of the situation by mail.

Dr. Gibson did send a copy of *The Medical Library Service – Review of a College Project.*[11] At the time when the first Sotheby sales of Edinburgh library material were taking place, and before he received the catalogues he had ordered, Dr. Hannah was again at work on the new library project, the central library. The new project appears to have been mentioned merely in passing at the Board meeting of 15 December 1968, for there is nothing to be found in the President and Managing Director's Report prepared for this session. Yet the minutes record this note: "CENTRAL LIBRARY – Dr. Hannah indicated another approach to the Medical Library question has come up for consideration. The need for a good Central Library in Canada is becoming increasingly apparent with good communication facilities with other libraries. The establishing and management of a Foundation for managing a central library may be a better approach than making contributions to a library at Queen's, Western or Ottawa Universities. Dr. Hannah is to canvass the situation further."

On 31 January 1969, Dr. Hannah wrote a letter to All Members of the AMS Board.[12] After first reporting on his recent disappointments – the Edinburgh library for Queen's, clinic-hospital setups, billing services at Queen's, and, above all, lack of recognition for what he had tried to do and had done – he went on to raise the problem, as he saw it, of the profession's need of a central library. He wrote,

> The Academy of Medicine Library is in difficulty, and unless it gets some means of support we are in danger of losing the only library that is recognized as being of suitable calibre for research purposes in Medicine. I am enclosing a draft proposal for consideration of the development and maintenance of a proper medical library in Toronto. Like all other projects that we have been con-

> sidering, I am not prepared to enter into this situation unless I can see a source of sustaining income adequate to take care of the situation. This, I believe, can be provided by the College of Physicians and Surgeons of Ontario, if they will accept my proposal as contained in the enclosed draft.

In the draft,[13] drawn by the President in the form of a quasi-legal document, he recognized three parties: the Academy, the College of Physicians and Surgeons of Ontario, and Associated Medical Services, Incorporated. The first-named had the library, but needed help to maintain and extend it, indeed to prevent its deterioration. The College, he said, was aware of the need for such a library and, moreover, was the only body that could legally assess its membership for maintenance of the standards of medical education and practice in Ontario. AMS was permitted by its charter to utilize its reserves to promote health and medical care in Ontario and in addition had the finances "to provide the necessary housing and initial capital not only for housing but for refurbishing and setting up a proper medical library". In the covering letter, he pointed out that AMS had an "unusual appreciation of the needs of the medical profession", and so was "prepared to assume the responsibility for promoting the concept set out in the attached document". He described his Draft No. 1 as a "white paper".

In the draft, he showed awareness that at the Academy there existed what he described as the best medical library in the province, the services of which had been made available to doctors provincially, not just locally. He recognized the extent of the Academy's property holdings; that it needed more space to carry on its library and other functions; and that it needed further funds for expansion of facilities and maintenance of the library and other services. Concerning the College, he stressed its legal powers and its future need for further accommodation. As to AMS, he wrote in the draft,

> AMS is prepared under suitable and proper conditions to make monetary contributions to properly-controlled and

financed facilities for housing and operation of a proper library in the Province of Ontario; and AMS will require additional accommodation to carry on its present operations and for future expansion.

The draft proposed the establishment by mutual consent of an Ontario Library Foundation, membership on whose board would consist of two representatives from each of the contracting bodies. The six would elect a vice-chairman from among themselves and, from outside their numbers, a prominent citizen or member of the College to be the chairman.

The arrangement Dr. Hannah put forward for raising the funds necessary for this whole scheme was quite complex. The Academy was to sell its property (described earlier in the draft as that land bounded by Bloor Street and Prince Arthur Avenue, and by Huron Street and a north-south line somewhere between Huron and St. George streets) to AMS for the sum of one dollar. At the same time, the Academy was to obtain suitable zoning rulings so that AMS could erect a first-class office building with sufficient space for the functions already described. AMS would then rent adequate space for its functions to the Academy for one dollar per year "until such time as AMS shall contribute either through cash donations or/and rental for the space at prevailing rates for similar type space in the immediate vicinity, a total of not less than one million dollars". In addition to the 20,000 square feet of space, free of charge, AMS would contribute to the Library Foundation board not less than $50,000 per annum for a period of five years. A review of the whole matter would take place after the five years. All of this funding was dependent on the College of Physicians and Surgeons of Ontario assessing from its members a sum of money equivalent to $25 per annum per registrant. The College's moneys were to be turned over to the Library Foundation board on a monthly basis.

The minutes of the Board meeting of 27 April record that the establishment of other medical societies was leading to dilution of membership in the Academy. The Board also foresaw a role for the Ontario Medical Association in the library project. The directors thought links could be established to computer programs in the United States, the United Kingdom, and continental Europe. The minutes also say,

> The question of increasing the annual fees paid by doctors through the College was discussed with the Registrar and the fee might be increased by $2.50 per annum. Dr. Hannah indicated that anything less than $25.00 per annum per licensed physician would be inadequate to establish and maintain a suitable financial base for a growing library service.

Dr. Hannah, at that time a member of the Council of the College of Physicians and Surgeons of Ontario, presented his plan to that Council 30 April and 1 May 1969. He presented a motion, which was seconded by Dr. Fielden and carried:

> That a committee be formed of representatives from the Association of Deans in Ontario and interested donors of funds re utilization of these funds in development of medical libraries' services in Ontario. And the College of Physicians and Surgeons of Ontario invite these representatives to to meet at 64 Prince Arthur Avenue, Toronto [the College's home] and that arrangements be made by the Executive Committee.

He next reported to his Board that he had presented another motion, again seconded by Dr. Fielden, but this time defeated:

> That this Council approves the Registrar-Treasurer to issue a cheque not to exceed $50,000 to match that issued to the College of Physicians and Surgeons of Ontario by Associated Medical Services Incorporated, both cheques to be utilized to promote the institution of the Academy of Medicine's library as a provincial library for the use of the medical profession in the Province of Ontario as a whole, subject to the approval of the committee appointed under motion 41-C-4-69 [i.e., the previous motion].

The archives, including the minutes, of the College of Physicians and Surgeons of Ontario have not survived or are not available. Therefore, we are dependent on Dr. Hannah's reasoning in his report to the AMS Board.[14] He pointed out to them that, as chairman of the Building and Finance Committee of the College, he had known of, advocated, and been involved in a program of building an extension to satisfy their accommodation needs. This had probably used up their reserves and was responsible for their cautious reception of his library plan. He went on to write, "It may be that some actual support for the Academy from AMS would not only be very acceptable, but sustain interest in this very worthwhile and much needed program." He thought some of the $300,000 research account might be used for the purpose and gave notice that, in addition, at the next meeting of the Board, 7 September, he would move

> That the Board of Directors of AMS instructs the President and Managing Director to continue negotiations with the College of Physicians and Surgeons of Ontario and the Toronto Academy of Medicine and hereby appropriate [sic] $50,000 to be used by him, in his best judgment, to support such negotiations.

He concluded his report with a statement of his belief that the Academy could not alone support such an undertaking. In addition he reiterated his feeling that the College was the body that should supply sure operating funds.

In many ways, this was a farsighted plan that could have made a very considerable contribution to continuing medical education. Yet, it seems very very clear that all the ramifications of such a scheme had not been thought out or studied before it was presented to the one body on whose support he himself knew he was dependent. Nor does he seem to have asked himself about the Academy's readiness, in any way, for such a role as that in which he would cast it. The committee approved by the College Council should probably have met and had the plan put before members for thorough discussion before it went to Council. Once defeated there, it would have been most difficult, if not impossible, to regain any momentum.

The concept of a central library, financed as proposed by Dr. Hannah, seems to have died a slow death in the months ahead, ultimately hastened somewhat when the opportunity was presented to buy the collection of the Medical Society of London. For two reasons apparently – government-AMS relations were strained, and there were no further reactions from the College of Physicians and Surgeons of Ontario to the Hannah assessment proposal – Dr. Hannah did not mention the concept of the central library in his reports to members of the Board.

Other Libraries

Nevertheless, two further library developments should be noted. First, Dr. Gibson drew to the President's attention the availability of a privately owned rare book collection in medical history in California. Nothing was done about it except to mention existence of the collection to the Board meeting of 14 December 1969.[15] Secondly, at the Board meeting of 12 April 1970, when questioned about the concept of the central library, Dr. Hannah mentioned a meeting with officials of the Academy of Medicine, Toronto, on 9 April, at which they noted their great need of funds to catalogue their own library holdings.[16] The Board approved a grant of $7,000 (paid in twelve monthly instalments) to aid the cataloguing function.

Thus began a closer relation with the Academy that was to become closer yet when the Medical Society of London library was purchased and needed a home.

CHAPTER III

Academy of Medicine – Toronto

To appreciate Jason Hannah's dealings with the Academy of Medicine, it is necessary to know something of the history, development, resources, and activities of what has been arguably Toronto's most important medical body.

The first decade of the twentieth century saw related developments in Toronto in the fields of medical education and professional organization. After medical teaching in the University of Toronto was abolished by the Hincks Act of 1853, there occurred the era of proprietary medical schools for approximately a third of a century. Hincks's legislation definitely favoured, at the expense of the universities, the private medical schools of Rolph and others. It was not until 1887 that the Faculty of Medicine was reestablished. Primrose tells us that the restoration of the faculty was "accomplished by an agreement between the then existent Toronto School of Medicine and the authorities of the University. The staff of the School became the faculty of Medicine of the University of Toronto."[1] It took another decade and a half to complete the reorganization satisfactorily, by which time there was serious consideration given to amalgamation between the faculties of medicine of the University of Toronto and Trinity University. In the summer of 1903, amalgamation was consummated. The inaugural address was delivered in the university gymnasium by Professor (later Sir) William Osler on 1 October 1903. It is interesting to note that Professor (later Sir) Charles Sherrington was present for the formal opening of the new laboratories, made necessary by the increased numbers of staff, and delivered that inaugural address. Among the many other distinguished guests on that day of celebration was Professor William Welch of Johns Hopkins.

The first medical society in Toronto, the Medico-Chirurgical Society of Upper Canada, was organized in 1834, the year that the town of York was incorporated as the City of Toronto. The College of Physicians and Surgeons of Upper Canada, successor to the Upper Canada Medical Board, was established by law in 1839, only to be disallowed by the British government at Westminster two years later. Confusion, not unlike that to be seen in medical education, and not unrelated to it, became the norm for a number of medical societies founded over the next five or six decades. Four of the medical societies were, however, to come together to form the Academy of Medicine within a few years of the amalgamation of the medical faculties of Toronto and Trinity.

Formation of the Academy of Medicine – Toronto

The stimulus for the Academy's emergence came from Osler – from a paper he published, *The Educational Value of the Medical Society*, and from a paper he gave on the subject to a meeting of the Toronto Medical Society in the Medical Building on 18 December 1906.[2] His idea was that Toronto needed a single strong medical society.

The four societies that came together to form the Academy of Medicine, Toronto, were the Ontario Medical Library Association (it had a good library), the Toronto Medical Society, the Toronto Clinical Society, and the Toronto Pathological Society. The library of the Ontario Medical Library Association, located at 9 Queen's Park since 1904 when the property was leased in perpetuity from the university, had by the time of Osler's address become an unofficial headquarters for all of the merging societies. From the beginning of the Academy's existence (the original Declaration for Incorporation of the Academy of Medicine was signed 26 February 1907 by executive officers of the four societies), the library was regarded not as a local but rather as a provincial resource, and of prime importance.[3] In 1907, there were 186 Charter Fellows and the library contained 4,062 volumes. In its first twenty-five years, the library was to grow fivefold.

By the time Jason Hannah was thinking of establishing an institute for the history of medicine in the early 1970s, the library had grown tremendously in holdings and in importance, particularly in a clinical sense. Dr. Hannah had been a Fellow of the Academy for a considerable period, and, as we have seen, AMS had made contributions to the Academy for the benefit of the library. The Academy was in possession of more than 2,000 volumes in its Rare Book Library alone, according to Dr. John W. Scott, a member of the Academy's executive.[4] Yet it seems, in the absence of definite proof, almost accidental that Dr. Hannah came to think of the Academy as a possible home for his proposed institute.

The Academy and Dr. Hannah

Before we examine the Academy as a possible home for an institute, it is necessary to review briefly certain activities mentioned. In 1969-1970, Dr. Hannah had initiated discussions with the Academy and the College of Physicians and Surgeons concerning conversion of the Academy's fine clinical library to a central library to be available to all Ontario medical registrants. This idea was, as we have seen, doomed to failure because of the inability of the various organizations to reach agreement.

Suggestions had also been made of a possible AMS grant to help provide a new wing for archives and museum in the new structure Academy officers hoped to build. The Board of Directors of AMS discussed this at their meeting of 18 October 1969, and passed the following motion:[5]

> That whereas AMS is desirous of establishing suitable and permanent testimonial to its President and Managing Director, Jason A. Hannah, B.A., M.D., C.M., C.R.C.P.(C); and
>
> Whereas the Toronto Academy of Medicine is desirous of establishing an arrangement to suitably house memorabilia in the contemplated new Toronto Academy of Medicine Building;
>
> It was moved by Mr. Hyndman and seconded by Mr. Barr and carried:

> That the Board of Directors of Associated Medical Services, Incorporated, authorizes a contribution of twenty-five thousand dollars ($25,000) to be made to the Toronto Academy of Medicine to assist in the establishment of such suitable arrangements; and
>
> That this contribution shall be used as a suitable testimonial to Doctor Jason A. Hannah, President and Managing Director of Associated Medical Services, Incorporated; and
>
> That this gift shall be made if and when the foundation for the said new structure has been put in prior to October 1, 1971.

Assisting in suitable arrangements is a Hannah euphemism for a partial contribution to an extension to the building being planned.

Dr. Hannah conveyed this information to the Academy by means of a letter to Dr. Mary C. McEwan, president of the Academy.[6] The turning of sod did not take place by the deadline given. However, the giving of the money to the Academy was authorized and carried out in December 1970. At no time in the discussions concerning a central library and a testimonial to Dr. Hannah, to be located at the Academy of Medicine, was a library for the history of medicine mentioned. Nor were the central library and testimonial linked in the sources left to us.

The Academy did have several links with history of medicine, however, as already noted. The most visible was Dr. John Scott's course in the Faculty of Medicine, which he planned to give to students in Art as Applied to Medicine (a sub-division of the Faculty of Medicine at Toronto) at the Academy in the spring of 1972. During 1971, Dr. Scott had been laying out his course and making arrangements for guest lecturers.[7] The very fine museum, featuring the Drake Collection in paediatrics, and the Rare Book Library were major assets for Academy activities in history of medicine.

The Library of the Medical Society of London

In a diary entry of 12 March 1971, Dr. Hannah, who was holidaying in Florida, notes a telephone call from Dr. William Gibson, who was in London. The purpose of the call was to inform Dr. Hannah that the Medical Society of London had put their library up for sale and part of it was already in the hands of Sotheby's. Dr. Gibson went on to say that the auctioneers were wondering if some university in Canada might like to acquire the books; he had told Sotheby's that he thought he might have a purchaser in Canada and he had asked them to stop the sale. Dr. Hannah told his caller that he would be prepared to take responsibility for saying that he, on behalf of AMS, would acquire the collection, but that he would have to wait until he returned to his office in order to do so. Dr. Hannah confided to his diary, "There are apparently 2,002 volumes [in retrospect, not the whole library Dr. Hannah believed it to be] and they are asking £65,000 for the library, despite that they feel that if it was split up, it would bring them £100,000 from Sotheby's." Dr. Gibson said he thought they would be prepared to hold up the sale, and they would be prepared to box up and ship the books to Canada wherever the purchaser should direct. Dr. Hannah wrote, "I indicated to him that I did not know where I would put the library at the moment, but he indicated that it would make an excellent start on an archives and medical history library which might be developed into something very much worthwhile."

The minutes of the Medical Society of London report that a private offer *had* been made for the books lodged at Messrs. Sotheby.[8] "The sum offered, £60,000, was considerably higher than that expected to be realized at auction (£30,000 to £40,000). A suggestion that a still higher price might be negotiated with the 'generous' purchaser was resolved by agreeing that he be asked to pay £60,000 plus the commission due to Messrs. Sotheby." Such commissions are normally paid by the vendor. A later entry in the society's minutes quoted Dr. T.C. Hunt as reporting that the sale of the books was being made to Queen's University, Kingston, Ontario.[9] Only on 25 October did the minutes disclose that the funds were provided by Dr. Hannah, who said that the society's library would form the basis of an institute of the history of medicine, to be established in Toronto.

Why did the private offer from Canada for the library of the Medical Society of London apparently originate at Queen's University? Why in October was Dr. Hannah's institute to be established in Toronto? How can we reconcile Dr. Hannah's belief that he was buying the complete library of the society with the statement of the treasurer of the society, reported in the minutes of 26 October 1970, that "the cream of the library was already deposited in the Wellcome Library and were seldom referred to by Fellows of the Society"? Dr. Ellis, a society councillor, was arguing that the same was true of the remainder of the books in the society's quarters and that therefore they should be sold "as a source of income" in order to improve the appearance of the building and to enhance its amenities. There are several anomalies here that it has proven impossible to explain – the date of agreement of sale, the reason for paying more than the vendor expected to realize, and Dr. Hannah's failure to know he was being offered second choices.

It is worthy of note that the Wellcome Institute completed the purchase of their books of choice from the Medical Society of London only in 1984.[10]

In a document dated 8 June entitled Acquisition of the London (England) Medical Society Library, and placed in the files of AMS, Dr. Hannah wrote: "My natural personal inclination was to place the Library at Queen's University so I placed a call to the Principal, Dr. John Deutsch, on April 28th but was not successful in contacting him. Since he had not returned my call by the morning of April 29th, I called again and was successful in contacting him and indicated that I had purchased the Library and that I would like to give consideration to placing it at Queen's University." The principal said he would have either the dean or assistant dean of medicine call Dr. Hannah. However, nothing further was heard from Principal Deutsch or anyone else at Queen's, according to Dr. Hannah, until 14 May. This time, Dr. Hannah stressed "my desire to put it at Queen's provided it could be properly cared for and there were people there with sufficient interest to make it the sort of thing that would be worthy of such an addition to the medical literature of Canada as a whole". What happened in future interviews with Queen's personnel, if indeed there were further contacts, is not known. During this time, Dr. Hannah was again quite ill, which may account for his or the vice-dean's failure to remember further contacts.

His illness did not prevent his writing to Dr. T.C. Hunt of the Medical Society of London about shipment of the books, the deal having been agreed to on 29 April.[11] In a letter dated 11 June 1971, Dr. Hunt wrote that the books would leave London shortly. He also displayed full knowledge of the plan for an institute. Dr. Hannah was by now determined the books would be associated with an institute for the history of medicine. Dr. Hannah wrote at some length about his illness in his diary, noting those times he received blood transfusions. The sequence of entries would thus seem to indicate that between 10 April and 3 June, he made the decisions concerning an institute and the Academy as a possible location for it.

During the intervals between transfusions (there were four such in that period of almost eight weeks), Dr. Hannah made initial contacts with officials of the Academy: Dr. William Ortved (chairman of the Building Committee), Dr. Douglas Snell (chairman of the Library Committee), and Mr. Trevor Alderwick (executive secretary), as well as Dr. W.E. Swinton, Honorary Curator of the Academy's Museum. A definite date, 2 June, is given for the first meeting with the president of the Academy, Dr. G.A. Pengelly.

Dr. Swinton deserves special mention here, since he was to play a most important role in the establishment of history of medicine in the province – as a historical adviser, as expert for the Academy's collection of museum artifacts and Rare Book Library, and as the individual who introduced Dr. Hannah to Dr. Robertson Davies, Master of Massey College.

William Elgin Swinton, a distinguished internationally known palaeontologist, was born and educated in Scotland. He spent many years of his brilliant career at the British Museum, before migrating to Canada in 1961. He served the Royal Ontario Museum in Toronto as Director, Life Sciences, and as Director until his retirement in 1966. He was Professor of Zoology in the

University of Toronto 1962-1966, and was made a Centennial Professor in 1966. He had already been named a Fellow of Massey College in the same year. His first interest in history of medicine appeared in the 1930s, when he learned of the International Congress of the History of Medicine in Madrid, and when he included a chapter on "Dinosaurs and Disease" in his first book. His interest in the subject grew from his renewed friendship with E. Ashworth Underwood, who had been appointed Director of the Wellcome Institute for the History of Medicine.

In conversation with the author, Dr. Swinton spoke of his role in history of science at the University of Toronto.[12] When making Dr. Swinton's appointment as Centennial Professor, President C.T. Bissell asked what he would now profess, to which the former replied, "Something you do not do at present." Dr. Bissell jumped up and asked, "What do we not do?" Dr. Swinton said, "History of science", and soon thereafter began to give lectures in the subject. He also started the Toronto Society for the History of Science, which gave way in 1968 to the Institute for the History and Philosophy of Science and Technology (IHPST) of the University of Toronto. Dr. John Abrams chaired a presidential committee (the second such) that included Dr. Maurice Careless, Dr. Tom Goudge, Dr. John Scott, Dr. Swinton, and the author, the purposes of which were to assess current activity in the subject and to determine how history of science should be organized on the Toronto campus. That committee made the recommendation that resulted in the establishment of IHPST.

In 1969, Dr. Swinton was introduced over lunch to Dr. Gerald D. Hart, chairman of the Museum Committee of the Academy of Medicine. Shortly after, he was appointed Consultant Curator to the Museum.[13] In 1970, he was elected to Honorary Fellowship in the Academy. It is not surprising, then, that Dr. Hannah sought to meet Dr. Swinton through Mr. Alderwick. Dr. Hannah questioned Dr. Swinton about the Academy, its library, history of medicine, and his interest in the subject. Immediately, Dr. Swinton became Dr. Hannah's second adviser concerning history of medicine, Dr. Gibson being the first. It is of interest to note that in May 1971, Dr. Gibson was making inquiries about the possible acceptance of what was to become the basis of the Hannah Collection by the National Library of Canada in Ottawa.[14] Dr. Hannah himself had written in his report to the Board dated 10 May 1971 (less than two weeks after the London purchase decision had been taken) that the Woodward Library at the University of British Columbia was "by far and away the most logical place for the Library and to endow such an Institute, if such should be approved or considered by AMS". He did, however, see as a major drawback the Woodward's location in Vancouver, far from Ontario, where AMS had made its money. Dr. Hannah first met Dr. Gibson at the Woodward Library and he was most impressed with both.

Where Should the Library Be Placed?

In the same report (10 May), Dr. Hannah had given consideration to the placement of the library in Toronto (geographically the most suitable location for such a library) and quite specifically to the Academy of Medicine as in some ways the best site. Yet he wrote at the same time and while beginning negotiations with Academy officers,

> There are, however, some compelling reasons why the Toronto Academy of Medicine is at this moment not entirely suitable for the project. First, they have not got the accommodation for the additional books (2,000 volumes) such that [they] would be displayed and perhaps utilized to the best advantage for at least some time to come. Secondly, it does not have, in my opinion, the personnel who are particularly interested in medical history to the extent that they might appreciate fully the Library which they would be given, and I am not at all sure the gift of the Library might stimulate this interest.

He said he would be consulting with Dr. Swinton the next day.

On 18 May 1971, the President sent another memorandum to all members of the Board.[15] It was concerned with what he perceived to be a lack of interest and an inability to cope with a library of this size at Queen's, and with revision to some extent of his thinking about the Academy. He wrote that

> it would appear that the Toronto Academy of Medicine, which is becoming more and more prominently connected with the teaching of medicine in Toronto, particularly in relation to the study of medical history, is the most logical repository for this library. I am particularly impressed with Dr. Swinton's approach to this problem.

In an accompanying document, The Origin of Sources of Finances,[16] Dr. Hannah gave more of the background of his thinking. He reported having made a study of the Wellcome Trust in Great Britain, the John and Mary Markle Foundation in the United States, and the Bickell Foundation in Canada. He realized that both the British and American organizations were much larger than AMS could ever hope to be. However, he was impressed with the Bickell Foundation, which, having begun operations in 1951 with a portfolio comparable in size to that possessed by AMS in 1971, had managed to make grants that exceeded the original funds in two decades while building the reserves to two and one-half times the original value. He saw this as an example of what he would like to accomplish with AMS. He also quoted some of the philosophy of Dr. O.M. Solandt, then chairman of the Science Council of Canada, with respect to a single granting agency that would help "break down interdisciplinary barriers in mission-oriented research and increase efficiency"; at the same time there existed a need for a Council for Lost Causes or Foundation for the Far-Out "where people could turn for support after they had been turned down by the main granting agencies". He met with Dr. Solandt to discuss these ideas.

He reminded members of the Board of the by-law approved in 1965, and amended in 1966:

> Should AMS for any reason be wound up, all its remaining assets after payment of all debts and liabilities shall, prior to dissolution be distributed or disposed of to promote medical education in the Province of Ontario; distribu-

tion of such remaining assets shall be made in manner and amounts to such institutions in Ontario and in such ratio to each of them, as the Board of Directors of AMS may in its sole discretion deem advisable, prior to such a distribution being made.[17]

He went on to say, "Although AMS has not decided to 'wind up', the time has come when we are able to lend support in a comparatively limited scope to various projects." He said McGill University and the University of British Columbia had good medical libraries and the housing and personnel to take care of the collection. He must have forgotten temporarily the restriction to Ontario that formed part of the 1965 by-law. He added, "There is need for a library and museum located where the largest amount of traffic occurs in relation to the study of medicine in Canada. This appears to be in Toronto, either in connection with the University of Toronto or in the Toronto Academy of Medicine which already has one of the best medical libraries in Canada."

An Institute for the History of Medicine

In his memorandum 18 May he continued to muse about the medical historical library he had purchased, the institute he desired to establish, the T.G.H. Drake collection at the Academy (consisting of artifacts and books on the history of paediatrics), and the finances that would be necessary to "establish an archives and museum programme in Toronto through which it would be possible for us to join in a circulating programme of exhibits including those from countries such as the United States, Great Britain, France, Germany, etc., etc.":

> Personally, I would like to see a Canadian institute for the study of medical history from which might emanate graduates and postgraduates who would give proper instruction to our medical students in this very valuable but much neglected part of their medical education.

> Therefore, I am proposing to my Board that we should delegate to their President and Managing Director the authority to proceed to the completion of the development as suggested in a motion of the Board of Directors under date of December 13, 1970 [which authorized the gift of $25,000 to the Academy's building campaign to create a testimonial to himself], and that AMS be prepared to give sufficient funds to construct approximately 2,000 square feet for archives and museum purposes in connection with the Toronto Academy of Medicine. Such a project must be capable of being expanded to meet future requirements. Further, I am suggesting to my Board that we indicate to the Toronto Academy of Medicine that AMS make available to the Toronto Academy of Medicine the income from at least $1,000,000 per year reckoned on the average percentage yield in respect of any one particular year and that this shall be established (all things remaining equal) for a period of at least five years.

Here he outlined for the first time the objectives of such an institute:

> 1) The Institute shall be known as *The Jason A. Hannah Canadian Institute for Medical History.*
> 2) The Institute shall be maintained as a suitable centre for the collection and storing and exhibiting and study of various documents, incunabula, museum pieces, and teaching as it or they pertain particularly to the history of medicine in Canada.
> 3) To encourage study and research into the history of medicine generally, but more particularly as relates to Canadian medicine.
> 4) To encourage and train suitable individuals to teach the history of medicine to students in medical faculties more particularly in Canadian universities.
> 5) For the above-noted purposes, AMS shall lend such financial and other support as in its judgment shall be within its competence.

There are several points that should be made about this statement of objectives – some positive, some negative, some not yet realized as possibly necessary to achieve these goals. In the last category, there is no mention of relations with universities. Positively, financial and other support would be provided; negatively, the word used was *lend*, a word that was going to cause much difficulty.

One of the many titles that would be ultimately proposed for the institute incorporated the word *Canadian* in the context suggested by Dr. Gibson in his letter of 21 May 1971.

In a later memorandum, dated 25 June 1971 and titled "Guidelines", Dr. Hannah spelled out what he thought AMS's negotiating picture with the Academy should be.[18] He wished the Board to authorize him to negotiate on these terms. AMS should should

(a) Retain a suitable and adequate site for the erection of a suitable structure and to house the Institute and its apurtenances [*sic*] in conjunction with the erection of a new Academy building to be located at the corner of Bloor and Huron Streets in Toronto.
(b) For this purpose, the Board authorizes the President and Managing Director to commit AMS up to but not exceeding seventy-five thousand dollars ($75,000).
(c) Negotiate a mortgage loan of one million dollars ($1,000,000) at the rate of 8% per annum repayable over a period of not more than twenty years, and that under conditions suitable and satisfactory to the Directors of AMS, the interest from such mortgage loan shall be utilized by AMS to establish prizes, fellowships and grants to suitable and deserving undergraduates and postgraduates, and to otherwise further the objects of *The Jason A. Hannah Institute for Medical History*.

The same document (which appears to have been, but may not have been, addressed to the directors) gave further guidelines to the effect that the Board reconfirm its approval of the purchase of the library from London, and that the library be placed in the

Academy "on indefinite loan on such terms as shall meet with the approval of the President and Managing Director of AMS". Actually, all of these terms and the negotiating position had been approved by the directors two days before, 23 June 1971, as recorded in the minutes of the meeting in Resolutions 19-22. On the other hand, a letter from Dr. Hannah to Dr. Pengelly, president of the Academy, with a copy to Dr. Swinton, refers to a 24 June telephone conversation between the two and appears to suggest release of the "Guidelines" document to Academy officials as a basis for further discussion.[19]

In a memorandum to the Board of Directors, dated 21 July, Dr. Hannah noted:[20]

> I have not received any very great encouragement in respect of the suggestions put forward at our last Board meeting, when I was authorized to discuss with the Toronto Academy of Medicine the possibility of making them a grant of at least $75,000 toward a building as well as making them a mortgage loan in order to enable them to retain their present holdings in property and construct a building which will be a credit to the medical profession and be useful to them for a long time to come, as opposed to doing further temporary construction and having to repeat the program in another 25 to 50 years.

In this same memorandum, he also wrote,

> I still hope it will be possible to convince the Academy of Medicine that, if given the London Medical Society Library, they will be prepared to do something towards supporting the development of a teaching and study centre for medical history.

It appears in retrospect that the Academy was giving serious consideration to Dr. Hannah's proposals. The evidence comes from two sources, Dr. John Scott and Dr. Hannah himself. Dr. Scott requested formal Academy approval to give at the Academy the History of Medicine course that Dean Chute had asked him to offer to students of Art as Applied to Medicine as well as to those from IHPST (it was expected to be an elective for medical students too). At the same time Dr. Scott forwarded to Dr. Pengelly a "Memorandum for discussion: Proposed Institute for the History of Medicine in the Academy of Medicine, Toronto".[21] This interesting document, well thought and well expressed, examined the current University of Toronto situation in history of science (i.e. IHPST), its relation to the School of Graduate Studies, its lack of strength in history of biology, and its absence of activity in history of medicine.

Dr. Scott went on to suggest the crucial point: that an institute for the history of medicine at the Academy would require the academic leadership and respectability that would make possible an association with the School of Graduate Studies. He wrote:

> There is a precedent for this in the Pontifical Institute for Mediaeval Studies, which is not part of the University of Toronto, yet several members of its staff hold honorary appointments within the university, and have academic status in the School of Graduate Studies. Consequently they can present their students for degrees to the University.

While Dr. Scott was analysing the previously neglected academic aspects and necessary university connections for Dr. Hannah's institute, Dr. Pengelly and his executive were apparently examining the financial implications to the Academy of the AMS negotiating position. In his memorandum to file dated 13 August, Dr. Hannah reported a long telephone conversation with President Pengelly on 10 August.[22] The Academy believed it was going to require a good deal more financial support than that already offered by AMS if the project were to go forward. The Academy did want the library, but in Dr. Hannah's dictated words,

> It is obvious that they are not prepared to pay the price that may be necessary to sustain such a project in a viable and healthy condition. It is certainly obvious from the discussions I have had in respect of this matter that the Academy has no concept of what might be involved

in the establishment of a *Canadian National Institute for Medical History*.

It is equally obvious Dr. Hannah had no idea what costs he was asking others to undertake for the institute he desired so strongly, nor why he should expect the Academy to bear any of the costs if they provided a home at relatively little expense to AMS.

The Library Arrives

In the same document, Dr. Hannah said he told Dr. Pengelly he would meet with Dr. Scott "who is heading up a new course on the history of medicine in the University of Toronto". He did so 12 August 1971. He also recorded in the memorandum that the shipment of the books from the Medical Society of London was at sea on the *Nordkap* and was expected to arrive 20 August and be delivered where he should so direct 23 August. In his conversation with Dr. Scott, he found him knowledgeable about the proposition and anxious to see such an institute go ahead. Dr. Scott and Dr. Hannah agreed there was a need for the discipline in the curriculum of medical students. In addition, they discussed both the Academy's building plans and Dr. Hannah's thought that the Academy might move to 615 Yonge Street (the AMS building) should it be vacated 1 July 1972. A handwritten note recorded Mr. Alderwick's observation that 615 Yonge Street would give the Academy less space than they currently had.

Dr. Hannah continued to dream of an even larger institute when he recorded:

> I intimated to Dr. Scott that the present presentation of the London Medical Society Library to Canadian medicine might well be just the beginning of a collection of the best medical history or science history books in the world, and that if other collections became available, it is possible that I would secure them for an institute if such was to be established.

Drs. Hannah and Scott decided it would be well for the former to meet soon with the executive of the Academy to facilitate delivery of the library with a minimum of handling in the light of the possibility that there should be a letter of intent exchanged between the Academy and AMS. Dr. Hannah proceeded to dictate the necessary letter to his secretary while Dr. Scott was still present. They also agreed that additions to the library or sale of books could not take place without AMS consent. It was also agreed that the library would never become an actual asset of the Academy; indeed the books would be on indefinite loan. This was to prevent the possibility of the library being sold and the proceeds used for other purposes if unexpected circumstances should occur.

It is not really surprising that Dr. Hannah's purchase should be on the ocean, en route to Toronto, with no designated site for its reception. The same thing was to happen again in 1975 when Dr. Hannah purchased another rare book library of some size.[23] That such a set of conditions should exist in 1971 when he was thinking of starting an institute for the history of medicine is almost beyond belief, and accounts for the use of the word *accidental.*

Dr. Hannah's letter of intent, sent to Dr. Pengelly, was returned bearing the signatures of Drs. Pengelly and Scott and Dr. Douglas Snell.[24] The purpose of the letter was stated very clearly:

> Until the matter is very definitely settled a letter of intent accepted by both the Toronto Academy of Medicine and AMS might clarify the situation so that when the books arrive, they may be delivered to the Toronto Academy of Medicine on the understanding that they are on indefinite loan and should it be necessary, arrangements for the further housing can be changed if suitable agreement, satisfactory to both parties concerned, cannot be concluded.

Dr. Hannah's next letter to Dr. Pengelly contained the points to be considered at a meeting with the Academy executive, scheduled for the Hannah home 17 August.[25] The agenda in the letter augured for a lengthy meeting. Among the subjects put forward for discussion were immediate housing of the library, scope and permanent housing, financing, insurance, conditions for disposal of any duplicates, access to the library, designation of ownership in the volumes, AMS right of inspection of its library, and development of an institute for medical history. In the rather long letter, Dr. Hannah threw out several more ideas. If the $1,000,000 loan were to be accepted by the Academy, the interest rate would indeed be 8% for a term of 20 years, but would rise to 9½% or 10% for 30- and 40-year loans respectively. Aware that even the lowest rate of interest would necessitate a very substantial increase in Academy dues, Dr. Hannah suggested he was prepared "to negotiate some method by which AMS will return the interest to the Academy (under continuing satisfactory circumstances) to assist with the staffing and continuing maintenance of the broader aspects of an institute." He expected the medical profession to make a reasonable contribution to the costs of an institute.

Dr. Hannah does not appear to have distinguished between the central (i.e., clinical) library about which he had previously negotiated unsuccessfully with other medical organizations – the Ontario Medical Association and the College of Physicians and Surgeons of Ontario as well as the Academy – and a library restricted to history of medicine. It is difficult to understand how he could expect the licensing body responsible for and to all physicians of the province to undertake special funding for a specialty library that would be used by a very small percentage of registrants. Should he have expected physicians, whether interested or not in the history of their profession, to pay a considerable share of the costs of the library and an associated institute, while non-medical personnel interested in the discipline in at least the same numbers did not pay?

Elsewhere in the letter concerning the agenda of the upcoming meeting with the Academy executive, he wrote,

> It is hoped that with this Library as a nucleus, we may be able to develop an institute for medical history from which may be graduated suitable individuals to fill chairs as Professors of Medical History at the various medical faculties.

Dr. S.B. Upper, Chief Medical Officer of AMS, was designated to attend the meeting as the second representative of the corporation. On his copy of the agenda letter, he wrote in the margin beside the foregoing excerpt, "Is the Institute to be a degree-granting institution or is it to be affiliated with a university which grants degrees?" He was obviously very much aware of Dr. Scott's statement (he may even have been the first to consider the problem of academic recognition[26]), that institute staff must have status with a university and its graduate school. Dr. Upper's comment about finances from the profession were, "how much? from where?" He also asked what would be the name for the library, once it had reached Canada.

The meeting between the Academy representatives (Dr. Pengelly, Dr. Snell, Dr. Scott, and Mr. Alderwick) and the AMS representatives (Dr. Hannah, Dr. Upper) took place as scheduled 17 August 1971. It was lengthy. Fortunately, the AMS archives contain a full set of minutes.[27] Each of the points in Dr. Hannah's proposed agenda was considered in turn, but the most time was spent on the Academy's finances and plans for building. The Academy executive had no problems with most of the agenda. They were prepared to receive the shipment and deal with it; to accept the books on indefinite loan; to deal with the increased insurance needed (they would add $175,000 to the Academy's rare book insurance at an annual cost of $475); to agree with the clauses dealing with disposal, designation of volumes, inspection; but they pointed out that the Academy rules with respect to access and use were more strict than those desired by Dr. Hannah. They agreed on the desirability of there being such an institute and with it being known as the Hannah Institute. In fact, both Dr. Pengelly and Dr. Scott claimed first credit for the name.

Dr. Scott again spoke at some length about the academic relationships of an institute and its staff, in particular with the School of Graduate Studies, but also with the IHPST. Dr. Hannah's reaction was that he wanted to avoid development of the institute being "lost in the well of the University of Toronto or government". The conversation shifted to appointment of a director, how this should be done, and what qualifications should be required. A number of suggestions were made but none were accepted.

There followed discussion of the financial backing required for an institute and more especially the effect of Dr. Hannah's suggestions concerning finances of the Academy budget and members' dues. The Academy's financial position was best expressed by Mr. Alderwick: "If the Academy wants to put up a building, they need $1,000,000 now for their own purposes, irrespective of any additional expenses for an Institute or an Institute program." To this and the specifics of the Academy's finances, Dr. Hannah said the discussion had given him a fresh perspective on the Academy's problems, and went on to suggest that one possible solution was for AMS to acquire the Academy property and develop it with the Academy getting benefits.

Mr. Alderwick informed Dr. Hannah by letter on 7 October that Dr. Pengelly had given his Council a full report of the meeting of 17 August, and that the library of the Medical Society of London had been received at the Academy. He expressed the Academy's promise to house and care for the collection properly and the hope of the executive that "the Library will fulfill the high hopes you have entertained for its role as a major influence for the study of the history of medicine in Canada".

AMS-Academy Disagreement

In the summer and early autumn, AMS went through a period of stress, which the President referred to as a crisis and which engendered some fear that AMS would not be able to continue its activities. Details need not concern us, but it should be noted that history of medicine and other diversification studies had less priority during this time. It is not surprising, then, that another meeting of representatives of the Academy and AMS to talk about the projected institute's being located at the Academy did not take place until 15 November. Again it took place at Dr. Hannah's residence, and again quite extensive minutes exist.[28] The Academy brought three more representatives to this meeting in addition to the four who had been at the August meeting. They were Dr. William E. Ortved, Dr. D.A. Sarjeant, and Professor W.E. Swinton.

Before the meeting, Dr. Hannah talked to the president, Dr.

Pengelly, by telephone 29 October, which conversation he reported in a memorandum to file.[29] Dr. Hannah wrote:

> I intimated to Dr. Pengelly that in my opinion, the Academy could not support the library even under present circumstances, much less if they had to make a loan of at least one million dollars to be able to house it in the future, and I felt that some other arrangement would be necessary if the whole situation is not be become [*sic*] a "cropper". I also intimated to Dr. Pengelly that in my opinion, I doubted whether or not there was enough of the "quality" interest to start up and sustain a medical institute. Dr. Pengelly admitted that financially he thought I was correct. He did hope, however, that they did have the "quality" to carry such a program through to a successful conclusion.

The principal conclusion of the meeting was drawn by Dr. Hannah in a long introductory statement. He had come to doubt that the Academy could afford a loan of $1,000,000. He said also,

> Even that is $1,000,000 short of what should be done for the situation in addition to what can be raised by the members. More money is needed to house things as they stand now and to meet the desires of the members.

He spoke of other medical societies' not being able to keep their libraries, let alone maintain them up to date. He felt the Academy might be declining to this position.

> Some other source of financing is already needed to maintain the library at its present state. That state is not good enough. The Academy will have to, if its library is to be in the forefront, be able to finance additions to it and add modern means of communication – both of which are expensive.

He then suggested that the 12,000 square feet of space at

615 Yonge Street could serve as the library for the Academy and the current Academy quarters could be refurbished for the social club desired by many Academy members. He was still anxious that the College of Physicians and Surgeons of Ontario be inveigled into contributing to the costs of the library. He still wanted the Academy's museum and clinical library, as well as his medical historical library, involved in whatever scheme should evolve on a provincial basis, paid for by the profession as a whole. He showed no signs of making a distinction between a clinical library, required by all members of the profession, and a specialist library, of interest to a small number of physicians only.

Representatives of the Academy pointed out that their building plans allowed for 20,000 square feet for the library, and that 12,000 square feet on Yonge Street would not permit expansion as required. The greater space was needed to ensure sufficient stack space over the ensuing fifteen years. Academy personnel seemed to agree on two points: that the Academy Toronto members alone could not keep up the library; and that the library, the museum, and meeting areas, plus club facilities, all provided in a new Academy building, would be far better than a plan that placed the library in a separate building, many blocks away. The question was asked, "Should we become the Academy of Medicine of Ontario rather than the Toronto Academy of Medicine?", to which several made the point that the Ontario Medical Association might object. Readers should appreciate that the Academy of Medicine, Toronto, serves as one of the branches (approximately sixty at that date) of the Ontario Medical Association. Dr. Hannah continued to insist that the profession, including the Academy, should be prepared to consider what it would give up "to accrue a greater benefit from combined efforts". As the meeting drew to a close, Academy representatives were still concerned with finances – those in which they found themselves at the time, and those that would result from extending services beyond Toronto. The need at that time for the clinical library was $75,000 per annum, of which two-thirds only was budgeted, to serve the present Toronto fellows. Dr. Hannah continued to see as essential an agreement on conditions whereby the temporary loan of his library to the Academy might be made more permanent as an "indefinite" loan. No agreement was reached.

There was a further meeting between Drs. Hannah and Pengelly at the Hannah home on 5 December, which is referred to but briefly in a long private and confidential letter.[30] Nothing substantial is reported from that meeting. The reason given for this failure was undoubtedly preparation for the 12 December Board meeting.

For the upcoming Board meeting, members of the Board received four appendices: two concerning Dr. Hannah's relations with the Academy, the file memorandum of 9 November, and the minutes of the meeting of 15 November between the Academy representatives and Drs. Hannah and Upper. These appendices were despatched 26 November.[31] The Report of the Managing Director was sent out also before the Board met.[32] It was a long report (twenty-five pages) and concerned a number of topics: the phasing-out of AMS as a designated agent for OHSIP (Ontario Health Services Insurance Plan); the necessity to continue using the present AMS charter for whatever the corporation should undertake in the future; AMS reserves and the future; the winding-up Board resolution of 1965, amended in 1966; a full answer to a question on the procedure for winding-up if AMS should feel compelled to take that route; and the alternatives to winding-up, of which the best, in Dr. Hannah's opinion, would be an institute for the history of medicine.

Part 5 of the document was entitled "The Toronto Academy of Medicine as a Vehicle to establish an Institute for Medical History". It related the history of the Academy and the organizations that had come together in 1907 to form the Academy. He wrote at some length about the importance of the library to the Academy over the years and of the burden placed on Academy operations by the maintenance of the library. He reviewed his attempt to create a central library in Ontario, a clinical library centred on the Academy, which, in his plan, would become provincial in operation and a charge against the profession as a whole. Again, he associated his medical historical library with the obligation he perceived for medicine in Ontario with respect to library resources. Then he stated,

> An institute for Medical History must have a broader outlook, function and acceptance than is possible in the Academy of Medicine, Toronto, or under the Health Council of Ontario. It must embrace the concept of the whole of Canada and perhaps eventually look to world recognition. Its primary function must be the dissemination of knowledge of the real history of medicine, free of local or political bias.

Part 6 of his report concerned an "Alternative to the Academy through which to establish an Institute for Medical History". Here he ruled out 615 Yonge Street for several reasons, saying "the possibility is mentioned only to dismiss it". The main reasons given were the need of a very considerable capital outlay if the Academy had been prepared to place its library at the AMS building, and the difficulty of AMS accepting an entirely new activity in which it did not have expertise. He also dismissed participation in government-supported projects.

For the first time, he now disclosed to Board members that he had met with Dr. Robertson Davies, Master of Massey College, 29 November 1971, at a luncheon arranged by Dr. W.E. Swinton. The sequence of events that followed on this meeting is detailed in the next chapter. It is worth noting here, however, that Dr. Hannah had begun negotiations with Massey College before he officially called off talks with the Academy. It should also be noted that Dr. Swinton had had no effect on the Academy's position even though he was Honorary Curator.[33] Dr. Swinton was to be an important participant in the relations between Dr. Hannah and Dr. Davies. Dr. Hannah raised with the Board in this document the question of the finances necessary to set up an institute for medical history at Massey College. The figures suggested in this report were at least $250,000 per annum "to assure continuing success", and an endowment of between $2,000,000 and $4,000,000 "to assure adequate and full support". Finally, he told his Board that "it is obvious that much more study and consideration will be required".

At the Board meeting of 12 December, members agreed with Dr. Hannah's decision, "which he had conveyed to Dr.

Pengelly", that the $75,000 gift, approved by the Board 23 June "to provide for the erection of a suitable structure to house the Jason A. Hannah Institute for Medical History and its appurtenances in conjunction with the erection of a new academy to be located at the corner of Bloor and Huron Streets in Toronto", would not be released until sod had been broken and the laying of the foundation had begun.[34] Dr. Hannah also reported that Academy staff had failed to locate 228 volumes of those purchased from the Medical Society of London and that he had ordered the withholding of some of the payment until the books should be located. He also is quoted in the minutes as having "concluded that the colloquial aspects of, and the limited human and financial resources of the Toronto Academy of Medicine makes it an unsuitable permanent repository for the Library of the London Medical Society recently brought to Toronto by AMS". As well, he reported to the Board in terms similar to those in his report concerning his initial talks with Dr. Davies and his first impressions of Massey College as a possible location for his institute. The Board gave approval to his proposal that he be authorized to continue to explore "the possibilities of working with Massey College in the University of Toronto in regard to the *Jason A. Hannah Institute for Medical History*, the London Medical Society Library, and the establishment of Chairs for Medical History in five medical schools in Ontario". The motion passed unanimously.

The minutes further record that Dr. Hannah stated that this resolution "may hold a good deal of the future of AMS". Dr. Hannah said that AMS should retain its charter as long as it was possible to do so and observe the charter in letter and spirit. He believed this was the most secure basis AMS had from which to develop its future. In regard to AMS reserves, it appeared more logical to use them to promote a limited number of projects of undoubted importance such as the establishment of an institute for medical history, the Ontario Geriatric Society, medical libraries, and the like rather than to deal with and sift out a multitude of applications, many of which would be for dubious purposes.

What remained for Dr. Hannah to do was to terminate his negotiations with the Academy concerning the possible placement of his institute there. He informed Dr. Pengelly and his executive officially of his decision, as ratified by the Board, in the letter marked "private and confidential" and dated 15 December. In this letter, he reviewed all his past relations with the Academy up to the receiving of the books from London by Academy staff and the many conversations about establishing the institute in a new Academy building. He repeated his previous conclusions and then added,

> This discovery has been a great disappointment to me. However, closer study of the Academy forces one to accept that those conclusions were inevitable but they have not lessened my appreciation of the Academy, nor my desire to continue to support it.

In a response dated 17 December, Dr. Pengelly acknowledged receipt of this letter. He went on to say he had read three and one-half pages before he realized he should read no more unless he had Dr. Hannah's permission to disclose it to and discuss it with the members of his executive. He wrote,

> I therefore stopped reading and placed all the papers in an envelope for return to you in the event I am not given permission to have the advice and opinion of the other members of the Executive on the contained matter, either in confidence or otherwise.

Dr. Pengelly then referred to the document he and members of his executive had signed authorizing Academy staff to receive on AMS's behalf the library of the Medical Society of London. He said indeed the word "temporary" occurred in the document, but he and his colleagues were

> persuaded that having fulfilled the requirements then specified in regard to insurance, disposal, access and use, designation and inspection . . . the books would be housed on indefinite loan. To be sure, indefinite may be temporary, but we felt sufficiently assured that we advised

> the Academy authorities to spend the sums needed to arrange for temperature and humidity control, and security in the area chosen for safekeeping.

He went on to assure Dr. Hannah it would be the latter's decision alone to move the books elsewhere. He made it perfectly clear that the Academy's first priority was the finding of sufficient sums of money for the immediate, if not long-term, housing of the organization. He said they would be delighted to have the institute established in the Academy, but that

> nothing, repeat nothing, can be done, nor can any firm commitments be made on either side until the financing is arranged for whatever housing is necessary, be this with or without the Hannah Institute.

Speaking of finances, he wrote,

> If you seriously want to house the Institute in the Academy, then an adequate long-term donation programme must be arranged by Associated Medical Services so that appropriate monies may be borrowed to build the needed space.

He went on to suggest AMS be prepared to give the Academy $125,000 to $150,000 from earnings each year for a period of twenty years. This would make it possible for the needed money to be borrowed readily, to house the Academy with all its departments for years to come.

In his reply on 21 December, Dr. Hannah asked for the return of the documents to himself. They form part of the AMS archives. One paragraph of the letter may be quoted.

> As I have no desire to allow what started out to be perhaps the "top" act of appreciation to my profession to degenerate into either personalities or an altercation with the Academy, or to tarnish in any way what has already been done, I shall in future respond or initiate only on a clearly written and defined document on behalf of the Academy.

The Last Act

One would have thought this the last act in the play with respect to the failure of AMS and the Academy to agree on placing the institute at the Academy. It was not. Dr. Hannah apparently felt it was necessary to convey his decision to the executive of the Academy as a whole at their meeting at the Academy on 19 January 1972. At the conclusion of the session, he handed each member of the executive a copy of a letter, dated that very date (hence prepared before the meeting), which put in writing the essentials of what he had just said to Drs. Pengelly, Scott, Snell, Sarjeant, and Box.[35] Two paragraphs sum them up:

> It is a matter of some regret to me that I have been forced to this conclusion after trying to arrive at some definite conclusions and to get matters moving in regard to an Institute for Medical History through the Academy over a period of the past six months. My conclusions are that such an Institute under the auspices of the Academy would inevitably lead to difficulties for the Academy in all respects, and to failure for the Institute. In short, I am of the opinion that it would be unfair to both the Academy of Medicine and the Institute to try to develop it further under the auspices of the Toronto Academy of Medicine, and I have therefore decided to make other arrangements for the establishment of the Institute and the placing of the Library on a more permanent basis.
>
> I recognize that the Academy has been occasioned some considerable expense in regard to storing the Library under suitable conditions, and would therefore be prepared to consider a reasonable contribution toward this expense in addition to the contributions already being made by AMS to the Academy for various other purposes.

At the time of the 19 January meeting with the executive of the Academy, Dr. Hannah asked Dr. John Scott, the most knowledgeable member of the executive with respect to history of medicine, to put his thoughts about an institute in writing. Dr. Scott did so the next day.[36] This is an important letter, and is reproduced in the appendices. It is not intended to suggest that this – or, for that matter, any other opinion – influenced Dr. Hannah in his actions. Nevertheless, the letter represents the thoughtful expressions of an individual deeply interested in steering Dr. Hannah's incomplete concept in a proper and academic direction. In notes on which the letter was based, Dr. Scott wrote,

> As you know, there is no institute for the History of Medicine, nor Medical Museum that is self-supporting. They are all supported by endowments, or receive government grants, directly or through universities.

Dr. Pengelly and his executive responded to Dr. Hannah's visit and letter two days after the meeting.[37] The executive wished its president to make the Academy's position very clear, and he did so.

He disputed Dr. Hannah's statements to the Board of AMS that the Academy would have to negotiate a loan of at least $1,000,000 in order to house the library properly, and that, to amortize the mortgage money, fees would have at least to be doubled. He wrote that he felt very strongly the Academy was by far the best place for the institute and attached an analysis by Dr. Scott that contrasted the institute's location at the Academy and at Massey College in favour of the former.

He stated most clearly,

> Our statement that the Academy could not afford to borrow a million dollars was *only* voiced after your suggestion and encouragement that A.M.S. might be prepared to loan this sum at 8% for 20 years in order that a much bigger project might be attempted.

He suggested that the amount of money required by the Academy from AMS would be in the area of $200,000 per year for twenty years. In addition, to pay for the proper administration of the institute, $150,000 annually would be necessary. (This figure was based on Dr. Scott's analysis.) A further budget of $50,000 could be used to strengthen the museum functions.

> As I said, the Academy, as well as providing a million dollars worth of land would produce three quarters of a million in cash, which would almost equal dollar for dollar. In order to provide funds for the continuing support of the Academy facilities, particularly the Library, the Academy would raise its dues slightly and institute an initiation fee.

He concluded with two promises: that the executive would recommend Dr. Hannah's election as an Honorary Fellow and that Dr. Hannah would, of course, be the first director of the institute.

It can be clearly seen by tracing developments during this period of negotiations that the purchase of the library of the Medical Society of London was the trigger for ensuing developments. As discussions were pursued, the idea of an institute for medical history, to constitute the memorial by which posterity would remember him, loomed larger and more important, until it became the *raison d'être* for Dr. Hannah's will to proceed despite frequent bouts of ill health and no period of really good health. It is very clear he did not appreciate, or would not accept, the need for academic links. It is also obvious he fully expected the profession, or specific organizations within the profession, to provide a considerable part of the costs of his desired memorial. He did not distinguish between a clinical library, necessary to the whole profession, and a specialty library of interest to a small fraction only. He did not seem to realize that he had no right to add to the financial problems of the Academy, which needed to and wished to expand, but not necessarily for the purpose of establishing an institute for the history of medicine. This despite the fact he had authorization from his Board to proceed to the establishment of his institute, which would require even greater expansion.

Thus ended any possibility that the institute might have been located at the Academy of Medicine, Toronto.

Why were the negotiations between Dr. Hannah and the

Academy unsuccessful? Was the period of approximately six months during which negotiations took place sufficient or necessary to come to the conclusions reached by Dr. Hannah? What was the exact relationship between the purchase of the library of the Medical Society of London, the need of a site and personnel to receive it, the opening of negotiations with the Academy concerning both the library and an institute? As a member of the Academy for more than three decades, was Dr. Hannah not aware fully of Academy building plans and difficult finances? Did he not realize, or did he not want to, that placing an institute he desired at the Academy would worsen the Academy's financial picture, unless he, negotiating with authority granted by the Board, paid both the costs of establishing an institute and the costs to be incurred by the Academy in housing it? What alternatives were available to him for location of the institute before he began conversations with Dr. Davies in late November, almost two months before the final break with the Academy?

Let us attempt to answer these questions, even though it may mean the indulgence in some speculation. It will be remembered that at the beginning of the concept involving the Academy, Dr. Hannah expressed doubts about the Academy, and still later he was not complimentary about the quality of staff and commitment. A period of six months for negotiations was not necessary. If the idea of an institute had preceded the purchase of the library, a most thorough investigation of the Academy could have been made. As it turned out, the library was almost in Toronto when the decision was made to place the books at the Academy; this then seems like a last-minute resolution of a difficult problem – where to put the books and have them cared for properly. Subsequently, Dr. Hannah was to buy other collections on impulse: one such library had to be received in his garage in January 1975. Dr. Hannah must have been aware of the Academy's finances and its building plans, for AMS was approached for help. We have seen how, in other diversification projects considered, he was always ready to shave budgets and look to other people to meet costs that really did not concern them. Too, there are never many alternative sites for an institute for the history of medicine. He himself had earlier noted that in Toronto the two possible sites were the Academy and the University of Toronto.

The Academy executive's letter was considered at the 22 January meeting of the Board of Directors – held, ironically, at Massey College, which for some weeks had been investigated by Dr. Hannah as a possible site for his institute. It is recorded in the minutes that copies of the letter were tabled to the directors, who read it and discussed it in detail, after which members agreed with Dr. Hannah's conclusions and passed unanimously the following resolution:

> That the Secretary-Treasurer be instructed to write to the Toronto Academy of Medicine and confirm that full responsibility was delegated to the President and Managing Director of Associated Medical Services, to negotiate in respect of locating the Library of the Medical Society of London (Eng.) as well as for the establishment of the Jason A. Hannah Institute for Medical History, and that all contacts in this regard must come through the President and Managing Director of Associated Medical Services, Incorporated and be in writing.

This not only confirmed the lack of strength in the Board, but also ended any chance that might have existed that the Hannah Institute would be established at the Academy of Medicine, Toronto.

The Board went on to discuss the negotiations under way with Massey College.

CHAPTER IV

Massey College

Massey College, the only graduate college in the University of Toronto, was planned, built, and furnished by the Massey Foundation. Years of thought and months of architectural planning preceded the official laying of the cornerstone by the Duke of Edinburgh in 1962. The Trustees turned over the title to the Master and Fellows at opening ceremonies 4 October 1963.

> It was the intention of the Founders to bring into being a College to serve a body of graduates limited in numbers but of high promise in scholarship and qualified to make of worth the fellowship to which they belong. It is the Founders' prayer that through the fulness of its corporate life and the efforts of its members, the College will nourish learning and serve the public good.[1]

The first Master, who served for many years, was Dr. Robertson Davies.

AMS and Massey College Begin Discussions

On 29 November 1971, Dr. Swinton, in his role as a senior scholar and Fellow of Massey College, introduced Dr. Davies and Dr. Hannah. A three-way conversation ensued about the possibility of associating Dr. Hannah's proposed institute for the history of medicine with Massey College. In the days immediately following this interview, and in anticipation of an approaching meeting of the Board of Directors of AMS, Dr. Davies wrote two letters to Dr. Hannah dated 30 November and 6 December. In the first letter, Dr. Davies said he felt he should repeat and expand the information already exchanged. In the second letter, he did so under the headings "What is Massey College?", "The Hannah Institute for the History of Medicine", "Practicalities", and "Continuity". He wrote at considerable length "in order to make clear what it lies in our power to do for the projected Hannah Institute, and also what lies outside our abilities". Under his first subheading, he wrote of the composition and governance of the College, its modest endowment, the fees paid by Junior Fellows, the annual payment received by the College from the University of Toronto for services rendered, and his hopes concerning the finding of funds to aid senior scholars in the costs of their research and publications.

Dr. Davies then wrote that he felt the institute of which Dr. Hannah had spoken would be a splendid addition to and an integral part of Massey College. He spoke of the concern expressed and work done within the College with respect to library preservation and bibliography. He also wrote of accommodation and privileges available to the director of such an institute. Under "Practicalities", he spoke in a preliminary way of the necessary financial support by AMS of the institute and its host, the College. He raised, as a question, the desirability of offering the University of Toronto a professor of medical history, to be called the Hannah Professor. He felt this step and consultation with the College concerning the appointment of a director would make the Institute acceptable to the university and remove any restrictions to the activities of the institute. What he foresaw was a cross-appointment for the director in the university, which would make all university benefits available to the appointee. He spoke of the need of a handsome room to be the home of the rare book library belonging to AMS.

The Master also wrote feelingly on the subject of continuity:

> I can say with a good conscience, and with the certainty that my colleagues are of the same opinion, that if you decide to place the Hannah Institute with us, it will continue its useful life and will perpetuate your name as its founder, for as long as scholarship itself; furthermore, in an autonomous institution like ours, it will not be the

subject of bureaucratic caprice. With opportunity, there is no telling how it might develop and extend its influence.

Speaking of continuity, he brought the subject back to financial independence and stimulation of quality research, indicating that the College offered in turn stability, expert services, and gratitude.

The meeting of the Board of Directors of AMS, for which Dr. Davies wrote the foregoing letters, was held 12 December. Within a few days, Dr. Hannah had delivered to the Master two copies (one for Dr. Davies and one for Dr. Swinton) of the Managing Director's Report of 12 December 1971, this being the report to the Board concerning his negotiations with both the Academy of Medicine, Toronto, and Massey College. He drew the Master's attention in this report to his studies and considerations of both organizations as vehicles "through which to establish an Institute for Medical History" in the covering letter.[2]

In his report to the Board as set forth in the minutes,[3] Dr. Hannah said he believed Massey College represented the most probable alternative through which to establish an institute for medical history and a repository for the London or other libraries. He noted, however, the need for more study on the part of both the College and AMS. He expressed the view that an endowment of approximately $4,000,000 would be required from AMS "to assure adequate and full support for an institute for medical history and libraries in Massey College". He expressed pleasure that none of the endowment would be required for construction since such facilities were already in existence.

Dr. Hannah went further – undoubtedly reflecting other thinking of his own and advice from others – and raised for consideration the idea that, in conjunction with Massey College, AMS might endow a chair for medical history in each of the five medical schools of Ontario. His estimate of the cost of such a plan was $250,000 for each chair, a total of $1,250,000 for the five universities. The same minutes go on to say that each of the currently existing universities would be eligible for an annual grant for an incumbent of a chair for the teaching of and research into medical history, but only with the approval of the institute for medical history. It was estimated the program outlined above would require approximately $5,250,000, which would still leave approximately $6,750,000 in AMS's reserves after all obligations would be met as of 30 June 1972 (the date on which AMS would cease to act as an agent for the provincial government).

The Managing Director did not see any reason why the balance of funds could not be used to make grants for "worthwhile projects with a sound basis", and also to add to AMS's reserves by appropriate management. The Board agreed, however, that it lacked sufficient information at that time to vote such large sums of money as had been mentioned. Nevertheless, the minutes record a unanimously approved motion:

> That the Board of Directors approves in principle Dr. Hannah's proposal to continue to explore the possibilities of working with Massey College in the University of Toronto in regard to the Jason A. Hannah Institute for Medical History, the London Medical Society Library, and the establishment of Chairs for Medical History in five Medical Schools in Ontario.

It is now necessary to raise some questions, not all of which will lend themselves to ready answers. Under what circumstances did the idea of multiple chairs in the history of medicine enter the picture? Which of Dr. Hannah's historical advisers – Dr. Gibson or Dr. Swinton, or someone else – was responsible for this scenario? How could Dr. Hannah think that Massey College, despite a very large measure of autonomy in its relations with the University of Toronto, could act in conjunction with AMS not only with that university but more especially with the other four universities to establish five chairs? How could he expect that Massey College could supply space for the library of the Medical Society of London and the other libraries he hoped to acquire, plus additional space to satisfy the needs of his proposed institute, without construction of new facilities and that at AMS's expense?

It is obvious in a number of ways that Dr. Hannah was much more comfortable running the affairs of AMS than he was in dealing with academia. A noteworthy illustration of this truth may be found in the discussion following on the motion just quoted.

> Dr. Hannah stated that Resolution No. 38, 12.12.71, may hold a good deal of the future of AMS. Dr. Hannah stated AMS should retain its Charter as long as it is possible to do so and observe the Charter in letter and spirit. He believes this is the most secure basis AMS has, from which to develop its future. In regard to AMS reserves, it appears more logical to utilize them to promote a limited number of projects of undoubted importance such as the establishment of an Institute for Medical History, the Ontario Geriatric Society, Medical Libraries, etc., rather than to deal with and sift out a multitude of applications, many of which will be for dubious purposes.

Dr. Swinton recalls the idea of a chair in the history of medicine being raised by Dr. John Evans (then Dean of Medicine at McMaster University, later to become President of the University of Toronto) in conversation when the two sat next to each other at a dinner they attended.[4] He does not remember talk of five chairs. In a letter to Dr. Hannah dated 14 February 1972, his other historical adviser, Dr. Gibson, strongly recommended one chair in the history of medicine, to be located at the University of Toronto and to be named after Sir William Osler. He wrote,

> In another generation of students, the Osler image will be getting a little fuzzy, because we will not have alive then teachers who actually knew Osler.

These two memories, then, along with the minutes referring to Dr. Hannah's meetings with officials of Massey College, seem to suggest rather strongly that Dr. Hannah himself was the source of the idea that there should be five chairs in history of medicine in Ontario. From a letter of 11 October 1972, it is apparent Dr. Gibson accepted the plan of the five chairs, for he wrote then, "I think the five chairs bearing your name would be, as Osler used to say, 'a great float to posterity'." In subsequent conversation with the author, Dr. Gibson corrected the quotation to the title used for the present history and also indicated he thought the five chairs represented the right decision, both academically and politically.[5]

Perhaps this is the point at which Dr. Gibson should be more fully identified. William Carleton Gibson, although born in Ottawa, was raised in Victoria. He entered Victoria College in 1929 and obtained his B.A. from the University of British Columbia in Vancouver in 1933. He received a Master of Science degree in 1936 and his M.D., in 1941, both from McGill; during that span, he also studied at Oxford for his D.Phil., obtained in 1938. He qualified professionally in both neurology and psychiatry.

His first academic appointment at the University of British Columbia came in 1949 (after war service and further post-graduate training) as Kinsmen Professor of Neurological Research. A decade later, he was appointed Professor and Head of the Department of the History of Medicine, and Research Professor of Psychiatry. In 1964, he also became Assistant to the President on University Development.

His interest in medical history thus was of many years' duration, whetted by a year as Visiting Professor in the subject with John Fulton at Yale, by service on the Wellcome Trust Panel on the History of Medicine, and by many international contacts. He was in an excellent position to give advice and to act as a sounding board. He is currently the Chancellor of the University of Victoria.

Dr. Gibson himself tells the story of his first meeting with Dr. Hannah, which took place in 1968 in the entrance to the Woodward Library at the University of British Columbia. Dr. Hannah was being given a campus tour by a former AMS employee who had moved to the university. Dr. Gibson happened along and was introduced to the visitor. There was a long pause, then Dr. Hannah said, "How much did this cost? I want one of these."

In early 1972, Dr. Hannah was at work on a proposed budget for his institute and chairs in a document entitled "Bursaries, Prizes, Fellowships, etc. for the Jason A. Hannah Institute in Medical History at Massey College."[6] He included a salary and travelling costs for a director, and a miscellany of other cost proposals that undoubtedly reflected conversations with Drs. Swinton and Davies, as well as his own thoughts. He made allowance for two annual fellowships with associated travelling costs ($6,000 stipend, $2,000 travelling expenses for each fellowship); two travelling fellowships at $10,000 each; five first prizes ($500 each) and five second prizes ($250 each) corresponding to the number of medical schools; the sum of $15,000 each for the five chairs and the costs of housing and maintenance and secretarial help. What the sums mentioned for prizes and for the chairs were intended to cover was not mentioned in the document. The total is compared in a questioning tone with the $250,000 that the Master had said the College would require.

Attached to this document was "Rules re Fellowships at the Jason A. Hannah Institute of Medical History". The Managing Director seems to have adopted Massey College nomenclature regarding fellows. Applicants would have been required "to hold a [bona fide] degree from a recognized and acceptable university". However, it is not clear what academic credit might be obtained by a fellow and who would control admission procedures. The last statement is most interesting: "Other considerations being equal preference shall be given to graduates in medicine who have practised medicine preferably for a period of not less than (5) five years." Such an applicant would indeed be a dedicated individual. Perhaps it is best not to consider this anything but musings, for on it is written "*not* sent to Dr. Davies or Dr. Swinton".

The Beginning of Disagreement

In a letter dated 17 December 1971, intended to summarize the previous discussions and to offer certain new ideas, Dr. Davies was unfortunate enough to put forward language and ideas against which Dr. Hannah exercised much prejudice – for example, the word "insurance", and the method of securing financial support for the institute and the College housing it and providing certain services to it. Dr. Hannah's written notes on the letter lend credence to the belief that this was the source, not necessarily the cause, of their first disagreement. One interesting suggestion from the Master concerned the title of the institute.

Dr. Davies put forward "The Hannah Institute for Research in the History of Medicine", noting "I have stressed the word *Research* in the title, as your Charter (c) specifies this as one of your aims, and lessens any objection that might be raised to your devoting funds to this project; *research* does not, of course, rule out teaching." An invitation was confirmed to hold a meeting of the Board of Directors of AMS in the Round Room of the College in January 1972.

A few days later, Dr. Hannah was at work on Draft No. 2 of a Memorandum of Agreement, in which the new name was "The Jason A. Hannah Institute for Research and Teaching in the History of Medicine".[7] Much of the Master's language of the 17 December letter was adopted, and the size of the necessary endowment was spelled out as $4,000,000. One change, however, is interesting. Dr. Davies had written, "*The First Director* of the Institute to be Dr. J.A. Hannah, in order that he may shape its character and set its course, and undertake himself a History of Medical Insurance in North America". In pencilled notes on the Master's letter, Dr. Hannah changed "Medical Insurance" to "Prepayment for Medical Care", and "North America" to "Canada". In Draft No. 2 the last clause was left out completely so that Clause 7 read "*The first Director* of the Institute shall be Jason A. Hannah, B.A., M.D., C.M., C.R.C.P.(C), in order that he may shape its character and set its course." The directorate that should oversee the institute would consist of four members, two appointed by the College and two by AMS.

> In case of a tie vote the four directors so appointed shall elect a fifth member pro tem from among the Judges of the Appeal Court of Ontario who shall, after presentation of the facts involved by any or all of the four appointed directors, determine the matter in dispute and his decision shall be final.

Dr. Hannah did append to this draft the statement,

> It is recognized that the foregoing is a draft only, to be used as a working basis only to refine and complete a finished agreement.

Dr. Davies' letter of 29 December 1971 found a number of difficulties with the draft; these included excessive director's powers not subject to the university or the College, and failure to appreciate that an institute could be established only after "careful scrutiny and consent of the Graduate School, and the assent of the Senate of the University". He went on to say, "The Director would have to be someone who held a professorial appointment if he were to do any teaching, and professorial appointments are not easily made." Dr. Hannah, desirous of being the first director, had no academic position. The Master again stressed what the College would bring to such a relationship and why it therefore deserved one-half the yield that would come from an endowment. He noted the length of time it would take AMS to plan and establish its own quarters.

To avoid problems that would be caused by the setting up of an institute or a centre (both academic terms of quite precise meaning) within the College, Dr. Davies proposed that the two talk of Hannah Fellowships, the chief of which, with a capital greater than the others, should be the Hannah Fellowship for Research in the History of Medicine. He emphasized that such fellowships could be established in Massey College without need to consult either the School of Graduate Studies or the Senate. This fellowship would be the appointment for Dr. Hannah, and with it would be associated the Hannah Library. In Dr. Davies' words, "I can assure you that a Fellowship with a splendid specialized library is uncommon." He felt the endowment necessary for such a fellowship would be $1,000,000, half of the yield going to the holder for living and research costs, and the other half to the College, in which associated or related studies would strengthen the rather narrow base of history of medicine.

A further letter of 7 January 1972 from the Master to the Managing Director spelled out how the College selected Junior Fellows and paid two-thirds of what it cost to keep a person in residence during term. There was further argument advanced concerning the splitting of income from the endowment equally between the College and the direct support of the Hannah Institute.

Dr. Hannah was still positive about the proposed location of his institute in his reply of 13 January, expecting that many of the remaining details – such as College representation on the AMS Board, minimization of the effects of inflation by annual grant (the customary way by which AMS made payments) rather than by the creation of an endowment, itemized costs for preparation of rooms for the institute – could be worked out by further consultation prior to the Board meeting scheduled for 22 January. (It should be remembered that he had still not closed off his negotiations with the Academy of Medicine, Toronto.)

On the same day, Dr. Hannah sent the Report of the President and Managing Director to the Board for the meeting to be held at Massey College 22 January 1972.[8] In his report, he included most, but not all, of his exchanges with Dr. Davies. Notable for their absence were the Master's comments about institutes, centres, directors, graduate school, and senate. To bring his Board into the picture with respect to required financing, Dr. Hannah said,

> It is your President and Managing Director's opinion that two million dollars ($2,000,000) should be set aside as an endowment for the College against unforeseen circumstances, etc. This should give a return of some one hundred and forty thousand dollars ($140,000) annually.

There is a paragraph in this report that supports a comment made to the author by Dr. S.B. Upper, Medical Director of AMS for a decade during the time when diversification was being constantly investigated. At the time and in retrospect, Dr. Upper thinks Dr. Hannah was not comfortable with any activity not part of prepaid medical care and that this is why so many well-investigated ventures were discarded before implementation.[9] In this same report in which he urged that not all AMS resources be tied up in one project, Dr. Hannah wrote,

> Furthermore, as the Board knows, it has been the hope of your President and Managing Director that some other form of non-profit prepayment for medical services may sooner or later be developed to replace our former doctors

services, and our capital be further enhanced through such activities.

One could then ask how the whole concept of the Hannah chairs and institute was permitted to begin and to grow. In all likelihood, Dr. Hannah's advancing illness and longing for immortality forced him to take decisions he would not otherwise have made.

In a letter dated 19 January 1972 and addressed to the Executive Committee of the Academy of Medicine, Toronto, Dr. Hannah had finally finished his explorations of the Academy as a possible home for his institute, in the following words:

> My conclusions are such that an Institute under the auspices of the Academy would inevitably lead to difficulties for the Academy in all respects, and to failure for the Institute.

This not only constitutes another example that supports Dr. Upper's view, but also foreshadows what was soon to happen at Massey College. The copy of this letter in the AMS Massey College file bears in the writing of Dr. Hannah's secretary the notation "Not given to Massey College. On file for information. 19/1/72."

Mr. Colin E. Friesen, Bursar of Massey College, supplied on 20 January 1972 a preliminary estimate of costs to be incurred by Massey College in preparing 2,350 square feet of space for the Hannah Institute.[10] These expenditures, for air conditioning, humidification, electrical work, a sprinkler system, removable ceiling, tile flooring, masonry, carpentry, cabinet work, furnishing, all to be reimbursed by AMS, totalled $45,525. Two letters dated 31 January at Massey College gave Dr. Hannah further information. One, from Mr. Friesen, discussed the services to be rendered to AMS by Massey College in return for the $125,000 annual endowment. The list included rent, bursary, library, and intangibles. In the other, Dr. Davies told Dr. Hannah that he needed a statement relating to the establishment of the institute for two formalities that he had shortly to observe. He had to report the proposal to establish the institute to the Standing Committee of the College and get its consent. Moreover, he had to disclose to the dean of the School of Graduate Studies what was going on. Consequently what he was seeking was a letter of intent.

The Board meeting held at Massey College 22 January 1972 discussed three major items. It also gave members of the Board an opportunity to view the facilities, particularly those the Master proposed to make available to AMS. The first matter discussed reflected the deteriorating relations between the Academy of Medicine and AMS. Dr. Hannah, according to the official minutes, spoke at some length on the subject, citing the letters exchanged 19 January and 21 January.[11] From his members, he gained unanimously a resolution:

> That the Secretary-Treasurer be instructed to write to the Executive Committee of the Toronto Academy of Medicine and confirm that full responsibility was delegated to the President and Managing Director of Associated Medical Services to negotiate in respect of locating the Library of the Medical Society of London (Eng.) as well as for the establishment of the Jason A. Hannah Institute for Medical History, and that all contacts in this regard must come through the President and Managing Director of Associated Medical Services, Incorporated and be in writing.

The second subject for report and debate concerned the continuing discussions between Dr. Hannah on the one hand, and Drs. Davies and Swinton on the other, about locating the institute and library at Massey College. Matters already described throughout this chapter were discussed by Board members for the first time, and in addition several seemingly new ideas appeared for the first time. The former included the directorship, accommodation and other costs, library, College representation on the Board, annual grant vs. endowment, and the need for further negotiations and for a legal agreement.

The Proposal for a Hannah Tower

The new matter introduced at the meeting demands a quotation from the minutes:

> Basement space in Massey College has been suggested as a location for the Library. This space was viewed by the Directors during their tour of the College and although it appears that it would be adequate after renovations, the Directors agreed with Dr. Hannah that it would be more desirable to be located above the ground level. Dr. Hannah reported that such space is not available at the present time, in the college, but it is his understanding that additional space can be added by building upwards in one of the towers. With the addition of more floors a small lift will be advisable. Indeed with frequent movements of books, etc., the need for such a lift is felt at present.

Here, then, is the first official intimation by Dr. Hannah to his Board of the idea that came to be known as the Hannah Tower, which would be located in the northwest corner of the College, and for which architectural drawings, dated 5 February 1972, exist. They were prepared by R.J. Thom, the architect who designed Massey College. The tower was intended to provide reception and display areas, offices, an elevator, and a library with carrels and a workroom. It seems clear that the College would have had to sacrifice some space to make the addition possible.

Although the Board authorized unanimously an annual payment of $125,000 to the College for maintenance costs, and an allocation of up to $45,000 "to provide immediate facilities to house the Institute in Massey College", it took no action on the Hannah Tower.

Dr. Hannah produced Draft No. 2 of a Memorandum of Agreement on 1 February 1972. For the first time, the library brought from London was referred to as "The Jason A. Hannah Rare Book Collection". It and any additions were to be maintained separately and were to remain the property of AMS. Another clause referred to the "Jason A. Hannah Tower" and stated it could be built, but only with the approval of the College and at the expense of AMS. One clause that must have disturbed the College was

> The relationship between the College, AMS, and/or the Institute may be terminated only after the expiration of six (6) full months following written notice given by either the College or AMS to the other party.

A lengthy clause dealt with publishing policy and assistance; it not only assumed that publications in the history of medicine would be profitable, but also dealt with the use of researched material in popular versions of medical history or in medical historical novels provided all such publications adhered to actual historical findings.

A Statement of Intent? – More Disagreements

Dr. Hannah responded to the Master's request for a statement of intent in a letter dated 8 February. This letter is rather difficult to understand clearly and perhaps shows the effect of declining health; he does state that he will have a transfusion on 10 February (in excess of twenty such since the previous April) and will leave for Florida three days later, to stay there as long as the effects of the transfusion should last. He summarized what he believed AMS would bring to an agreement. This included the library and its cost of housing; the opportunity the College would have to develop an institute; the cost of accommodation for the director, his secretarial staff, and up to six research assistants; the salaries of all the foregoing; the sum of $2,400 towards the cost of maintenance of resident Junior Fellows; and an annual grant, in an amount not yet determined, to support intangible services and benefits. It could be argued, with good reason, that most of these were benefits that would accrue to AMS rather than to Massey College.

Dr. Davies' letter of 9 February dealt with a number of continuing matters – date of AMS taking possession of its quarters, equipping and furnishing of the space allotted, privileges desired by the President for his staff, and the way in which the annual grant should be paid – and then went on to raise two subjects never or little discussed previously. The first is best expressed in Dr. Davies' words:

> In discussing the possibility that in future either the Board of A.M.S. or the Hannah Institute might found chairs of the History of Medicine in a number of Ontario universities, we did not reach any decision as to whether the professor so appointed at the University of Toronto should also be the Director of the Hannah Institute. I hope that this is what you have in mind, as I can see problems arising from any other decision.

After that comment, which would almost surely be seen by Dr. Hannah as a threat to his control of AMS interests, the Master went on to raise the future of the Hannah Tower should it be built. He felt there should be agreement that the tower should never be used for other than institute business by AMS. Undoubtedly he wished to protect the College's tax status. Dr. Davies also expressed himself as happy that the College and AMS were "moving into the final stages of an agreement about the establishment of the Hannah Institute here".

About this time, Dr. Swinton became ill. It seems in retrospect that his absence from the picture made communication between Dr. Hannah and Dr. Davies somewhat more difficult. Dr. Hannah's long reply to Dr. Davies, dated 11 February 1972, dealt generally with the Master's letter of 9 February, but especially with the two newer concerns raised in his letter. With respect to the one, Dr. Hannah wrote,

> I regret that there might be some problems "if the professor so appointed at the University of Toronto should (not) also be the Director of the Hannah Institute". I can foresee problems with four other universities if he was so appointed. This would virtually place control of such appointments outside those other universities. I have no doubt that such an arrangement would be as unfavourable

> as was the case with Bishop Strachan's concept in the 1830's or the insistence of Trinity College regarding the acceptance of the thirty-nine articles before they would graduate medical students. My proposal is that grants would be made available to all universities alike – including the University of Toronto – to support chairs in the History of Medicine and whether or not any one or none of the medical schools chose to utilize such grants would remain a matter of choice and all such appointments would have to be acceptable to the Institute before the grant would be made. I am unable to understand why the University of Toronto should be given special consideration or exercise control over any such appointment except in the University of Toronto.

In the same letter, he had more to say about the Hannah Tower. He wanted to be sure AMS could carry on the management of the portfolio in the tower, if it should be built, in order to produce the funds necessary to support the medical historical and other plans. But it is in this section of his letter that he begins to develop the theme of how very much the institute, and the parent AMS, would bring to the College, for which reason any grant made to the College for tangibles and intangibles should be rather less than had already been discussed. The seeds of final dissent were being sown. He also made the argument that the presence of the library, as well as activity in the history of medicine, would not prove a narrow role but would rather strengthen the field of history and philosophy of science, of which he felt history and philosophy of medicine would be an integral part.

Several telephone conversations apparently took place before the next clarifying letter from Dr. Davies came to Dr. Hannah's desk. It was dated 21 February 1972. The Master wished to "hammer a few brass tacks". He wrote,

> If I do not misunderstand you, you propose that AMS should make a grant to Massey College in return for tangible services rendered, and provide also an endow-

> ment as recognition of intangibles, as evidence of the goodwill of AMS toward the College, and the desire of AMS to *encourage medical research* as stated in part (c) of its Charter . . . When you asked us for figures that would justify an annual grant of a certain sum, we did not understand that this was intended to cover maintenance and services, and that the endowment sum was additional . . . May I propose, therefore, that we forget about *two* grants, and discuss *one* only, which would take care of such expenses as the College would incur because of the Institute's presence here, and also provide monies for endowment.

In addition, Dr. Davies clarified his position vis-à-vis the directorship and a professor of the history of medicine in the University of Toronto. He expressed the opinion that whoever became the director would have also to hold a professorial appointment in the University of Toronto, or else the Hannah Professor could "make the Director's life a misery". He found no disagreement with the majority of matters discussed and welcomed Dr. Hannah's suggestion of a meeting to be composed of themselves along with Dr. John D. Hamilton, Vice-President (Health Sciences) of the University of Toronto, and Dr. John W. Scott, who would represent the Academy of Medicine, Toronto. Dr. Scott, a professor of physiology in the University of Toronto, had been charged at this time with setting up a course of lectures by a number of individuals interested in the history of medicine.[11]

In the interval during which the Master was considering how he should answer Dr. Hannah's previous letter, the latter wrote again to express agreement in principle that the institute should be established in the College, and to say each must then deal with his Standing Committee or Board concerning details of the agreement to be sent to the lawyers.[12] He said he did not anticipate any disagreement from Board members. Up until this time, he had indeed experienced little or no disagreement from any of them. In this letter, he expressed some of his philosophy about the subject and its relationship to medicine and its practice.

> It is my personal experience that my profession (medicine) lacks appreciation of their history and background and consequently, fall into many unfortunate errors in their relationship with other disciplines and others in general. Neither I nor many other graduates from other medical schools with whom I have discussed the matter were inducted into this very important and interesting realm of human relations. Consequently there are all too few of us who appreciate the extent to which we depend on the accomplishments of our predecessors.

To combat the frequent argument that most medical progress has occurred in this century, he put forward the names and activities of Lister, Simpson, Jenner, Reed, Krebs, and Loeffler. In a derogatory sense, he spoke of the Ph.D. candidate who said that "science has no history". He then wrote,

> The corollary to this, however, is that the general public accepts that this history is the background against which the profession parades their abilities. The discovery that this premise is false has led to an unfortunate degree of cynicism between the professions and the public. The misinterpretation and popularization of scientific half-truths by the media, and the inability or failure of the profession to counteract this tendency has led to some very unfortunate results, particularly in the field of medical care.

Here he comes full cycle back to what he knows best, prepaid medical care.

Dr. Davies was able to report on 9 March 1972, in a letter to Dr. Hannah, that the previous day the Standing Committee of the College had approved a motion:

> That the proposal of Associated Medical Services, Incorporated, as conveyed to the College by its Managing Director, Dr. J.A. Hannah, be accepted in principle pending the provision of further detail which can be laid before the College Corporation at its meeting in May.

He commented that a motion could not "convey anything of the keen interest of the Committee which discussed your proposal in great detail, both in its implications for the University and its implications for the College".

The Master also wanted Dr. Hannah to know that he had spoken with Dr. A.E. Safarian, Dean of Graduate Studies of the university, about the AMS proposal. He reported that the dean was greatly pleased with the proposal and could not foresee any difficulty with the university's implementation of it, especially since it was warmly approved by Dr. John D. Hamilton, Vice-President (Health Sciences). It must be remembered, however, that Dr. Davies' version of the project continued to be quite different from Dr. Hannah's. How the latter's plan would have been received by the university and its representatives may very well never be known.

The Master went on to remark that the Standing Committee was quite curious about the financial terms that Dr. Hannah was proposing. He said he had no authority to discuss the size of a grant and understood Dr. Hannah's inability to discuss this matter before the April Board meeting. He did, however, wonder if he might have some information that he would regard as confidential.

The End of Negotiations

The next series of letters brought about the demise of the whole scheme that would have placed the Hannah Institute physically within the structure of Massey College. One has to speculate what lay behind the letter that Dr. Hannah addressed to Dr. Davies on 17 March 1972. Was he even more ill? Was he afraid the initiative for his memorial would cease to be his? Did he realize he was deep in an area quite different from prepaid medical care, which he understood so well? Perhaps too deep for his liking! Perhaps he would have to seek advice and help from other sources! Perhaps he thought he should "swim for shore"! We shall never know for sure, since he gives no clue. What he wrote, whatever the reason, was, however, more than sufficient to sabotage the working relations that had grown up between Dr. Davies and himself, with the aid of Dr. Swinton.

He sought to apply business principles to all aspects of the proposed agreement between the College and AMS, to intangibles as much as to tangibles. He compared the area for which he was negotiating in Massey College with the total space he had at the AMS building at 615 Yonge Street, in terms of a rental figure per square foot, salaries and wages, cleaning supplies, heat, insurance, light and power, repair and maintenance, taxes, and sundry other expenses. The comparison was most unfavourable and unfair to Massey College, a prestigious structure. He regarded both the proposed library and tower as features AMS would be providing to the College rather than as structural changes he had suggested in the first place as necessary for the operations of the Hannah Institute. He downgraded the offer of a grant for intangibles from $150,000 to $50,000.

Under the sub-heading "Alternative Costs and Considerations", he analysed what it would cost to establish the institute at 615 Yonge Street or at another university, to which the institute would bring its own "sustenance". He concluded by saying,

> All told, it will cost AMS at least $200,000 per annum and such sum as may be required *to sustain the Institute* which may eventually prove even more costly, exclusive of the cost of construction of the Tower, to bring the Institute into existence at Massey College. In fairness to the situation as a whole, it appears that AMS is not being less than generous. It is hoped that success will result in which there can be satisfaction to both parties.

He added a postscript to the letter: "If AMS constructs the Hannah Tower, it will be necessary to reconsider the item for rental of space." He invited discussion with Dr. Davies before the Board meeting scheduled for 16 April.

It is difficult to see how satisfaction for both parties could be achieved after receipt of this letter by the Master of Massey College. Certainly, Dr. Davies could not foresee any successful future relations; nor could Mr. Friesen, with whom the Master had discussed Dr. Hannah's letter.[13] They were, he wrote, unwilling to take the Managing Director's latest offer to the College finance committee. Perhaps one excerpt from this letter will summarize the differences between business and academic attitudes. This is not meant to suggest business attitudes have no place in academia, but it must be noted that academic life does contain many intangibles. Dr. Davies wrote:

> Nor, if you choose to found an Institute, do we see why we should be penalized in terms of what its expenses would be. We regard the Institute as potentially a fine addition to Massey College, but also as your creation and your monument, which we undertake to keep alive, and an honour to your name for as long as the University lives. Understandably we do not value in terms of square footage or any other commercial scale of values.

He then listed once more the intangibles offered AMS by Massey College.

Dr. Hannah's response of 27 March 1972, rambling in nature, offers a possible explanation of his ill-written letter of 17 March, when he remarks that he had required another blood transfusion 23 March. He concluded his letter and the whole plan to establish the institute at Massey College in these words:

> I regret that AMS and Massey College will have to forgo the many obvious advantages which might have accrued to both of them and the Institute if I had been personally acceptable to you and had the amount of *academic experience* you deemed essential, and you had accepted at least a relative equality between the various factors involved. I shall regretfully have to proceed to prepare my report and recommendations to my Board and Annual Meeting on April 16, 1972, in light of the attitudes contained in *all* your communications.

He did so in a document entitled "To All Members of the Board of Directors of A.M.S.", dated 28 March 1972. He advanced arguments, including his long-past relationship with the Banting

Institute, to support his recommendation that negotiations with the College be terminated, and that the institute be established at 615 Yonge Street. The Board approved the recommendations at its meeting, which had to be postponed from 16 April to 30 April. Dr. Hannah at that time reported fully on a variety of matters concerning his institute, including the present state of the Medical Society of London library, relations with the Academy, termination of negotiations with Massey College, and the future use of the premises at 615 Yonge Street when the agreement with government should end 30 June 1972.[14] The minutes also reported that he gave the directors further information on the background of Professor W.E. Swinton, Dr. Henrietta Banting, and Mr. Howard Shillington and of Drs. Deborah Levy and Peter Clarke of the Ontario Geriatric Society. He said that the work of this group of people would be definite activities that could be supported by AMS as a start toward the development of the Hannah Institute. How work in geriatrics and medical economics could contribute to an institute for medical history is indeed difficult to appreciate. In any event, grants totalling $69,000 were approved.

At this meeting, one of the directors, Dr. John B. Neilson, raised a question that must have concerned the Board as a whole for some time: What *were* the objectives of the Hannah Institute? Dr. Hannah replied that they had not yet been specifically put down, but went on to say that they would be brought to the Board in due course. Here we have proof he did not yet know what his institute would be.

Conclusion

Why did the negotiations between AMS and Massey College fail? Immediate reasons are cited in the exchanges of letters between Dr. Hannah and Dr. Davies. These include the costs of tangibles and intangibles that the College would provide for the Hannah Institute or would incur on behalf of AMS, and the status of the institute as well as the qualifications of its director academically.

These, however, are not causes. They are rather symptoms – symptoms of Dr. Hannah's deep feeling that he would not willingly yield any of his – and his Board's – control of AMS and its finances to any other body. After all, he had built AMS to a quite remarkable status since 1937. Both Dr. Upper, the AMS Medical Director for nearly a decade, and the author, Executive Director of the Hannah Institute for more than a decade, agree on this conclusion.

It seems very strange that, despite their disagreements detailed in this chapter, Dr. Hannah and Dr. Davies resumed relations in 1973 when, having sold the premises at 615 Yonge Street, Dr. Hannah required quarters for his institute. Not only did he acquire space, he was also made a Senior Fellow of the College.

It does not seem strange, however, that once again disagreements should disrupt the resumed relations.

CHAPTER V

An Institute and Five Chairs

By the end of the discussions and negotiations that had involved Massey College and AMS, it was clear where the institute would not be established (the Academy or Massey College) and where it would probably not be established if Dr. Hannah were to have his way (at the University of Toronto). Talk had been heard about coupling from one to five university chairs in history of medicine in some sort of relationship with the library purchased from the Medical Society of London and with the proposed Hannah Institute. Much advice had been given Dr. Hannah on these subjects, but little, especially of that involving academic matters, had been heeded.

Developments after the break with Massey College were rather slow for several reasons. Among the delaying factors were the necessity to close out the AMS relationship with the Ontario government by 30 June 1972. What the relationship of AMS and the provincial government had been before that date should perhaps be summarized here. AMS had operated since 1937 under a provincial charter as a private purveyor of prepaid medical care plans until 1969. At that date, AMS became a government agent for a period of three years, during which time the province would establish its own apparatus. Staff and the space owned by AMS at 615 Yonge Street became much less needed during this time. Ultimately either the accumulated resources had to be turned over to the general provincial treasury or AMS had to find alternative activities compatible with the 1937 charter. Having begun to create alternatives, the Board now needed to consider where the London library and the institute should be established, what activities should concern AMS *in toto* and how they should be funded, and whether all or part of 615 Yonge Street should be retained by AMS. There were other matters that should have been given top priority, such as the possible need of supplementary letters patent to the charter, and the very real necessity of determining the status of the corporation with the Department of National Revenue in Ottawa.

For the next meeting of the Board, scheduled for 16 April but because of Dr. Hannah's illness postponed until 30 April, the President prepared his usual report.[1] The first part, somewhat nostalgic, made a statement that is now difficult to substantiate:

> I have a good deal of material written on what I propose to call, *The Rise and Fall of Prepayment for the Cost of Medical Care in Canada.* Writing and assembling of material on this subject will be my *opus major* in *The Hannah Institute for Medical History.* As this progresses, it will be placed in your hands as a lingering and nostalgic study and presentation of what, in light of government action, might be considered a "wasted lifetime".

Later in the report, he disclosed a grant to Howard Shillington as a research assistant to himself in preparing the development of the papers and history of the Trans-Canada Medical Plans (TCMP). Mr. Shillington was also expected to write the history of the other provincial plans. Mr. Shillington did indeed produce a manuscript, which did not meet with Dr. Hannah's approval but which is part of the AMS archives. It should perhaps be considered for publication now.

An Alternative Site for the Institute

An alternative approach for a location for the institute was now advanced. It was to be at 615 Yonge Street, the AMS building, a portion of which would be utilized for the new enterprise. Dr. Hannah was aware that this building did not and could not have the "intangibles" possessed by Massey College (or the Academy of Medicine, for that matter), but he pointed out that a capital outlay and grant such as was demanded by Massey College could permit a great deal to be done instead in the AMS building.

In addition to restating the grants approved by Board for Dr. Swinton, Lady Banting, Mr. Shillington, and two young geriatricians working with Dr. Robert Laird and Dr. Irwin Hilliard at the Toronto Western Hospital, Dr. Hannah spelled out again a proposed AMS policy with respect to subsidizing suitable publications in the history of medicine. He wrote,

> AMS will have prior claim on all receipts from all publications up to the amount of the subsidy made. After such subsidies have been recouped, AMS will have claim on one-half of all receipts received from royalties on any and/or all publications or otherwise howsoever.

He did foresee the possibility that such books would not make a return, and might even create a deficit, but he expressed the view that one good seller might cover a number of books suffering deficits. Before the end of the report, Dr. Hannah also indicated there could be further library purchases.

At the 30 April Board meeting, discussion included matters of interest to the history of medicine program.[2] Thirty-five volumes in the library bought from the Medical Society of London were still missing, and the suggestion from Dr. Gibson that the society be permitted to supply substitutes was accepted. It would seem from later developments that the substitutes came from another portion of the total society library. The Board agreed to the establishment of the institute on two floors of 615 Yonge Street. The remainder of the space there was to be rented. The grants asked for by Dr. Hannah were approved and authority was given to take the funds from the Medical Research fund of $350,000. As noted earlier, it was at this meeting that Dr. Neilson's query about institute objectives did not achieve a definitive answer.

When next the President reported to members of his Board on 15 July, the AMS/OHSIP relationship was winding down (the agreement had lapsed 30 June) and there were but twelve AMS employees at 615 Yonge Street, six of whom were about to be severed.[3] The last AMS audit was in process and was to be followed by the last OHIP audit. Another three AMS employees (they might be needed later, depending on future plans and functions) would leave when that audit was completed approximately mid-August. The long-time Secretary-Treasurer, K.W. Atcheson, who had stayed on a year past his normal retirement date out of loyalty to AMS, was to complete his duties at the time of the September Board meeting. There would then remain only three AMS employees: Dr. Hannah, President and Managing Director, Dr. Upper, Chief Medical Officer, and a secretary.

In this report, the President wrote at some length about the Jason A. Hannah Institute. He said that proper management of a portfolio exceeding $12,000,000 in value would "put AMS up among the top, a responsibility of no mean proportions". He gave further information about "projects arranged or under way". That undertaken by Professor W.E. Swinton was to be a book to be called *The Doctors and the Sciences.* An outline by chapters was included in the report. Dr. Hannah reported having received a manuscript, *The History of Health Insurance in Canada,* from Mr. Shillington, to whom he promised publication support on a 50-50 basis. He said grants had been made over the past two years totalling $14,000 to the Academy of Medicine, Toronto, to assist the library there to sort out the papers of the late Major-General J.T. Fotheringham, Director General of Medical Services. He suggested that a portion of the grant might have been applied to the salary of a librarian. He also told his directors that in June 1972 he had talked with Dr. Pengelly, president of the Academy, once more about AMS help to the Academy to "finance the construction of a suitable building to house their rare book collection as well as the AMS library and museum". He also proposed that AMS might finance upkeep costs. It is not surprising, in the light of past experiences, particularly those of January 1972, that Dr. Scott reported to Dr. Hannah during the course of one of the latter's blood transfusions that the Academy executive was "not enthusiastic". Dr. Pengelly, about the same time, went further. He ended a conversation with Dr. Hannah by saying, "If you have anything to propose, put it in writing and send it to the Executive."

Institute and Chairs

Chairs in the history of medicine were discussed also:

We still have in mind the necessity to establish and support chairs in the History of Medicine and related sciences in each of the medical faculties in Ontario. This will require considerable negotiations and time. It has therefore been deemed advisable to postpone these developments until after the complete conclusion of our AMS/OHIP relationship and we get the Institute settled in at 615 Yonge Street. Such a program really is a part of the whole development and it could be used as part of a program for those studying toward their doctorate in the History of Medicine. This, of course, involves the problem of "academic pride" and "local autonomy"; neither of which are easily reconciled.

This raises again the problem of a suitable academic connection, which is very important for continuity. I am informed that the Wellcome Foundation [i.e., Wellcome Trust], as well as other endowed and worthy projects, have and are becoming increasingly limited in their usefulness because they have not had the connections with other academic institutions. If I should live so long, it might be that permanence could be established. It appears, however, that it is very difficult for an idealist to find successors who can keep even an established concept viable, let alone develop a concept for a new approach to an old problem.

Of course, the Institute is a bit different in that it will be composed largely of post-academic people working together, financed and controlled by AMS – the primary purpose of which will be to finance and keep viable the Institute in which older, select and mature academics will be given the privilege to record their experiences. Basically, it will be a centre of information which may be tapped by those who know its value. It will not attempt to "teach" in the sense that a university "teaches". I hope it will become a centre where good talk, good writing and good associations may be developed.

This hope seems to relate to one of the Wellcome Institute's major attractions he had found during a sabbatical year spent there.

> This, of course, represents a totally different concept from institutions which feel they must "teach" the inexperienced how to make a living. Rather the Institute will be a centre for intercommunication. This, hopefully, will become and remain self-perpetuating – a place most acceptable to those who wish to learn and combine this with their ability to communicate.

This is quite a different concept of an institute to that investigated with the Academy and with Massey College. First, chairs in the subject are mentioned, but it is never made clear what their relationship is to the institute. The latter does not sound as if it is intended to have students in the normal age bracket; it rather seems to be populated by physician practitioners writing and exchanging their own stories. There is talk of academic connections and of considerable negotiations being needed, but also of no attempt to "teach in the sense that a university teaches". The self-perpetuating centre that will exist for intercommunication sounds very much like a professional medical society or academy. It is not at all clear that Dr. Hannah's understanding of an institute for the history of medicine has advanced; in fact, it may even be thought by some readers to have regressed, or never to have developed in the first place. There is no doubt the pressure of closing off the AMS/OHIP relationship was the dominant activity at this time, but this task was assigned to and was carried out by Dr. Upper.

When one asks "Why these changes in an institute?" one is faced with the belief that Dr. Hannah was determined to be the head of the Jason A. Hannah Institute, and that whatever structural and administrative changes were needed to achieve this goal would be incorporated into his planning. If academic credentials such as he himself did not possess were required for the institute's director, then the institute would have to change to permit him to be its director. His Board can be seen not to have been sufficiently strong to check his domination.

A Second Purchase from the Medical Society of London

Speaking at the Board meeting 10 September 1972, Dr. Hannah noted that while the London library was still located (less the missing volumes) at the Academy of Medicine, it should be realized AMS had a written agreement that the library could be moved at any time, and it was his intention to move it to 615 Yonge Street as soon as facilities should be in order.[4] The balance of payment for the library was also released, since the Medical Society of London had agreed to substitute for the missing books in accordance with Dr. Gibson's suggestion. Here he disclosed another surprising action: he had agreed to buy a second collection of some five hundred books from the society for £25,000. This startling move, again completed without appraisal, added to the collection books that would require much repair and rebinding. Again, one must question the role of the Board, whose approval was not sought.

A Committee of COFM Is Established

Although not reported in the corporation minutes and although there do not seem to exist (or survive) in the AMS archives all presidential reports concerning the chairs proposed for the five universities, nevertheless developments were going on behind the scene. Dr. Hannah was undertaking discussions with officials of the five universities having medical faculties.

In a letter dated 20 September 1972, Dr. John D. Hamilton, formerly Dean of Medicine and then Vice-Provost (Health Sciences) at the the University of Toronto, wrote to his successor as dean, Dr. A.L. Chute, about a proposal made to him by Dr. Hannah. The fact that copies of the letter have been found in archives of some of the other medical faculties indicates the importance attached to, and the attention paid to, the proposal. Dr. Hamilton wrote:

> The Associated Medical Services purchased a major collection of historical medical books during the past year.

> Since then Dr. Hannah has been exploring with various universities, how he may promote the study of the history of medicine. He indicated to me that his interest was in the establishment of five chairs in the history of medicine in Ontario, one in each medical centre. Where the collection of books would be remains in doubt. I pointed out that the Robarts Library in Toronto was a Provincial resource with a transportation service operating with all the university libraries in Ontario. Dr. Hannah indicated that the collection of books could be deposited in a library, but he gave no indication that he would be willing to make a gift of the books to any library. In other words, the conditions under which he would award custodianship of the books remains obscure. The only positive statement he did make was that he would be willing to provide up to $20,000 per annum to support one medically qualified medical historian in each centre. He would be interested in the creation of a graduate training program in the history of medicine.
>
> If the Council of Ontario Faculties of Medicine is interested in this proposal and in developing a joint proposal where each Faculty would have access to the books, a common graduate training program, and even possibly utilizing all the professors in the development of courses in each medical centre, then Dr. Hannah would like to discuss the matter with the Council.

At the bottom of this letter he had received from Dr. Hamilton, Dean Chute, who was serving as chairman of the Council of Ontario Faculties of Medicine (COFM) at that time, displayed sufficient enthusiasm for the proposal that he wished it considered by a representative small committee that would make recommendations to the Council regarding the matter. One can imagine a series of telephone conversations having taken place with his fellow deans prior to his letter to Dean Jacques Lussier of the University of Ottawa, dated 26 September. In his letter, Dr. Chute asked Dr. Lussier to chair the small committee, which he suggested could include Dr. F.L. Holmes (Chairman, Department of the History of Medicine and Science, Faculty of Medicine, University of Western Ontario), Dr. A.A. Travill (Department of Anatomy, Queen's University), Dr. William Spaulding (Department of Medicine, McMaster University), and Dr. John Scott (Department of Physiology, University of Toronto). Apparently, Dr. Spaulding could not serve, and Dean Lussier substituted the name of Dr. C.B. Mueller (Department of Surgery, McMaster University). Dean Chute had suggested the proposal be on the agenda of the deans' meeting (i.e., COFM) at the end of October. In letters dated 13 October that mention telephone conversations the previous day, Dean Lussier set the date and place of meeting as Friday, 20 October, at 10:30 a.m. at the University of Toronto.[5]

The committee met as scheduled and Dr. Hannah was invited to take part in a portion of the meeting, presumably in order to answer questions. That evening, Dr. Hannah entertained to dinner the members of the committee (except Dr. Mueller, who was unable to attend). Also at the dinner were Dr. Hannah's two historical advisers, Dr. Gibson and Dr. Swinton, as well as G. Eric Barr, a director of AMS. Minutes do not survive for these most important meetings, but participants have left behind or made available for the author's use documentation written before and/or after the meeting; and, of course, Dean Lussier's report, and comments on it, survive. Together, these documents give us a good review of the session and the aftermath.

Dr. Hannah placed before the meeting a document dated 18 October 1972 and entitled "Memorandum of Agreement re the Jason A. Hannah Institute for the History of Medical and Related Sciences made and entered into this ________ day of ____________________ A.D., 19____". It was a curious document, most probably because it was written in what has come to be known as "Hannahese" (quasi-legal language), modelled on the original charter granted to AMS by the Government of Ontario in 1937 for the provision of medical care on a prepayment basis. It is true the original document had additional clauses that would permit the establishment of activities in the field of medical education, and it is true Dr. Hannah always maintained the extra clauses were obtained to protect AMS reserves for such causes should the protection be required. However, it is equally true that the original charter did not lend itself to an imitation agreement establishing something quite different from prepayment of medical care, à quite different experiment in medical humanities, one involving five universities, each possessed of a different tradition and personality.

In the draft, Dr. Hannah spoke of the subscribers to the agreement that would establish and maintain the Hannah Institute as "members". There would be twelve members, one each representing the five universities and seven representing AMS. The latter were the current members of the AMS Board, which would be dissolved and replaced by the twelve-member committee of management of the institute. The members would have all the powers normally possessed by Board members and, in addition, would be responsible for "the co-ordination and teaching of the History of Medical and Related Sciences in each and all of the universities subscribing to this Memorandum, or who may subscribe thereto in the future".[6]

Supplementary to the original charter, presumably to be attached legally by supplementary letters patent, was Article VII, containing a preamble and four clauses. The former was the AMS Board statement of intent to support the Jason A. Hannah Institute for the History of Medical and Related Sciences, and the four clauses were the objects of the institute, expressed as follows:

> To assist financially and otherwise the medical faculties of the various universities in Ontario and others, to advance and disseminate knowledge of the History of Medical and Related Sciences; and more specifically to establish and maintain a suitable centre through which acceptable persons may advance their personal knowledge through study and research.
>
> To establish and maintain and make available to suitable students a comprehensive library of original background, the nucleus of which, the Library of the London (Eng.) Medical Society of some 3,000 to 3,500 volumes and folios has been purchased and imported into Canada by AMS to which suitable additions may be made from time to time.

To provide financial assistance through grants and otherwise required by individuals or others to advance and disseminate knowledge of the History of Medical and Related Sciences.

To do all such legal acts as shall advance the Objects of the Institute.

Dr. John W. Scott, in comments prepared 18 October (i.e., before the meeting of the committee with Dr. Hannah), identified some of the clauses that could prove troublesome. He thought it would be necessary to plan for participation by non-medical personnel and by members of the general public, perhaps through appointment of *ad hoc* committees and sub-committees. He felt sure the universities would not agree to a non-academic body coordinating and teaching, although it might be permitted to assist. He thought provision should be made for AMS to receive other bequests. Then, as he had earlier, he put his finger directly on the most contentious academic principle, in this case the 1972 climate for establishing new fields of graduate study. He thought some mechanism would have to be developed for a joint effort among the five universities. In a letter to Dean Lussier, he wrote, "I think the matter should be pushed forward as rapidly as possible for the longer Dr. Hannah has to consider the matter the greater the possibility of new terms of reference."[7]

During the morning meeting, Dr. Mueller sketched out a plan that found favour with his fellow committee members. He labelled his plan "Guidelines". He believed the purpose of the meeting was to establish a Hannah Institute, chartered as a non-share-capital corporation. He thought that the board of management should contain representatives from the College of Physicians and Surgeons of Ontario, the Ontario Medical Association, AMS and COFM, and perhaps other groups. It should have authority to propose budget, to receive moneys, to expend moneys, to employ staff, to employ professional personnel, and to provide grants to the medical schools for faculty and graduate and undergraduate students. It should also, in his opinion, be enabled to rent, own, and operate library facilities, or to lease these functions. It should support publications, receive funds and grants from sources other than AMS, organize support meetings, and manage operational funds but not develop the capital investment portfolio. The institute, Dr. Mueller emphasized, should be concerned with medical history in its social context, with the education of all health professionals *through contact with duly authorized educational institutions*, and should provide resources for all schools and colleges in Ontario for research in and education for medical history.[8]

In a letter addressed to Dean Lussier and copied to the other members of the deans' committee, Dr. Hannah expressed himself as pleased with the portion of the meeting he attended 20 October.[9] He said he thought the same spirit and interest was obvious at the dinner he had hosted that evening. He wrote:

> It was my understanding that you and your Committee are favourably impressed with the whole concept, particularly that the Institute is to be established as a co-operative effort between all the Medical Schools in Ontario and also that the members of the Institute who come as representatives of their university and faculty, will assume primarily the role of advisors as set out in the draft Memorandum of Agreement and Objects of the Institute. On the other hand, it was agreed that the control of finances shall remain with and be the responsibility of the remainder of AMS – the whole project to be a working partnership. I shall look forward to receiving your report to your Principals, the Deans Committee.
>
> To expedite and facilitate matters, I am preparing amendments to the AMS Constitution and By-Laws which it appears to me will be necessary in order to bring the Institute into being under the AMS Charter and effect certain other changes occasioned by our new status. When completed, this may be the simplest and most expeditious method of making progress.

The Report from the "Ad hoc" Committee to Study a Proposal from Doctor J.A. Hannah, Director of Associated Medical Services, concerning History of Medicine was dated 2 November

1972. In it Dean Lussier summarized the discussions, morning and evening of 20 October, and comments received from all members thereafter. He noted that the proposals made 20 October to the committee by Dr. Hannah were more specific than those outlined in the earlier letter from Dr. Hamilton to Dean Chute, and would result in the establishment of the Jason A. Hannah Institute for the History of Medical and Related Sciences as a cooperative effort. He reviewed the institute's objects: financial assistance to the medical faculties from AMS to advance and disseminate knowledge in the field, "to establish and maintain a suitable centre through which acceptable persons may advance their personal knowledge through study and research", to make the acquired library available, to provide grants to individuals and others for the aforementioned aims, and "to do all such other legal acts as shall advance the objects of the Institute".

The committee did note some deficiencies, for example the lack of clarity with respect to the legal status of the institute (was it an entity or a division of AMS?). The committee was in favour of AMS's continuing to control the finances subject to the rest of the report, and were in unanimous agreement that the proposal was attractive. As a result, the members thought the concept of the institute could be pursued. One member, not identified, suggested the name "The Hannah Foundation" be substituted for "Institute". It was very clear to members that the medical schools could not be party to any legal agreement, since this would usurp the role of the universities. Dean Lussier went on to say that "members of the Committee applied themselves in identifying a set of guidelines which they would like to be followed in the establishment of the Institute". These were essentially those suggested by Dr. Mueller. One clause, "that the Institute be an institute-without-walls", was not his; it originated with Dr. Gibson and derived from an early description of the Royal Society of London.[10] It was remarked that Dr. Hannah's intentions with respect to the placement of the library he had purchased were not at all clear, although he had mentioned the possibility of its location in an independent building, which the committee concluded could be "the walls within the institute-without walls". Lastly, the committee expressed Dr. Scott's view that there would have to be modification of the document presented to them because the most such an institute could do was "to assist in the co-ordination and teaching of the History of Medicine and Related Sciences, etc.".

The report of Dean Lussier's *ad hoc* committee was of course first presented to COFM, which then referred it and all relevant documentation to each of the five medical deans individually.

An AMS Committee to Look at the Future

Coincident with these developments were a series of meetings of a special committee of the Board of AMS, which was appointed at the Board meeting of 10 September 1972. This committee consisted of Dr. Hannah, Mr. G.E. Barr, and Dr. J.B. Neilson and was "to consider the future of A.M.S. and to bring in a detailed report on their findings to the Board of Directors at an early date". Meetings were held 12 October, 10 November, and 1 December. At the first of these, Dr. Hannah had placed before the special committee "A Confidential Report re the Future of A.M.S.", which contained much information about AMS's past, about members of its staff, and about a number of the studies concerning diversification. A report on the AMS portfolio was also made available.

The special committee concluded it could not see at that time any unexplored, possibly productive avenues of diversification. The grants, already begun, were thought likely to provoke other requests. The committee thought the major and immediate activity for financial and other support from AMS should be the physical establishment of the Jason A. Hannah Institute for the History of Medicine and Related Sciences as soon as possible and practicable. The report went on to comment about the Managing Director's health, suggesting the need for immediate steps to be taken to procure an assistant or associate director to be responsible for developing and managing the institute. Members saw no continuing need for the position of Chief Medical Officer. They also thought definite steps should be taken to ensure that the AMS assets would be made available for the support of the institute. The recommendations of the committee that concerned history of medicine were as follows:[11]

(c) That the Managing Director continue to develop plans for the Jason A. Hannah Institute and in discussion with the Deans of the Faculties of Medicine, and Presidents of the Universities in Ontario and the Government of Ontario to receive their endorsement of the Institute to be financed entirely by A.M.S.
(d) That the Managing Director pursue the legal requirements for establishing the Institute with the Department of the Provincial Secretary and to arrange as necessary for establishing the Institute by means of a private bill submitted to the legislature of Ontario.
(e) That certain possibilities relating to the location of the Institute continue to be followed by the Managing Director so that a reasonably early decision can be made as to the most advantageous and desirable location for the Institute, the decision not necessarily being that the Institute be housed in a separate building.
(f) That the Managing Director take early steps to interview and recommend for appointment as Assistant Director a suitable candidate for the position.
(g) That arrangements be completed by the Managing Director with the Toronto Academy of Medicine, on whatever terms are necessary, to continue to house the rare books purchased from the London Academy of Medicine [*sic*] in England until such time as they can be moved to the library of the Institute.
(h) That the Managing Director continue, with as much expedition as possible, recently-opened discussions with representatives of the Provincial Department of the Attorney [General] with the object of ensuring that the assets of A.M.S. can be used in pursuit of its objectives and that the Managing Director keep the Board of Directors informed on this matter so that any necessary steps may be taken to ensure that the assets of A.M.S. can be used for the desired purposes without tax implications.

Government and Other Contacts

There were no meetings of the directors of AMS as a Board between 10 September 1972 and 30 May 1973. Beyond doubt, the latter meeting was delayed by another serious illness suffered by the President. There was, however, much activity in that interval.

Dr. Hannah made a number of approaches to members of government and to other parties whose interest he wished to engage during this period. Some of these letters were despatched in advance of his approach to COFM; some were coincident with the October meetings and November developments; some followed on Dean Lussier's report from the *ad hoc* committee. As was customary with Dr. Hannah, he started at the top. He wrote to Premier W.G. Davis on 5 October 1972.[12] In his presentation, he dealt with his personal and early AMS history, and commented on the present belief that all very great advances in medicine were twentieth-century developments (a point with which he did not agree). He used his viewpoint on this matter as a justification for his desire to found the Jason A. Hannah Institute for the Study of the History of Medicine and Related Sciences. He then wrote of the grants already made both for the promotion of history of medicine and for other medical research purposes.

The last four paragraphs of this presentation to the Premier summarize his thinking at that date:

> Throughout my professional life in association with universities, etc., it has appeared to me that co-operation between all our medical schools might produce better results than a narrow competitive attitude. Also the situation would benefit from a return to a greater interest in medical education by the profession at large.
>
> With this in mind, I have contacted the Deans of the Medical Faculties in Ontario universities and, at a meeting held on Friday, September 22, 1972, they appointed a representative from each of the universities to act as a committee with which we hope to discuss and develop this programme. It is hoped to eventually draw the College

> of Physicians and Surgeons of Ontario and the Ontario Medical Association into this co-operative effort. It is, however, our concept that our independence from *all* outside sources is essential for continuity and future developments.
>
> AMS proposes to retain its non-profit charter and manage its portfolio, the income from which will be sufficient to support and develop the activities as briefly outlined herein.
>
> In view of the support and co-operation given by the Ontario Government to AMS at its inception, we are seeking approval and moral support from you, as Premier, and your Government in the Province of Ontario. With the projects already under way, and your support, we believe that a great benefit can accrue to the training of medical doctors and the practice of medicine. It is hoped to make the Institute we propose a *mecca* for the study and development of the History of Medical and Related Sciences.

There is no evidence that a reply was received by Dr. Hannah from the Premier. However, the former did meet with other officials of government, generally civil servants, in the near future. It is possible, then, to assume that Dr. Hannah was not discouraged by not receiving an answer.

Dr. Hannah exchanged letters with Dr. F.N.L. Poynter, Director of the Wellcome Institute of the History of Medicine in London, England.[13] Dr. Poynter was to be a guest speaker at the Academy of Medicine, Toronto, 19 November 1972. Dr. Hannah hoped to see him then. From Dr. Hannah's letter of 19 October, we learn some more of his current thinking.

> As you know, I am endeavouring to get an Institute set up here for the History of Medical and Related Sciences. I am endeavouring to involve all the faculties of the five universities in Ontario as a co-operative effort in co-ordinating the handling of the History of [*sic*] Chair in

> that subject, until such time as there is evidence of sufficient interest to warrant the risks involved in financing such a project. I think there is a much better chance of success if the efforts are centralized and co-operation exists in such a manner as will be possible to bring outstanding authorities in the subject on tours of lectures over a period of time in each of the universities. In due course, however, it may be possible there will be sufficient interest generated, and sufficient people trained to take on the equivalent of a Chair and the direction and securing of the interest of the medical profession in the university centres. It may be possible when that time arrives that a full time occupant of a Chair will be warranted.

He went on to say he thought he had pretty definite assurance that the Ontario government would back up his efforts.

It should be noted that this letter, containing this philosophy, was written 19 October, just one day before the meeting of Dr. Hannah with representatives of COFM. Are his views and actions on two successive days consistent? The working draft (No. 3) of the proposed Memorandum of Agreement with the five medical faculties, dated 18 October, did not mention chairs and concentrated solely on an institute. Nor did his letter to Dean Lussier, dated 23 October. Yet, the idea of five chairs had been discussed on a number of occasions previously. It is rather difficult to understand where he hoped to obtain chair occupants if he did wish to establish a chair or chairs for training purposes at the beginning of his project.

On the suggestion of Dr. Ian Urquhart, retired chairman of the Ontario Hospital Services Commission and a friendly acquaintance for many years, he went to see the McMichael Gallery at Kleinburg, in which is displayed the marvellous collection begun by the McMichaels of the works of the Group of Seven. Apparently, Dr. Urquhart suggested the visit because of the relations between the McMichaels and the Government of Ontario. Dr. Hannah acquired a copy of the 1965 agreement with government from Mr. McMichael, who was most enthusiastic at that time about the value of his agreement and relationships with provincial authorities. Dr. Hannah was seeking a parallel for the relations he desired with government, the source of the AMS charter and of any supplementary letters patent that would be needed.

On the same day he met Dean Lussier's committee, Drs. Hannah and Gibson also met Dr. John W. Abrams, Director of the University of Toronto's Institute for the History and Philosophy of Science and Technology (IHPST) and two other members of Dr. Abrams' staff at lunch.[14] The luncheon was a social event in honour of Dr. Gibson's lecture to IHPST that day, but Dr. Hannah took advantage of the opportunity to confirm there would be no conflicts of interest between IHPST and the institute he proposed. Indeed, he expressed the view that the meeting cemented relations in post-graduate work in history of medicine.

Dr. Hannah produced two more documents, both dated 1 November 1972. The first was Draft No. 5 of the Memorandum of Agreement concerning the establishment of the Jason A. Hannah Institute for the History of Medical and Related Sciences. In this draft, he incorporated some but not all of the points discussed 20 October and subsequently; but it did, it should be observed, precede the report of Dean Lussier's committee. The second was Draft No. 2 of "An Act to confirm an Agreement between Associated Medical Services, Incorporated, and the University of Toronto, Queen's University, University of Western Ontario, Ottawa University, McMaster University, and such other bodies or persons who may from time to time subscribe to and be accepted under such Memorandum of Agreement". Obviously, at this time, Dr. Hannah still believed an act of incorporation passed by the legislature of Ontario was required to establish his institute. The AMS charter still served as his model. The Memorandum of Agreement was to be appended as Appendix A. Members were to be AMS Board members, deans of medicine, Dr. Swinton, Judge R.J. Cudney (a longtime legal adviser to Dr. Hannah), and Dr. Urquhart. The first director of the institute was to be Dr. Hannah. Members of the AMS Board and representatives of the subscribers were to constitute the committee of management, but the latter must never exceed the total number of Board members less two. The objects and powers of the incorporated institute were spelled out in the rest of the draft act, which would come into effect on the day it received Royal Assent.

Again, Dr. Hannah wrote to Premier Davis, asking for his support and saying,

> to lend permanency and continuity to this development, our proposals have been presented to various departments of your Government involved and they have expressed their appreciation of the concept. It is hoped that you, as Prime Minister of Ontario, will also find merit in our proposal and support its establishment by a special Act, similar to that which established Massey College.[15]

He attached copies of the two documents above and, seemingly at the same time, sent copies also to Judge Cudney for advice. He went, with Dr. Urquhart, to see Dr. Douglas Wright, the Deputy Provincial Secretary, at Queen's Park, on 2 November. In his memorandum to file concerning the meeting with Dr. Wright, dated the following day, he referred to Dr. Urquhart as having acted as his liaison officer with the government up to that date, contacting many officials and even Premier Davis himself. According to the memorandum, Dr. Wright had "an overall command in respect of education as well as a number of other fields". The two visitors presented copies of the two documents to Dr. Wright for discussion and later opinions. Dr. Wright was reported as having been very receptive to the idea, saying that perhaps the government would also be very happy with the concept and mentioning that the government would probably require some assurance that it would not be saddled with some expense in the future that did not appear on the surface at the moment. The magnitude of AMS reserves seemed to allay this fear. Dr. Wright is quoted as thinking government might require some changes in the working draft, but this did not prevent conversation closing on a pleased note.

The Nature of the Institute and Location of Its Library

On 7 November 1972, Dr. Hannah sent a letter to the members of the *ad hoc* committee of COFM, including sufficient copies for deans not serving on the committee.[16] In the letter he raised, as one of the first problems to be solved, determination of the site for the institute's library, which he wanted to be used, but not excessively used. It should rather be inspirational. He also posed the problem of the nature of the institute. Moreover, he expressed the opinion that "another advantageous approach might be to co-ordinate the consideration of the historical background in any particular disease or operation at the time the matter is under consideration with the students", while still expressing preference for helping medical practitioners rather than students (he did not like the idea of didactic lectures to the latter). Dr. Holmes of the *ad hoc* committee has confirmed this preference to the author.[17]

Dr. Holmes responded 14 November 1972 to Dr. Hannah's letter to himself and the other committee members. He agreed with the priority of locating the library in an accessible site having flexible policies. Then he proceeded to make a case for the teaching of history of medicine to the future medical profession – that is, to the medical undergraduates. He wrote:

> I would like to suggest that there should be a high priority on teaching within the medical schools, and especially on teaching history of medicine to pre-medical students. The reasons are first, that attitudes toward history formed early in one's career are likely to exert a deeper influence on the individual, so that he will be more apt to maintain such an interest through his later life; and second, because there are still too few well-trained historians of medicine. It is through the teaching of the subject in medical schools that a student here and there decides to devote himself to the history of medicine, and we need more of them if we are to build up the body of information and interpretations to be imparted to a broader public. One way of combining both goals, I believe, would be to support chairs in the history of medicine at the Universities, but with the stipulation that the usual teaching load be reduced by one third or one fourth and that the holder be expected to use the extra time to hold public lectures, to

speak at medical societies, or otherwise reach outside the academic world.

Dr. Holmes mentioned too that Western was going to incorporate the history of medicine lectures into a course called Medicine and Society, which would also include other topics such as health care systems and medical ethics. In his letter of acknowledgement, Dr. Hannah noted that pre-medical students should be less pressed for time and therefore more able to appreciate the teaching of medical history.

The Meeting with COFM

On 16 November, Dean Chute wrote on behalf of COFM "to assure you there is very great interest in your proposals to establish a foundation to support work in the study and teaching of the History of Medicine". At the same time, there was agreement that the next meeting of Dr. Hannah and COFM would take place 28 November.

In preparation for this meeting, Dr. Hannah had a very long letter delivered by hand to each of the five deans – Dr. A.L. Chute (Toronto), Dr. J.J. Lussier (Ottawa), Dr. Douglas Bocking (Western), Dr. D.O.W. Waugh (Queen's), and Dr. Fraser Mustard (McMaster) – and to Dr. J.B. Neilson, who, with Dr. Hannah, would represent AMS at the meeting.[19] In the letter, he outlined what may be seen as an agenda.

He wrote that there were three organizations "which must be brought into understanding, appreciation and accord": the Government and Legislature of Ontario, the five medical faculties, and AMS. He said he thought there was general agreement on principle between the latter two, and that he had it on good authority that the plan was "acceptable to the senior Deputy Ministers at Queen's Park" and indeed that it had been well received by the Premier.

He enclosed with his letter Draft No. 6 of the Memorandum of Agreement and Draft No. 3 of the proposed Act, saying his purpose in so doing was to receive suggestions and criticisms. In his letter to the deans, he listed the matters on which he desired reaction as:

1. Where will the Institute be located?
    (a) Within a university, or
    (b) Separately located?
2. The appointment of a Director and his staff.
3. How best can the library be made most accessible?
4. What will be the status of the Institute?
    (a) How will candidates be accepted by the Institute?
    (b) Will candidates' studies be acceptable for post-graduate degrees?
    (c) How can the Institute best "disseminate" knowledge of the history of medical and related sciences?
        i) to undergraduates?
        ii) to the practising profession?
        iii) to the public in general?

Under the heading "accessibility of library", he wrote at some length about mailing, handling, and shipping of fragile books, and about the availability of modern technology used in libraries. What he seemed not to appreciate were the procedures employed by libraries in storing, handling, and lending (or not lending) books in different categories.

In another paragraph of his letter, he indicated the draft act named himself as the first director. He said he thought "someone younger, more erudite in the history of medicine must become his chief advisor and probably have the title of Assistant Director. The Director will require other assistants with specialized knowledge in various fields, e.g. finance, personnel, office management, etc."

He assured the deans that AMS possessed sufficient funds to support the development of such an institute, and asked for their continuing cooperation.

In this agenda, there is no mention of chairs in the history of medicine in the five universities. Yet, it must be remembered that some months earlier, on 11 February, he had written to Dr. Robertson Davies, the Master of Massey College:

> My proposal is that grants would be made available to all universities alike – including the University of Toronto –

to support chairs in the History of Medicine and whether or not any one or none of the medical schools chose to utilize such grants would remain a matter of choice and all such appointments would have to be acceptable to the Institute before the grant would be made.[20]

It did not take long for the deans to respond after the meeting of 28 November (for which no minutes appear to exist). On 30 November, Dean A.L. Chute, in his capacity as chairman of COFM, wrote to Dr. Hannah:

> This generous and farsighted offer was eagerly endorsed in principle by the Deans of all the medical schools. They are now seeking endorsation from their respective Academic and Governing Councils. It is our hope that this endorsation may come very shortly in order that you may proceed with the necessary legislative and other arrangements as expeditiously as possible.

University Acceptances in Principle

On the very same day, Dr. John R. Evans, President of the University of Toronto, wrote:[21]

> I am pleased on behalf of the University to accept in principle this most generous offer pending development of detailed arrangements which could be submitted for formal review and approval by the Governing Council of the University of Toronto.

In this letter, he recapitulated his understanding of the agreement reached 28 November: that AMS would support studies in the history of medicine by complete financing of the institute for a guaranteed minimum period of five years, and that "membership of the Institute would consist of representatives from the five medical schools and their respective universities, together with representatives from A.M.S. and its nominees". He also spoke in his letter of the library acquired by AMS, "which would be available for study under conditions to be established by the Institute when it is formed".

A similar letter was received from Dean of Medicine Douglas Bocking on behalf of the President of the University of Western Ontario, Dr. D.C. Williams.[22] In a meeting held in Dr. Hannah's room at the Toronto General Hospital on 1 March with Mr. G. Eric Barr also present, Dr. John Deutsch, Principal of Queen's University, accepted the broad principles previously enunciated by Dr. Hannah, on behalf of his university, as well as personally.[23] This meeting was a long, detailed one, characteristic of Dr. Deutsch's thoroughness. He made a number of suggestions, one of them subsequently adopted after the establishment of the Hannah Institute. This was that there should be an advisory committee of the deans to deal with the AMS Board on budget recommendations and all other relationships between the parties (i.e., AMS and the five universities). Dr. Deutsch outlined the steps necessary, in his view, to implement the President's dream.

a) a firm proposal from AMS.
b) acceptance of same or agreed to amendments by the various academic and administrative bodies at Queen's (Faculty, Senate, Board of Trustees).
c) sign a memorandum of agreement with AMS.
d) set target date for recruitment of Professor of Medical History.
e) Dean of Medicine to prepare a budget of expenditures for first year indicating when first monthly draw required.
f) set target date for preparation of courses.

This is a most concise summary of necessary university procedures concerned with the acceptance by its governing bodies of the gift of a chair. All five universities would be bound by similar protocol and procedures. What might appear to some to be a time-consuming process was, of course, a series of measures required to ensure academic quality.

Before receiving indications of willingness in principle on the part of the other two universities to be involved in his plans, Dr.

Hannah on 10 May despatched to all five university heads a draft copy of what he proposed as the basis for an agreement (Draft No. 1, 24 April 1973) between AMS and each of the universities.[24] In his reply of 16 May, Dr. Evans of the University of Toronto remarked,

> There are certain elements of the agreement which I believe we should discuss further, since they could well present an obstacle to acceptance of this arrangement at this university, and possibly others in Ontario. However, before making these suggestions I shall confer with my colleagues who are much closer to the situation.

In his 17 May response to President Evans, Dr. Hannah displayed some impatience, expressing the view that it should be possible to work out "as many obstacles at the top level of administration before the matter would be placed before colleagues". Undoubtedly, this impatience led to the method adopted by the five universities subsequently in their dealings with Dr. Hannah. It must be remembered that some of the impatience might well have been due to several periods of severe illness and hospitalization suffered by Dr. Hannah during the first half of 1973.

On 31 May, President A.N. Bourns of McMaster University replied in a manner quite similar to that of Dr. Evans' letter, and went on to suggest he would like to propose that Dr. Fraser Mustard, the university's Vice-President of Health Sciences and Dean of Medicine, should meet with Dr. Hannah at the latter's convenience to discuss rewording that seemed to be needed in a few of the individual clauses in the draft agreement. Dr. Bourns did report that McMaster was "very enthusiastic about the proposal and we find the general tenor of the draft agreement satisfactory".

In another letter addressed to the university heads, 13 July, Dr. Hannah wrote,

> To date we have received only acknowledgements of receipt of some of these documents from all but one university. We have not, however, received any proposals, amendments, deletions or additions toward the furtherance

> of the advance of the establishment of the proposals offered.[25]

This complaint would have crossed in the mail a letter and attachment from Dr. Deutsch, written 12 July. Principal Deutsch wrote:

> I am pleased to advise you of the warm support and appreciation of the Faculty of Medicine and the University for the generous action of Associated Medical Services Incorporated in financing the cost of maintenance of *The Jason A. Hannah Chair for Medical and Related Sciences.*

He attached eight recommended amendments that came from an April meeting of COFM and that had been approved by the Faculty of Medicine at Queen's. He then wrote:

> The amendments do not alter the spirit of the agreement. They merely modify it to conform more closely with academic policy and make available to all students of the university educational programmes in the history of medicine and related sciences.

The principal then disclosed that Dr. John Evans had agreed "to collate the responses of each university in order to simplify the preparation of an agreement satisfactory to all universities and to A.M.S.".

Dean Bocking again responded on behalf of President Williams on 23 July. He noted that Draft No. 1 had been reviewed by Dr. F.L. Holmes and by the chairman of the Advisory Committee to the Department of the History of Medicine and Science, and certain comments regarding the agreement had been forwarded to President Evans, "who was asked by the Presidents to collate the responses from the various medical schools". Dr. Hannah's reply to Dean Bocking still indicated some discontent with this procedure agreed to by the presidents and by COFM:[26]

> As indicated in my communication under date of July 13,

> 1973, I am still of the opinion that in order to arrive at a satisfactory solution for this situation it will be necessary for each of the medical schools in Ontario to have contact and communication with Associated Medical Services.
>
> It was for this purpose that I wrote to each of the Medical Schools individually hoping that they would communicate directly with me rather than "collate" all the concepts into one broad overall plan. I am quite sure that it will be most difficult to arrive at a conclusion that will satisfy everybody concerned and that in the long run it will be necessary to deal directly with each of the Medical Schools.
>
> I am already in possession of certain comments from the Medical Schools and these comments, although claimed "not to change the principle of my proposal", succeed in doing so and reversing matters to the place where the history of medicine and related sciences has throughout the years been relegated to an entity in so far as their relationship to obtaining a medical degree is concerned. I am convinced that the same will happen again and the funds may well be utilized for purposes other than originally intended, unless there be assurance in writing and unless the funds can be cut off if such occurs.

He went on to say in this letter that he had no intention to try to influence medical curricula, but he was very much concerned that the universities not permit what he called "deadwood" from "obstructing the free flow of research and study".

Did the suggested changes alter the nature of his proposal? The universities wanted funding for individual chairs to begin on the date of appointment of a professor. This is just. The same title, History of Medical and Related Sciences, should be used consistently throughout the agreement. No problem can be seen with this request. The universities wished to participate in the development of the institute rather than being charged with developing and establishing an institute. This seems appropriate. The five universities wished to provide the funds for suitable housing and administrative and other costs from the annual grant, rather than from other revenues. This surely could have been discussed and a compromise found. Eventually, there was. Dr. Hannah in his draft agreement wanted clause 7(a) to read: "within two years of the signing of this agreement [the university shall] make a full course in the study of the History of Medical and Related Sciences a requirement to obtain its medical degree". The universities wished to replace this with a statement saying: "each university would agree that within a period of time agreed upon by each university and the 'Institute', to make available a program in the History of Medicine and Related Sciences for Students of the University as a whole (and not limited to medical students alone)". Anyone professing to know universities, as Dr. Hannah said he had since 1921, should realize that curricular changes, and especially changes in degree requirements, cannot be effected within two years. Indeed, a curriculum committee represents many competing interests and requires much horse-trading to accomplish agreement for changes. Nor is it likely that history of medicine rated highly enough in more than one or two of the five universities to be thought of as a degree requirement. Nor would it ever likely be thought of as such. This proposed change then gave promise of controversy. At the same time, however, it is easy to understand why Dr. Hannah would think the universities were not the slightest bit interested in history of medicine but very much interested in AMS finances.

The next change suggested by the universities actually would strengthen the agreement in that it would require the fund recipients to "design a five-year Program". It would also provide for "an over-all review of the program at the end of three years". Dr. Hannah would have required an annual budget and an annual reconciliation for the grant. This, then, should occasion no disagreement. The universities asked for two years' notice, rather than Dr. Hannah's "forthwith", if, in the opinion of AMS, the agreement had been abrogated by the university or if its agents or servants failed to fulfil the terms. Two years would certainly give time for a university to effect changes felt to be necessary for the continuation of the chair. Lastly, the document appended the statement, "A joint COFM response be made to the Presidents of the five Universities concerned, and that they might choose to make a collective reply". It has been noted that Dr.

Hannah objected to this when the procedure was put in force. Yet, surely it was sensible if only to relieve the drain on Dr. Hannah's health. Summing up, then, it seems the major – perhaps only – disagreements between Dr. Hannah and the proposals of the five universities were curricular and procedural. It is difficult to see them as threatening to eventual agreement if goodwill were exercised and if one spokesman negotiated for the five universities.

On 18 July, Dr. Evans had written to Dr. Hannah to say he would collate the responses of the five universities as soon as possible but he had heard from only four of them to date. He wrote also, "There are certain aspects of your proposed draft agreement which would be difficult for certain of the universities, and I believe that in these institutions there has been a great deal of discussion of the proposals during the last two months"; and "I personally believe that the extra work at this end is fully warranted in order that the universities are in a position to respond to this important proposal." On the same day, Dr. Bourns, President of McMaster University, wrote: "The Deans of the five Faculties of Medicine came to the conclusion that a single response which carried the support of all of the universities would be more productive than having each university come forward with its individual suggestions." It is possible to disagree with this procedure, for it did inevitably result in a standardized agreement for five universities. That there was no variation to accommodate local circumstances may have resulted in some of the problems later experienced in several of the universities.

President Evans wrote again on 30 July and 10 August, to indicate to Dr. Hannah that Dr. John Hamilton would bring to him the amendments proposed by the five universities, since Evans himself would be out of the country. On 13 August, Dr. Hamilton wrote, forwarding the collated response and saying he would seek an appointment by means of a telephone call. Drs. Hamilton and Hannah met 14 August. Their meeting preceded by one day a scheduled meeting of the AMS Board. Consequently, Dr. Hamilton wrote again on 15 August, the letter being addressed to Dr. Hannah and intended to be read by all Board members at the meeting. He confirmed the conversation of the day before, in which he had conveyed the agreement of the five medical deans with the concept of establishing five Jason A. Hannah Chairs for the History of Medical and Related Sciences, and said this agreement was also supported fully by the three presidents, the rector, and the principal of the respective universities. He wrote:

> The fact that the Deans are in agreement about the desirability of establishing five chairs for the history of medicine and about the conditions, ensures that there will be, as you have suggested, co-ordination in the development of educational programs and especially in optimizing the contributions of academic staff that is, in this discipline, in short supply.

He also expressed the view that the minor changes and additions suggested did not alter the spirit or the intent of the concept. Dr. Hannah acknowledged Dr. Hamilton's letter two days later,[27] after receiving Board approval 15 August.[28] He said he and Dr. Hamilton had reached general agreement in their 14 August meeting, but there remained several university proposals that required further consideration. He was concerned that if courses in the subject were thrown open to all university students, medical students would be crowded out. He also was worried that expenditures for making the courses more widely available might exhaust the annual grant. He reminded the heads that the AMS charter stipulated that the corporation's assets should be utilized to advance medical education. He wanted also to be assured that in the agreement, when signed, chair appointments should be full-time.

On 24 August, Dr. Hamilton wrote to say he saw no difficulty in answering Dr. Hannah's concerns, but, to be sure, would take up the points with President Evans and Dean Chute when they should have returned from vacation. He did so and wrote 13 September to say all was in order to complete university agreements directly with Dr. Hannah.[29] Dr. Roger Guindon, Rector of the University of Ottawa, wrote 24 September of his university's pleasure concerning the agreement. All were by this time in agreement about signing a formal document. It was to be Draft No. 3, dated 3 October 1973, that would become the official pact between AMS on one hand and each of the five universities on the other.[30] (See Appendix 4.)

Agreements Signed

We have reached the point where there was agreement with respect to the funding of five chairs. It should be remembered that this successful exercise really began with the idea of founding an institute, even though the thought of five chairs had entered the picture earlier. We must go back to trace developments within the AMS Board during the two meetings, 30 May and 24 June, preceding the August meeting that received the conditional agreement with the universities. It was, of course, Dr. Hannah's serious illnesses that prevented meetings of the Board between 10 September 1972 and 30 May 1973. We have seen that illness did not deter Dr. Hannah from certain activities on behalf of his dream, some of them even carried on from his hospital bed.

One of the more interesting ones was the first research grant in medical history. This consisted of a $1,200 award, on the advice of Dr. J.W. Scott, to Mr. Michael C. Wills, a second-year medical student. The summer fellowship enabled Mr. Wills to "produce . . . an historical treatise from the records of two Hillary brothers who practised medicine in the Aurora, Ontario area in the 19th century". The award, made 3 May 1973, was administered for Mr. Wills through the Office of Research Administration of the University of Toronto.[31]

The first application for a Hannah Professorship had been received by Dr. Hannah in March 1973 (its acknowledgement was delayed until May by the President's illness; the acknowledgement merely stated no agreement yet existed between AMS and any of the universities).[32] Appropriately, the letter of application had come from Dr. Paul Potter, who was to be the first historian of medicine appointed to a Hannah Chair, that at the University of Western Ontario. (Strangely, the advice that he write Dr. Hannah was given him by Dean Chute of the University of Toronto.) Many other would-be applicants for funding also wrote Dr. Hannah or Mr. Barr at this time.

Perhaps more important to the ultimate establishment of the

five Hannah Chairs and the Hannah Institute was the decision made between January and June 1973 to place the library collection in the Fisher Rare Book Library of the University of Toronto. It was becoming obvious to Dr. Hannah that 615 Yonge Street was not, and could not be made, the place to establish the Hannah library. It would appear that the initial contact between Dr. Hannah and Mr. David Esplin, Associate Librarian of the University of Toronto, was made 31 January 1973 at the Hannah home. According to Dr. Hannah, "We are anxious to get the library placed, so that we can get on with other details in respect of the *Institute for the History of Medicine and Related Sciences,* in which we are trying to interest all the medical schools in the province."[33] The librarian was given for study copies of the catalogue cards of the books still held at the Academy of Medicine, Toronto. On 6 February, Miss M.E. Brown, Head of the Rare Book Library, sent a memorandum to Mr. Esplin, in which she wrote:

> This is a very good collection of early medical works which lacks some of the top classics in the field (e.g. the 1543 Vesalius) but contains little duplication of what is already in the library collection. It certainly would be an admirable start for an outstanding collection in the history of medicine.

She also asked Mr. Esplin in her memorandum if there might be a "possibility of receiving salary for a cataloguer for, say, two years to catalogue the collection to make it more readily and quickly available".

Mr. Esplin and Dr. Hannah met again 9 February at the latter's home.[34] Mr. Esplin gave Dr. Hannah a copy of Miss Brown's memorandum, assured him the collection would be kept intact if deposited in the Fisher Library, and said that Toronto had the greatest supporting collections, which would be of great advantage to researchers. This latter remark was in reply to Dr. Hannah's suggestion that the other universities might like to have the collection deposited in their libraries. Dr. Hannah would not commit himself at this time to depositing his library at Toronto.

Mr. Esplin had already made it quite clear that the Fisher Library had space available for the Hannah Collection and any additions to it, that Toronto was not interested in deposit on indefinite loan, that the Fisher Library was not part of the Ontario library plan envisaged in the Spinks report, that Toronto was interested in acquiring the collection under a trust agreement, acceptable to both parties, on a permanent loan basis. If so acquired, Toronto would take responsibility for cataloguing, indexing, repairing, and housing services, but would be most pleased to receive a grant for these purposes even though the availability of the grant would not be a condition of deposit. The Fisher Library would also supply research space, and make the collection available for examination and referencing on the premises, and by inter-library loan to any university.[35]

As was his custom, Dr. Hannah now began to draw up an agreement, which would be signed by AMS and the University of Toronto with respect to the deposit of the Dr. Jason A. Hannah Rare Book Collection in the Fisher Rare Book Library. Successive drafts paved the way for continuing conversations between Mr. G. Eric Barr and Mr. Esplin, acting on behalf of Dr. Hannah and the University of Toronto respectively.[36] Mr. Barr was acting for Dr. Hannah because of the latter's continuing illness. Indeed, it is conceivable that his illness forced a decision with respect to the site of deposit, and even the terms of deposit, of the Hannah Collection. It was Mr. Barr who recommended to Dr. Hannah that his library be so deposited, and who gave excellent reasons for doing so.[37] It is ironic that, just at this time, came an offer of sale from the Medical Society of London of another 300 books for approximately £3,000.[38] These, as noted previously, were the books that would ultimately require the most repair and rebinding. A fourth draft agreement, dated 25 May 1973, altered slightly, was signed 12 June 1973 by Dr. Hannah and Mr. Barr on behalf of AMS and 6 June by D.F. Forster, Vice-President and Provost, and Richard Smith, Assistant Secretary, on behalf of the University of Toronto.[39] This concluded the travels of the portion of the library of the Medical Society of London from England to a final resting place in Canada, for the University of Toronto soon managed the removal of the two parts of the library from the

Academy of Medicine, Toronto, and from 615 Yonge Street to the Fisher Rare Book Library. The Board of AMS had authorized the transfer of the library by motion passed at its 30 May meeting.[40]

At this same Board meeting, members approved the offer of $50,000 per annum per university for the costs of the five Hannah Chairs for the history of medicine. This was at the time that Dr. Hannah had begun negotiations with the five university heads.

Dr. Hannah's plans were of interest to parties outside the five universities concerned. One of the interested parties was the provincial government, in particular the Department of the Attorney General. The principal concern of the Department was the proposals involving disposition of surplus funds. It is important to note that Dr. Hannah had always been aware of the need to keep government informed of his planning, because of the nature of the AMS charter and its tax-free status acquired from the federal government in the 1940s. It has been previously mentioned that he utilized the services of Dr. R. Ian Urquhart as a conduit to appropriate departments and levels of provincial government, right up to the office of the Premier.

It is not then surprising that in December 1972 Dr. Hannah had a discussion concerning his planning, and the draft act he then thought necessary to change AMS activities, with the Assistant Deputy Attorney General. There occurred an exchange of letters[41] and the despatch of the documents of interest to the Department. Nor is it at all surprising that, when Dr. Urquhart returned to Toronto from Florida, Dr. Hannah conferred with him about a letter received from the (newly styled) Ministry of the Attorney General,[42] which stated, "We have put our file in abeyance for the time being until our principals have considered our reports" – a statement that seemed to revive Dr. Hannah's generalized dislike of governments, as shown in his file report of his lengthy talk with Dr. Urquhart on 9 February.[43] Out of the discussion, which considered an unofficial approach to the Ministry "to find out what had gone wrong", came a decision that it was essential that AMS disburse some of its money. Here was where Dr. Hannah suggested the giving of $50,000 each year for a period of five years to each of the five universities in Ontario that had medical schools: that is, the firm decision to establish five Hannah Chairs for the History of Medical and Related Sciences. When his adviser seemed to hesitate about this move, Dr. Hannah pointed out he thought AMS needed to spend some of its accumulated funds, and if it accepted his plans for the history of medicine it had to leave the actual expenditure of funds in the hands of the universities, but did not need to endow the chairs. He wrote, "the giving of this $50,000 a year was not the same as endowing chairs to produce $50,000", and went on to suggest that control of the funds would remain with AMS, who could just not renew the agreement if members of the Board should be dissatisfied with the performance of an individual university. He said, "We were in agreement that such a programme be started in order to forestall any questions about what we intend to do with our income." This seems to indicate greater concern about the subject than he had shown when it was raised in the Board by Dr. Neilson.

In any event, matters proceeded as described. In September, he felt able to write to Dr. Douglas Wright, the Deputy Provincial Secretary for Social Development, to describe the developments that had taken place and of which he was now quite justifiably proud.[44] He also mentioned that he had been responsible for placing the AMS portfolio in the hands of the National Trust Company, under the guidance of the Board, in order "to bring some degree of continuity into the picture". He noted that he would be obliged if Dr. Wright were to inform other interested persons at Queen's Park of the AMS developments. He was endeavouring to make sure the government approved of the arrangements in the process of completion.

A second interested individual was Dr. T.H.B. Symons, head of the Commission of Canadian Studies, established under the auspices of the Association of Universities and Colleges of Canada. Dr. Symons, a distinguished academic and administrator, wished to know more about the plans for history of medicine in Ontario. He said any information that could be given him would be of interest and assistance to the Commission in its work.

Other Questions and Advice

Of all the members of the *ad hoc* committee established by the deans of medicine under the chairmanship of Dean Lussier to examine Dr. Hannah's proposals, the one who tried to maintain closest contact with Dr. Hannah after that committee had reported to COFM was Dr. F.L. Holmes of the University of Western Ontario. His interest seems quite natural, for Dr. Holmes, a very fine historian of biology and biochemistry, was the relatively recently appointed chairman of the Department of the History of Medicine and Science in the Faculty of Health Sciences. It would be in this department that an appointee in history of medicine would find an academic home. On 7 March 1973, Dr. Holmes wrote to Dr. Hannah, since a visit with him, which he had previously contemplated, now seemed impossible for some time owing to the President's illness and hospitalization.

In his letter, he expressed some of his hopes and concerns. He very much wanted those holding Hannah Chairs to "participate in programmes designed to disseminate knowledge of this subject among the public and the practising profession" and therefore felt that in "the terms of the donations" there should be specified a percentage release time from normal academic activities for that purpose. He also felt there should be periodic meetings of holders of the chairs to plan such coordinated efforts. He went on to ask, "Do you intend to wait until all five universities have agreed to participation in the Jason A. Hannah Institute for the History of Medical and Related Sciences, or do you plan to go ahead with those who have indicated their interest in the hope that getting started will induce the others to join in?" This was a very good question, but Dr. Hannah was too ill to answer until 2 May. At that time, he wrote that he did not intend to tell the universities how to disseminate medical historical knowledge to the general public: "All that will be expected is a satisfactory effort and result on the part of the departments and individuals involved." He went on to say that, when the institute was established, he proposed "that it shall be the responsibility of the combined effort of all the medical schools in the Province of Ontario at the present time".

Another interested academic was Dr. Lloyd G. Stevenson, the most distinguished director of the Johns Hopkins University's Institute of the History of Medicine in Baltimore, Maryland. By reason of his position in the university, he was also editor of the *Bulletin of the History of Medicine*, a publication of the Johns Hopkins Press that is also the official organ of the American Association for the History of Medicine. In a letter dated 30 May, which initiated a series of exchanges, Dr. Stevenson expressed interest in the plan for five chairs and in the acquisition by Dr. Hannah of the Jason A. Hannah Rare Book Collection, and asked for material that he could publish in the *Bulletin*. He also told Dr. Hannah that he had a special interest in developments since he was a Canadian who had graduated in both Arts and Medicine at Western. Since the date of this letter was but a few weeks after the Association's 1973 annual convention in Cincinnati, one can readily imagine that there would have been considerable comment about the happenings in Ontario. Dr. Stevenson proposed to make it absolutely clear in the *Bulletin* that the plan was for Ontario only so that applications from other jurisdictions would be precluded.

Dr. Hannah replied quickly, saying he did not think anything should be written about the establishment of the chairs until the current negotiations had been completed.[45] With respect to the library he had purchased, he did not feel qualified to write about its contents. When Dr. Stevenson wrote again within a week, he had two things on his mind.[46] He wondered if he might meet Dr. Hannah and see the collection when he came to Ontario during the summer. Also, he wished to put forward the name of a medically qualified medical historian, as a candidate for the chair at his alma mater. He felt that his nominee, who was scheduled to complete his Ph.D. at Johns Hopkins in the fall, was the type of medical historian who would be in quite short supply, and therefore quick action was really necessary. Again, Dr. Hannah responded with little delay in a letter dated 18 June. He suggested that Dr. Stevenson's candidate might contact Dr. Holmes at the University of Western Ontario.

In this letter, Dr. Hannah complained about the lack of speed with which universities dealt with such matters, and about the possibility of diversion of the funds to other purposes. He wrote,

> I propose to pay the money directly monthly to the university rather than endowing a chair with a large sum of money, which when once out of our hands, would no longer be subject to our control in any way, shape or form.

This indeed was the way in which money was sent to the universities to pay for the chairs. When, a number of years later (conditions possibly having become different), the universities were asked by Dr. Hannah's successors if they would prefer endowment to the monthly payments favoured and instituted by Dr. Hannah, unanimously they said no. In 1973, however, on the basis of long experience in the field, Dr. Stevenson picked up for discussion in his next letter the proposed method of funding the chairs in the universities.[47] He wrote that he was coming to the Toronto area in mid-July in the role of a medical journalist gathering information for the *Bulletin* in order to run "a couple of brief news items, one about the Collection and hopefully a longer one about the great good fortune of medical education as a consequence of the great good fortune of the history of medicine" (referring to it, he said, not as a discipline but as an area of intellectual interest). He went on to express grave doubts that the second plan would work out: it would make tenure arrangements impossible and would destroy university autonomy. He wrote,

> the plan appears to me to be self-defeating. It comes to this – that you are suggesting an innovation the medical schools cannot be said to be eager to have on terms that their parent universities cannot be eager to accept.

He stated quite firmly that if Dr. Hannah persisted in this proposed method of payment to the universities, he hoped the Ontario universities, as a matter of principle, would refuse an otherwise splendid offer. He himself, he said, would advise any applicant to go elsewhere. He concluded the body of his letter by suggesting Dr. Hannah might well not wish to meet with him in

July. In his postscript, he did ask if it was intended that appointments might be made in the medical schools only. Further, he wondered if Dr. Hannah would require that applicants be medically qualified.

When Dr. Hannah replied, he reassured Dr. Stevenson that he would hope to meet with him.[48] He wrote that he felt Dr. Stevenson had some misconceptions and that he had never had any desire to have anything to do with university appointments to the chairs. He said he did not wish to provide a "crutch . . . for some doctor to go through the motions of holding a lecture or demonstration or a class once a week and who has no more interest in the subject than the cheque that goes with it":

> Indeed my proposal to the Deans of the medical schools and other authorities has been that the funds will be available for a period of five years and the only time there might be any interference with the "autonomy of the universities" would be when some "restful" individual has found a desk on which to place his feet without danger of having either the desk or his feet removed.

He did hope, however, that any appointee would be medically qualified, even though he was aware there were very well qualified historians of medicine who were not. He also remarked (this thought is not found elsewhere in the archives) that it had been his hope "that the selection for the head of the Institute might be chosen through a co-operative effort on the part of all the universities". He was beginning to doubt there was enough initiative around to realize this.

Drs. Hannah and Stevenson did meet one day for two hours in July.[49] No record exists of the content of the meeting, but it is not apparent that either changed his mind. One can reasonably assume, however, that they did discuss monthly payments vs. endowment, and that Dr. Hannah made very clear his constant view that he would maintain control of AMS funds. Subsequently, Dr. Hannah at least gave thought to the possibility of offering Dr. Stevenson the directorship of his institute, if we are to believe the comments of several Board members of the time. No written record that supports this belief remains.

It seems wise, at this time, to try to appreciate all the tasks a very ill man was trying to carry out in 1972 and 1973. In late 1972, he made an offer to the deans of medicine that would initially have resulted in cooperative establishment of an institute for the history of medicine, but that eventually gave rise to five chairs in the subject, one in each of the five Ontario universities having medical faculties, as well as to an institute. He met with COFM to discuss his idea. He kept provincial government officials informed of his planning. He sought or was offered advice from a number of individuals, such as Dr. Gibson, Dr. Poynter, Dr. Urquhart, and Dr. Stevenson, about his hopes for AMS. He drew up for discussion and revision a number of drafts of an agreement between AMS on the one hand and the five universities on the other. He recommended to his Board the first grants in history of medical and related sciences. He negotiated the transfer (with the help of Mr. Barr) of the several portions of the library of the Medical Society of London that he had purchased to the Fisher Rare Book Library, where it became the nucleus of the Hannah Collection. He drew up a number of versions that would in time produce an agreement, between AMS and the University of Toronto, governing this transfer. While Dr. Upper had day-to-day responsibility for the winding-up of the health care relationships of AMS and the Government of Ontario, it was Dr. Hannah who had ultimate responsibility to his Board for the completion of this phase of AMS activities as well as for the initiation of the next. He arranged to sell the AMS building at 615 Yonge Street (Dr. Upper managed the disposal of equipment) and to acquire smaller, more suitable quarters for the new activity in history of medicine. That the new quarters were not satisfactory was not particularly important except that it required another activity, the buying out of the lease. Most important, after giving in to the wishes of the five universities that they present a combined answer to the AMS offer, he achieved the signing of the agreement by the heads of the five universities individually by January 1974.

For a well man to have achieved all this would have been most remarkable. For a very sick man to have done it almost surpasses belief. He had to be stubborn and obsessive, and to "have a mission". He did, of course, have the goal of writing his name in history. In this he has undoubtedly succeeded. To complete the work associated with bringing his second great idea to reality, however, required the work and dedication of many other persons.

CHAPTER VI

Organization of the Hannah System

By January 1974 the agreements between AMS and the five universities in Ontario with medical faculties had been signed; as a result there was in place a framework for five chairs in the history of medicine and the Jason A. Hannah Institute for the History of Medical and Related Sciences. However, no chair was occupied, and the institute consisted of Dr. Hannah himself. The books purchased by AMS from the Medical Society of London had been given to the Fisher Rare Book Library of the University of Toronto in June 1973, and there constituted the Hannah Collection. Dr. Hannah had maintained his position that AMS (i.e., its President) would retain control of the accumulated funds. He was determined too that he would have a great deal to say about the relations with the five universities and the five Hannah Chairs established. The Hannah Chairs along with the Hannah Institute would constitute the Hannah system that would be his memorial.

In the early days of developments described, Dr. Hannah's two most important advisers (not members of the Board) were Dr. William C. Gibson, then Professor of the History of Medicine at the University of British Columbia, and Dr. William E. Swinton, then a Senior Fellow of Massey College.

They were important primarily because they were historical advisers. The former had worldwide connections in medicine and a substantial knowledge of the international trade in rare medical books, both of which he made available to Dr. Hannah. Libraries bought on his advice and embodied in the Hannah Collection included two purchases from the Medical Society of London (Dr. Swinton was also involved in the second acquisition) and the first of two libraries bought from Dr. Thomas Lambo, Deputy Director-

General of the World Health Organization. Later he would recommend that AMS buy the second Lambo library and the Rucker collection in the history of obstetrics and gynaecology from Henry Schuman-New York. By the time the latter two libraries, as well as the working collection of the late Henry Schuman, were bought, appraisal requirements had been adopted by Board. We have seen that the first purchase from the Medical Society of London triggered the development of the whole Hannah system. Dr. Gibson once suggested in passing that he would be willing to help Dr. Hannah in Toronto, but there is no indication this offer meant day-to-day involvement in Toronto or elsewhere in Ontario with the Hannah Institute or Chairs.[1] Certainly, nothing developed from the suggestion.

We have seen that Dr. Swinton played a role in the obtaining of the second London library, and particularly in the relations with Massey College. Dr. Hannah suggested to the Queen's University authorities, after they signed the agreement in the fall of 1973, that Dr. Swinton might be available as first Hannah Professor or at least as a visiting Hannah Professor.[2] For a number of reasons, among them the lateness in the academic year, Dr. Swinton did not go to Queen's.[3] During the negotiations with Massey College, there was an indication that Dr. Swinton might serve the projected institute as assistant to the director.[4] All that resulted from this liaison was continued advice about the future of the institute and the chairs.

Quarters at Massey College

Late in 1973, considerably more than a year after the break in relations between AMS and Massey College, Dr. Swinton again brought the College and Dr. Hannah together. The latter had disposed of the AMS building at 615 Yonge Street, and finding the offices he leased at 43 Eglinton Avenue East unsatisfactory for his purposes, he was seeking a more prestigious location where he might work toward establishing the institute and the chairs. It appears that Dr. Swinton suggested office space might be available at Massey College, where he himself had office facilities.[5] Space was available, and Dr. Hannah reached agreement with College authorities to occupy three rooms from November. The Master, Dr. Robertson Davies, expressed his delight that the founding of the Hannah Institute would go ahead. He invited Dr. Hannah to establish it in Massey College, but the latter was interested in the space only. Dr. Davies thought that Dr. Hannah should be the first director of the institute and asked Dr. Hannah to allow his name to be put forward for election to a Senior Fellowship in the College at the annual meeting on 23 November.[6] On 9 November, Dr. Hannah wrote to accept the offer of a Senior Fellowship but made it clear the AMS Board would decide where the institute would be established.[7]

Replying several days later, Dr. Davies said the Fellowship was in no way contingent upon the establishment of the institute at Massey College.[8] On 26 November, the Master was able to inform Dr. Hannah that he had been elected a Senior Fellow.[9] It was then possible for the College and AMS to reach agreement concerning provision within the College of "suitable accommodation for the *Director of the Institute* and his staff, and Assistant(s) in *The College* as shall be mutually satisfactory". The 19 November draft went on to say:

> This agreement shall in no wise affect the independence of A.M.S. or *The Institute* as to policy, economics; or the right to make or withhold grants, determine salaries of its staff or to hire or fire staff; or in any respect whatsoever.[10]

At its meeting 13 December, the Board of AMS expressed the pleasure of members that their President had been elected to the Senior Fellowship, and authorized a grant to be paid annually to Massey College for the provision of accommodation. They also approved funds with which to obtain secretarial assistance and equipment for Dr. Hannah in his new location.[11] At this same meeting, members dealt with the designation of the National Trust Company as financial agent for AMS, with the President's Interim Report containing "Constitution and By-Laws, as amended, to establish THE JASON A. HANNAH INSTITUTE ______",[12] and with whether Dr. Hannah's health was such that he could continue in office as President and Managing Director. The minutes paraphrase a typical statement of Dr. Hannah's as: "Dr. Hannah pointed out that in his opinion there are circumstances under which health, and even life itself is secondary, and that while he appreciated the solicitude of the Board about his health it remains his prerogative to decide which course he chooses to follow." This answer did not please some members of the Board, but after a considerable discussion in his absence, members saw no alternative to his completing his contract until the end of the calendar year, if establishment of the institute were to be achieved. Institute offices remained at Massey College for a time.

An Assistant for Dr. Hannah

While quartered at Massey College, Dr. Hannah made his first approach to the present author about his need for assistance at the institute. Since I did become his assistant, I shall henceforth have to present the story from a more personal point of view. Dr. Hannah and I had met once only briefly on 13 March 1974, at the reception given Dr. Hannah at the Fisher Rare Book Library by the University of Toronto to mark the gift of the Hannah Collection. Our 23 April meeting at Massey College was a two-hour wide-ranging discussion of AMS history, with many questions and answers about the proposed institute and its relations with the five universities.[13] I remember that Dr. Hannah complained at length about the divisions in the Board of AMS. Later, I was to learn that the Board had begun to become more vocal (about Dr. Hannah's health and his plans for his memorial, which were difficult to understand) in its opposition after the library purchase of 1971. This meeting was a prelude to several more before I went overseas at the end of May for research and a holiday. I left behind my schedule while away and was not surprised to come home and find a message that Dr. Hannah wished to see me the next day (26 July).

It became clear during a number of meetings that the President would like me to give at least half my time to AMS in the upcoming academic year, which possibility depended very much on the attitude of the Dean of Pharmacy, Dr. William E. Alexander. The arrangement proving to be acceptable to the dean, it then became apparent the next obstacle, in Dr. Hannah's mind, was the 18 September meeting of the Board, a Board that he described graphically as "obstructive". Dr. Hannah had offered me a position as his assistant (part-time, because I made it clear that I had obligations to my faculty and my dean) in late July, and there were several weeks during which I had to turn multiple factors over in my mind. The decision to offer the position was relatively easy for Dr. Hannah: his health was precarious, he had to demonstrate progress to his Board, and he needed someone with an understanding of academia. To put it bluntly, he also needed a pair of arms and a pair of legs.

As for me, I had already expressed my desire for a change and a second career by applying for the Hannah Chairs at Queen's and McMaster. Queen's never replied, but McMaster set up a series of appointments for early August. It should be noted that Dr. Hannah did not know I had made these applications until I told him. There was, of course, no guarantee that I would be offered a chair. I believed I had administrative abilities as well as a considerable love for and knowledge of the field of history of medicine. Moreover, I believed that fleshing out Dr. Hannah's second idea would present a very big and welcome challenge. My wife agreed with me. Therefore, I told Dr. Hannah I would accept the position if Board members extended an invitation to me to do so when they met 18 September. I believed that common prudence required that I should be so invited, and that request was accepted by Dr. Hannah.

Perhaps I should now introduce myself and my qualifications. I was born in Hamilton, got my first bachelor's degree at the University of Toronto in 1942, and served in the Canadian Army until the spring of 1946. I received my second bachelor's degree in Pharmacy and a master's degree in Pharmaceutical Chemistry (Phytochemistry) at Saskatchewan in 1947 and 1948 respectively, and my doctorate at Wisconsin in 1954 in Phytochemistry. The doctoral studies included a very extensive minor (more like a second major) in history of pharmacy and related sciences; Wisconsin had not only the first chair in history of pharmacy in the Western world (Dr. George Urdang), but also an excellent historian of medicine (Dr. Erwin Ackerknecht), a very fine historian of chemistry (Dr. Aaron Ihde), and a strong department of the history of science.

I returned to Toronto in 1951 to teach at the Ontario College of Pharmacy. (The educational function of the College was transferred to the Faculty of Pharmacy of the University of Toronto in 1953; before that date the College had been an affiliate of the university.) I was given the opportunity of teaching a newly required course that was essentially history of medicine and pharmacy, for pharmacy students in their senior year. I did so for sixteen years, during which time I also directed a number of undergraduate historical theses.

When I was approached by Dr. Hannah in 1974, I thought I must have been recommended by Dr. Swinton, a friend for some years. This he has confirmed.[14] He told me his reasons for making such a recommendation were my teaching record, active membership on President C.T. Bissell's committee that brought about the founding of the Institute for the History and Philosophy of Science and Technology, activity (as an Associate Fellow) on the Museum Committee of the Academy of Medicine, and, above all, the role I played in establishing the Niagara Apothecary in the town of Niagara-on-the-Lake.

The invitation came from the Board at its stormy 18 September meeting.[15] It does not appear that the invitation was the cause of the dissent: Board members had been telling Dr. Hannah for some time that one of his difficulties in his medical historical planning was the lack of an expert assistant. Nevertheless, after the contentious meeting, several Board members resigned and the President had to seek replacements. On 1 October 1974 I began part-time work for AMS leading to the elaboration of an institute. AMS was to reimburse the faculty one-half my salary for the balance of the 1974/75 year, and it was believed I could obtain a leave of absence 1 July 1975 to serve AMS if I proved to be a satisfactory assistant.

At this same meeting of Board, members were informed that Dr. Hannah had given up his quarters at Massey College because of a disagreement about more space and the time of its availability. He had, indeed, given notice to the Bursar of the College on 25 July.[16] Although special events were on occasion held at Massey

College in the years ahead, the 1974 action ended any chance that the institute might have been established at Massey College.

Search Committees and Other Committees

After the signing of the individual agreements with the universities, the faculties of medicine were free to set up search committees. The two most active universities in this regard in 1974 were the University of Western Ontario and Queen's University. The latter had earlier negotiated unsuccessfully with Dr. Swinton and Dr. Hannah to have the former appointed either the first Hannah Professor or at least a visiting Hannah Professor. As it turned out, it was Western's chair that was the first to be occupied (September 1974) and Queen's the second (January 1975). Toronto (December 1976), McMaster (July 1977), and Ottawa (September 1977) followed. Thus, the five chairs were filled in a period of three years.

Brief *curricula vitae* of all the Hannah Professors are given in Appendix I. The initial appointees were as follows: Dr. Paul M.J. Potter (Western); Dr. Ruth Hodgkinson (Queen's); Dr. Pauline M.H. Mazumdar (Toronto); Dr. Charles G. Roland (McMaster); and Dr. Toby Gelfand (Ottawa). Dr. Hodgkinson resigned at Queen's in 1978 and was replaced in 1979 by Dr. Samuel E.D. Shortt, who remained until 1984.

The brevity of reference to the Hannah Professors here is not because they haven't contributed mightily to the dissemination of history of medicine in Ontario. They have. It is because this is a history of AMS.

Early in 1975, Dr. Hannah was able to obtain the agreement of Dr. William C. Gibson to serve as chairman of a grants committee, which I had argued was needed because of increasing numbers of requests. When I attended a meeting of the American Association for the History of Medicine for the first time in May 1975, I was able to persuade Dr. Lloyd G. Stevenson (Johns Hopkins) and Dr. C.G. Roland (Mayo Clinic) to serve as the other two members of this important committee. Both were Canadians by birth and still by citizenship; and Canadian background was regarded as a requisite at that early time. It is fair to say Dr. Roland became interested in himself filling McMaster's Hannah Chair because of his experience on the Grants Committee of the Hannah Institute during its early years of existence.

At the 9 January 1975 meeting of the Board, two of the new members and one who had served almost a decade were named to a special committee of Board to examine the future of AMS.[17] The chairman of the committee was Dr. John J. Deutsch, formerly Principal of Queen's University and at that time Professor of Economics at that institution. The other members were Mr. Justice Walter Little and Dr. John B. Neilson.

In preparation for the meeting of directors of 9 January and for the work of this special committee that he proposed to establish, Dr. Hannah prepared a notice of motion.[18] It set out the steps already taken to establish the institute and the chairs, reviewed the charter and accomplishments of AMS that would make possible these new directions, and listed what the President saw as the objectives of the institute. It should be noted that the institute foreseen in the agreements signed by AMS and the universities differed rather markedly from that which would develop after staff was in place; Dr. Hannah really did not know what kind of institute he wanted or what kind would be appropriate to the necessary relations with five universities. The clauses in the draft that were pertinent to the format of the institute at the time of those agreements were:[19]

4. The individual appointed as Professor and Director shall devote his full time to the objectives of *The Jason A. Hannah Chair for the History of Medical and Related Sciences.* Such appointee shall, however, co-operate in the establishment of an overall *Institute for research into the History of Medical and Related Sciences;* and
5. the universities herein indicated have agreed to participate in the development of an Institute to be known as *The Jason A. Hannah Institute for Research Into and Study of the History of Medical and Related Sciences*, which shall be for the purpose of extending the purposes of the Jason A. Hannah Chairs beyond the confines of the universities . . .

It will be obvious that one reason why incumbents of Hannah Chairs could not participate in establishing the institute was their disqualification from judging their own grant applications. Too, they had enough to do at their own universities in promoting the discipline.

In his motion prepared for the 9 January meeting – the 38th annual general meeting of the members of the corporation for the fiscal year ended 31 December 1974 – Dr. Hannah expressed the objectives of the institute (fourteen months after the university agreement) as:

> *Generally,* to advance and disseminate knowledge of the History of Medical and Related Sciences; to purchase, receive, own and preserve medical objects of historical interest; to value, acquire and hold property and sites related thereto; to receive gifts and donations which may advance and enhance the objects of A.M.S. and/or the Institute; and
>
> *In Particular,* to co-operate with established Medical Faculties in Ontario (as of 1975) in establishing and maintaining suitable centres in which suitable persons can advance their knowledge, and that of others, in the History of Medical and Related Sciences, through study and research; to establish, maintain and make available to suitable persons, comprehensive and other facilities and resource materials for such study; to evaluate applications for financial and other assistance, and, in acceptable cases, to grant such aid; and to organize and carry out such other legal acts and procedures as will advance the interests of A.M.S. and the Institute.

Dr. Hannah advanced in this document a category of individual called a "Trustee of the Institute". All Board members of AMS would be trustees, and one of the deans of medicine should serve each year as an ex-officio medical member of the Board, and hence a trustee, voting on all matters except those affecting finances. The order of service of the deans in this capacity from

1975 to 1979 should be Queen's, Western, Toronto, McMaster, and Ottawa.

Although the institute never had trustees (the term lapsed because it proved unacceptable to the universities), two deans did serve a year each on the AMS Board: Dean Waugh (Queen's) and Dean Bocking (Western). In Dr. Hannah's scheme, trustees were to be eligible for re-election annually, but could not, with the exception of the Managing Director, serve more than ten years or be elected past a seventieth birthday. With the consent of the trustees, the Managing Director could do both.

After 1 October 1974, because the quarters at Massey College had been given up, Dr. Hannah carried on his work at his home, 5 Douglas Drive, and I used my Faculty of Pharmacy office for both faculty and AMS purposes, with the permission of Dean Alexander. Many of our meetings were held at the Toronto General Hospital during Dr. Hannah's treatment. We agreed on the hiring of Miss Mary Wildridge as secretary of AMS and the institute as of 2 January 1975. She too had to be flexible concerning the sites of her duties (Dr. Hannah's home and my office) during the first several months of her employment. When it became very apparent that office space was really necessary, it was sought first on the campus of the University of Toronto and, when that proved impossible, at a site nearby. In February 1975, eight hundred square feet of space were found at 50 Prince Arthur Avenue, one block from the Toronto campus. Our being off the Toronto campus was most important to the other four universities. Being near the Toronto campus was important to the institute because of activities there and visits of personnel in the discipline.

Restructuring AMS; Structuring the Institute

The Board gained new members: Dr. Deutsch, Mr. Justice Walter Little (a Queen's alumnus), and Dr. William B. Spaulding (Professor of Medicine at McMaster University). The special Board committee of Dr. Deutsch (chairman), Mr. Little, and Dr. Neilson was set up to look at the future of AMS, in particular its relations with the universities and the chairs via the institute. The committee reported at the 17 July meeting of the Board in the following terms:[20]

1. Dr. Hannah be requested to continue in his appointment as Managing Director of Associated Medical Services until December 31, 1975.
2. Dr. G.R. Paterson be appointed Executive Director of the Hannah Institute for the History of Medical and Related Sciences as of July 1, 1975; the term of appointment to be a period of five years; subject to review by the Board of Directors upon completion of one year's service, when the appointment may be terminated at the discretion of the Board upon giving one year's notice as of July 1, 1976.
3. Dr. Paterson be requested to prepare, before April 30, 1976, a plan of development of the Hannah Institute for the next five years; this plan of development to include in particular a plan of development of each of the five Hannah Chairs in the History of Medical and Related Sciences in the five Medical Faculties in Ontario after consultation with the Deans of these Faculties; this five-year plan of development to show the details of annual expenditures to be provided from A.M.S. funds; this proposed plan of development to be submitted for consideration of the Board of Directors of A.M.S.
4. Proposals for expenditures on libraries or for any other purpose from A.M.S. funds in excess of $25,000 be submitted to the Board of Directors for approval before commitments are made.
5. When the term of office of the present Chairman of the Board of Directors [i.e., Mr. K. Hossick] expires at the end of 1975, a new chairman be appointed with the qualifications required to advise the Board regarding its responsibilities for financial and investment policies and to act as the chief executive officer of the A.M.S.

Some parts of this report require elaboration. Dr. Hannah was not able to attend the Board meeting of 17 July,[21] and consequently he made known later a number of personal objections to the report and its contents. The second clause served to protect the Board, who did not know me (the President had kept me in purdah), and myself in that two years was the minimum leave of absence I could have from the university. This protection was crucial to me and to Dean Alexander in June 1975, when Dr. Hannah was strangely reluctant to accept the university's terms concerning leave of absence and Dean Alexander needed to know my plans in order to work out teaching schedules. Almost ready to return to the university, I obtained the President's permission to visit Dr. Deutsch in his capacity as chairman of the special committee. A frank talk, contents of which he shared with his committee, resolved the problems.

The third clause, reflecting some of the June conversation between Dr. Deutsch and me, constituted necessary planning for the institute's role in the future, and certainly a test of a new executive director's abilities. The fourth clause reflected my concern about the earlier acquisition of substantial libraries without benefit of expert appraisals. The Board, of course, also had reason for concern in this field. The last clause referred to the continuing restructuring of the Board. At the time the Board received this report, it was not clear whether Dr. Hannah would find it acceptable, even though he had been consulted. The members passed a motion that, if he did not choose to continue in office until the end of the year, I would also serve as acting Chief Executive Officer until Dr. Hannah's successor as Managing Director and/or President of AMS should be appointed. In our conversation, Dr. Deutsch and I agreed that the executive director of the institute should not be a member of the Board, and that the institute should be the creature of AMS, with the executive director in attendance at Board meetings to report on the carrying out of assigned responsibilities. I would, of course, also have the duty of offering advice to the Board on matters concerning history of medicine.

On 16 April 1975 Dr. Hannah had written to Dr. Deutsch as chairman of the special committee, enclosing a copy of the

Interim Report of the Hannah Institute for the History of Medical and Related Sciences, prepared by me (April 1975). In his letter, the President told Dr. Deutsch he had over the years always kept the Board informed of developments by means of reports from himself or his assistants. In this instance, he said, he had asked me to prepare the report because of "the necessity to evaluate Dr. Paterson as my successor". He expressed pleasure with the report.

My report summarized briefly developments towards actual establishment of the institute both before and after my arrival on the scene up to the date of the report. The latter only need concern us here. I referred to the two motions that approved the President's annual report and the special resolution concerning the reorganization of AMS, passed at the annual meeting of members and by the Board at the 6 February 1975 meetings,[22] as the Magna Carta of the Hannah Institute for the History of Medical and Related Sciences.

In late 1974, I noted, each of the universities had been told that AMS would sponsor, soon after the filling of the individual chairs, "an inaugural lecture, reception and invitational dinner to make the existence of the Chair and the Institute, and the Hannah Professor, as widely known as possible to campus and community". At the inaugural celebration of the chair at Western, 30 January 1975, the guest speaker was Dr. Lloyd G. Stevenson, Director of the Johns Hopkins Institute of the History of Medicine (he had early in his career taught history of medicine at Western), who spoke on the subject "No Time Like the Present" to an audience of 110-120. Two-thirds that number attended the dinner at which Dr. Hannah spoke about his long struggle to establish the program.

At Queen's University, the inaugural celebration was held 25 March. Dr. Hannah was again the dinner speaker. According to custom at Queen's, Dr. Hodgkinson gave her own inaugural lecture on the subject "Breadth of Vision: The Social History of Medicine". Her lecture attracted a large audience of approximately 250, of whom 65 were present at the dinner. It became customary in future inaugurals for the newly appointed Hannah Professor to profess his or her credo as it would be interpreted in teaching and research.

The arrival of the first Lambo library purchase at Dr. Hannah's home in December 1974 was noted in the report, as was the deposit of the majority of the books acquired in the Hannah Collection at the Fisher Rare Book Library. It was also recorded that the University of Toronto had applied for special funds to repair and rebind some of the books in the growing Hannah Collection. Of very great importance, it was reported that AMS had deposited "the files, documents and other materials related to the operation of Associated Medical Services, Incorporated" in the University of Toronto library system. Ultimately, they would be housed in the Fisher Rare Book Library and a summer student hired to index the materials.

Suggested library policy formed an important part of the report. Physical accommodation and arrangements were discussed in some detail. Initial contacts with the Ontario Medical Association, the Ontario Medical Foundation (where it was considered history of medicine could play a part in continuing medical education, a concept not realized unfortunately), the Academy of Medicine, Toronto, the Canadian Medical Association, and the Société Canadienne d'Histoire de la Médecine were noted. The last-named, originally a local medical historical society founded in Quebec City in 1950, had in 1972 extended an invitation to the International Society for the History of Medicine to hold its XXV Congress at Quebec in August 1976. It became national by charter and by recruitment of personnel from across the country. One of the recruits, with the permission of the Managing Director, was myself, who became vice-president (Ontario) of the national association. Dr. Hannah is quoted as saying, "It is hoped by this liaison to know of speakers who may be available for a Hannah Institute Symposium on History of Medicine in one of the five Ontario centres soon after the Quebec meetings."

The possibility was mentioned of having Alan Fleming (chief designer of the University of Toronto Press, who had created the logos for Canadian National Railways, Ontario Hydro, and the Canadian Broadcasting Corporation) update the AMS message concerning its new activities. It is sad that this idea did not come to fruition. The longtime AMS logo was modified by substituting "HANNAH INSTITUTE" for "MEDICAL CARE BY PREPAYMENT".

The grants committee, previously noted, was discussed with reference to structure (I was to serve as the non-voting secretary of the committee). It was promised that application forms, probably based on those of the Canada Council, would be placed before the new committee soon. The need for expert appraisers of applications was also commented upon.

Lastly, the subject of videocassettes concerning the history of medicine was discussed. Thirteen medical videocassettes, made by Dr. William C. Gibson in 1973 for the CBC, had been obtained for teaching purposes. The Instructional Media Services of the Faculty of Medicine, University of Toronto, had been engaged to produce two videocassette prototypes, one on Dr. William Boyd, one on Dr. Hannah. The videocassettes were expected to play a dual role in the future: to stimulate young medical students, and to be resource material for history of medicine courses.

In concluding this interim report, I expressed my hopes as follows: "I believe there is much to do in the future that will be of great benefit to Medicine and the Related Sciences. I anticipate a satisfying future for both the Institute and myself." This interim report undoubtedly served to persuade the Deutsch committee to give me a chance as Executive Director.

Other matters dealt with at the 17 July meeting of the Board concerned the structuring of the Hannah Institute and the restructuring of the parent organization. The special committee of the Board was continued (consisting of Dr. Deutsch, Mr. Little, and Dr. Neilson) to "pursue the matter of the appointment of a new Chairman and Chief Executive Officer and report to the next meeting".

The Board decreed that the *ad hoc* grants committee be continued "to review grant applications and to recommend terms of reference, appointments and procedures for a standing grants committee for the Board". It was also agreed that an *ad hoc* committee be set up "to review publications assistance requests, and to recommend terms of reference, appointments and procedures for a standing publications committee for the Board". Before long, this committee would consist of Dr. Murray L. Barr (chairman), Dr. Arthur D. Kelly, and Dr. D.O.W. Waugh. Dr. Barr had had a distinguished career in anatomy teaching and research at the University of Western Ontario. Dr. Kelly was the most highly respected senior diplomat of Canadian medicine. Dr. Waugh, who had served on the Board representing the deans, was about to become the chief executive officer of the Association of Canadian Medical Colleges.

As new Executive Director of the Institute, I reported having already made preliminary inquiries on site about the holdings of the libraries of the five universities in history of medicine. I was given Board permission to complete the purchase of the Dervis Collection in Internal Medicine and Psychiatry from Dawson's of Pall Mall for Queen's, whose Hannah Professor had recommended its acquisition. I was also permitted to continue the investigation of a library offered for sale in California. I informed the Board that videocassette films of Dr. William Boyd, famous teacher and author in pathology, and Dr. Hannah, because of his pioneer work in prepaid medical care, had been completed and would be shown to the Board at a subsequent meeting. Lastly, I reported that Frances Gage, the fine Canadian sculptress, had made a head of Dr. Hannah. I asked that Board commission a series of six such so that each of the five chairs and the institute might be readily identified with Dr. Hannah.

Between the Board meeting of 17 July and that of 22 September, efforts went on on several fronts to organize the institute and to reorganize AMS, the latter because of the impending resignation of Dr. Hannah as Managing Director on 31 December 1975 (although he hoped to continue as President past that date). The former involved initial study of library needs in the Hannah system as well as the investigation of committee structures and procedures in other granting agencies, and acquisition and examination for suitability of the application forms in use by the other agencies. These activities, of course, were also related to the five-year plan the Board required for April 1976. Plans were also under way for the series of visits to the five campuses for necessary consultations, now realized to be very much wider than talks with the deans of medicine only. It had early been realized that a number of individuals, different ones at different universities because of the different personalities of the five schools, would have to be met and consulted with in order to proceed with a thorough analysis of desirable relations and preparation of a plan acceptable to AMS and to the universities. There was also a need to identify carefully the representative office holders in the universities who would speak to AMS and the institute in the name of their organizations. I was also of the opinion there had to be a better way of obtaining valuable university knowledge and points of view than by having one Board seat allotted in rotation to a dean who would represent all five schools while being limited in his Board activities. To set the stage, then, for the important interviews that would precede the writing of the report required many telephone and other contacts, and the presentation at September's Board meeting of a plan of attack, as well as a progress report.

At the 22 September Board meeting, a Report on Libraries set forth the beginning of a library policy for history of medicine in the five universities when AMS finances would be involved.[23] Initial classification of needs for a chair and its occupant were assessed as: (a) a working library whose content was in no way dependent on the identity or research interests of the Hannah Professor, (b) library materials bearing on the research interests of the Hannah Professor and on the Canadian studies AMS wished to promote, and (c) a rare books collection, which had been already begun with the purchases of Dr. Hannah. With respect to the last, the report said, "It is considered less expensive and more secure to move properly accredited scholars to rare books than attempt to send such books to readers requiring access to them." It was also less expensive to have one rare book library only. The report also included a detailed analysis of what had been seen in a first viewing of the California collection with Dr. Gibson – the Prinzmetal collection, ultimately sold by Jacob Zeitlin, which consisted of works on cardiology, psychiatry, and Osler. Permission was sought from the Board to bid for a portion of the library up to a maximum bidding position. This permission was given by Board on 22 September.[24] The Osler portion of the library was later obtained from Zeitlin, and was duplicated on fiche for the Ontario medical libraries.

The report also spoke of other libraries offered for sale to AMS. In addition to the Dervis Collection previously mentioned as intended for Queen's, there were two more in the area of London, England, and its environs. These were to be seen in January. One of these was not bought, for there proved to be too many obstacles to its purchase. The other, the personal library of the late Lord Brock, in the field of his specialty, cardiovascular surgery, was subsequently acquired and placed in the library of the appropriate department of the Toronto General Hospital on loan. It was further reported that a short list and detailed inventory of the AMS Papers (archives) had been prepared by Mr. Ian Crellin during the summer, and that the Thomas Fisher Rare Book Library had been authorized and funded to hire a cataloguer and a bookbinder to give necessary attention to the Hannah Collection. Lastly, availability of the main library of Dr. Thomas Lambo, Deputy Director-General of the World Health Organization, was made known to the Board. Within months, this library was seen in Geneva, appraised as required by the new Board rules, and acquired, with most of the books being added to the Hannah Collection. Appraisal saved many thousands of dollars.

A Report on the History Videotape Project was also presented.[25] A continuing commitment to such a program was suggested, and permission was sought to have a videotape made of the career of Canada's great medical missionary, Dr. Robert McClure. Another report presented concerned the sculpted head of Dr. Hannah and an awards program in which a medal using the Hannah head would find a place.[26] Board gave permission for implementation of these reports; an analysis of costs of preparing a Hannah Medal was included in the report, the purpose of the medal being to serve as a stimulus for creative writing in the history of Canadian medicine. Similar awards given by other organizations were described, including conditions attached. It was suggested, and accepted, that an AMS *ad hoc* committee be established to determine conditions for a Hannah Medal. Miss Gage was to be commissioned to cast the medal, using the Hannah head as a model. Ultimately, an *ad hoc* awards committee, chaired by Toronto's very distinguished historian, Professor Maurice Careless, recommended that the medal be given through or by the Royal Society of Canada. Arrangements were worked out that this should be the method and route of honouring an author of a book or series of articles within the last ten years in a field described as "history of medicine which is Canadian"; the medal was to be called the Jason A. Hannah Medal of the Royal Society of Canada.[27] It was first offered in 1978.

Other reports presented to Board were those of the *ad hoc* committees for grants and for publications. The former had considered three grant applications. The publications committee presented two reports, one concerned with terms of reference for the committee, and the second with an application for a subsidy to effect publication of a book that would not otherwise be published. This first book subsidized was *The Miracle of the Empty Beds*, by Dr. G.J. Wherrett (University of Toronto Press, 1977). In my roles as Executive Director and as the newly elected secretary of both committees, I presented the reports to the Board, which I had drafted and had approved by the respective chairmen, Dr. Gibson and Dr. Barr. Thus was established another procedural pattern for the institute. The Publications Committee at this time became the first standing committee of AMS associated with the support programs of the parent body. Indeed, this succession of reports and procedures established patterns for institute activities and relations between the Board and myself.

There was considerable discussion at the 22 September Board meeting, led by Dr. Deutsch, chairman of the special committee of the board that had pursued the matter of appointment of a new Chairman and Chief Executive Officer of AMS. The President continued to see a parallel between the role he had played for years as President and Managing Director and the new situation in which AMS had placed itself in promoting history of medicine. The author must confess to being pleased that other members of the Board did not agree with the President. They and I felt I would be busy enough with the affairs of the Hannah Institute without taking on the responsibilities of Chairman and Chief Executive Officer of AMS. To the suggestion that National Trust was supplying the business acumen – the need for which in the opinion of some Board members would be an overloading factor in joining the position of Chairman to that of Executive Director – Dr. Deutsch is quoted in the minutes as having said, ". . . it is the Board that sets down policies and makes decisions.

The role of the Trust Company is to keep the records and carry out instructions." Several names were placed before the Board but no decision was made except that the committee was to continue its work.

Tax Status of AMS

Before the Board was scheduled to meet again, the warning made several times in the past by some members, in particular by Dr. Neilson – that AMS's longtime tax-exempt status was threatened by the corporation's loss of its function in prepaid medical care – was proven to be sound. The Chief Examiner of the Office of the Superintendent of Insurance in the Ontario Ministry of Consumer and Commercial Relations, Mr. R. Brewerton, asked to have a copy of the 1974 financial statement of AMS. Dr. Hannah chose to deliver it in person, taking with him myself and Mr. P.J. Sewell of National Trust, serving AMS as Secretary-Treasurer, to explain the projects in history of medicine being undertaken by AMS. In his letter of 24 October 1975,[28] Mr. Brewerton said he appreciated the summary "of the excellent projects which your association is undertaking", but then went on to say, ". . . we believe that you should give careful consideration to the tax status of A.M.S. We draw your attention to Sections 149(1)(g), 149(1)(h) and 149(1)(j) of the Canadian Income Tax Act, which make provision for exemption from income taxation under certain conditions for certain non-profit corporations and charitable trusts":

> It would appear to us that A.M.S. as it is presently operating would not qualify for exemption under these provisions of the Income Tax Act. We would therefore recommend that you seek independent legal advice in this matter in order to avoid a potential tax liability which could reduce significantly the funds available for your worthwhile research projects in the field of medical history.

At its 9 December meeting, the Board interpreted this letter as a very clear warning that should be heeded and that made expert advice essential within a very short time.[29] Dr. Hannah seemed to think the advice should be obtained from the lawyers who had advised "Blue Cross in continuing its position of exemption from income tax". The majority, however, thought that since AMS was no longer, unlike Blue Cross, functioning as a provider of prepaid hospital care and other related plans, the advice needed should come "from a legal firm with experience in setting up charitable trusts and foundations".

It was therefore determined that legal advice should be sought from Mr. John Hodgson, QC, of the legal firm of Blake, Cassels and Graydon and that a Board committee of Dr. Neilson as chairman, Dr. Hannah, and Dr. Deutsch should meet with Mr. Hodgson and then follow whatever procedures were required to establish AMS as a tax-exempt corporation. The Board noted that AMS was facing an indefinite period of reorganization, the length of which would depend on the speed with which the required legal processes could be realized. Members therefore moved:

> That pending the conclusion of legal discussions respecting AMS and its future tax status, that AMS continue to function with its present Board of Directors; that Mr. K. Hossick continue as Chairman of the Board and that Dr. G.R. Paterson be the Acting Administrative Officer following on Dr. Hannah's resignation as Managing Director on 31 December, 1975.

Continued Reorganization

The most important action taken by the Board at the 9 December meeting on institute matters was receipt of the report of the *ad hoc* grants committee, which had met under the acting chairmanship of Dr. Stevenson (Dr. Gibson was ill) to discuss a position paper prepared by me to encourage full discussion of the structure of a standing grants committee, its procedures and duties, its scope in a support program, payment of grants, and publicity of its support programs. It also considered one grant-in-aid application. The committee decided it should define the term "Medical and Related Sciences" (as had the Publications Committee). It suggested as the definition *the human healing arts and professions, and ancillary sciences and humanities related to these professions.* This definition was also adopted by the Royal Society of Canada for the Hannah Medal. Some years later, both AMS and the Royal Society broadened the definition to include veterinary medicine.

It was recommended and passed by the Board that the first standing Grants Committee consist of the three members of the *ad hoc* committee, and that they establish a plan of rotating membership, of three-year terms, and of maximum periods of service. Future appointments to the Grants Committee should be made by the Board acting on the advice of the Executive Director, who should continue to serve the committee as secretary.

As Executive Director, I had explained to the *ad hoc* committee that I wished a wide-ranging discussion of my position paper with respect to the scope of support and to whom it should be made available, in order to have expert advice for purposes of preparing the five-year plan, which Board wished to receive by 30 April 1976. Receiving, rather than receiving and adopting, the report gave Board members time to consider my initial thoughts on the subject before they should be presented with the more formal document in the spring. The most important thing in December was that AMS now had two standing committees, Grants and Publications, to deal with the quality of applications before they should come to the Board for funding decisions.

When the Board of Directors next met on 10 March 1976, members passed the report of the Grants Committee with a few minor changes. As a result, the method was now defined by which the applications for support, which were coming to AMS in increasing numbers, would be considered. Applicants could now be given information with respect to dates and forms of application, and information as to when they might expect to learn the fate of their requests. It became possible also for the Executive Director to schedule meetings of both standing committees.

Resignation of Dr. Hannah as Managing Director

The two most important matters dealt with at this meeting

both concerned reorganization of AMS.[30] Dr. Hannah told the directors present that "he had reached the stage where he was prepared to step aside entirely if the Board so wishes but he did agree that administrative assistance in carrying on the affairs of the Corporation was needed because it was evident that Dr. Paterson was required to devote almost all of his time to the affairs of the Institute". He went on to say that, having met several times recently with Dr. Neilson, he was now convinced the latter "would be suitable to take on these responsibilities". As a result, Board approved a motion that Dr. Neilson be appointed Acting Managing Director, effective 1 January 1976 to 31 December 1976, subject to review at the end of the period and with a commitment of a minimum of two days per week to the administrative affairs of the corporation. When Dr. Hannah stepped down as the President and Managing Director of Associated Medical Services, he had served since 1937 as the corporation's only Managing Director and since 1965 as its President.

At this same meeting of the Board, Dr. Neilson, as chairman of the Committee on Reorganization of AMS, presented a written report and promised more details for the committee for 19 March. Dr. Neilson and his committee had met with Mr. Hodgson on several occasions and at their 19 February meeting had received the legal adviser's initial report. In it, he dealt primarily with three subjects, which were reported by Dr. Neilson as follows:[31]

a) *The Charter of* A.M.S. – Mr. Hodgson was of the opinion that the present charter of A.M.S. could be amended in a form which would acceptably reflect the non-tax liability status.
b) *The Income Tax liability prior to and after September, 1972* – The legal opinion expressed by Mr. Hodgson was that income tax exemption for A.M.S. ceased when A.M.S. ceased to be a hospital and medical plan carrier in September 1972. He said that an approach would have to be made to the Department of National Revenue to seek income tax exemption from September 1972 and he was optimistic that this approach could be successful.

c) *Future Exemption from Income Tax* – The exempting sections of the Income Tax Act which A.M.S. could operate under were presented for discussion all being under Section 149 of the Act – the possibilities being "an operating charity", "a charitable foundation" and a "non-profit corporation for scientific research". It was agreed by the members of the Committee that the most appropriate designation for A.M.S. would be that of a "charitable foundation".

The committee had instructed Mr. Hodgson to proceed with the necessary revisions of the charter and with by-law changes that would reflect the new activities of AMS in history of medicine. They also asked him to meet, as soon as possible, representatives of the federal income tax department to seek regularization of the corporation's income tax status from September 1972.

At this time AMS suffered a severe loss in the death of Dr. John Deutsch, who passed away 18 March 1976. It is true that Dr. Deutsch did not serve long on the Board of Directors, not even a complete term; but in a relatively short time he had a considerable effect on the future of the corporation and on the planning for the program in history of medicine. This influence, of course, was exerted because of his past distinguished record and experience in government and academia, in the position of chairman of the special committee on the future of AMS. AMS never had a better Board member, and I could not have had a more effective colleague as I came into the position of Executive Director of the Hannah Institute.

At the meeting of the Board held 25 March 1976, Mr. Hodgson's report concerning necessary revisions of the charter as shown in the report of the special committee was approved in principle.[32] It and any other changes submitted in the interval were to be placed in a draft for the annual meeting in April 1976. Also at the March meeting, National Trust suggested the formation of a finance committee of the Board to work with portfolio managers on investment policy. Dr. Neilson pointed out the relationship of investment policy to the Paterson Report due at the end of April.

An annual meeting of members is always preceded and followed by meetings of the Board of Directors. This order is of importance because members elect directors and the latter elect members. Usually the members are greater in number and constitute a questioning body for the actions of directors, although by this time Dr. Hannah had allowed the number of members to decrease by attrition so that the members and the directors were now the same people. For 1976, these three meetings took place 24 April. In the first Board meeting that day,[33] a draft special resolution for consideration of changes in Letters Patent was considered at some length. Making very minor changes only, the Board

> resolved as a special resolution that the Corporation be and is hereby authorized to make application to the Lieutenant Governor of the Province of Ontario for the issue of Supplementary Letters Patent.

This resolution was passed on to the meeting of the members for their action.[34] At the Board meeting of 25 March, Dr. Spaulding had given notice of motion "that AMS pay the full cost of a major book collection when such is donated to a university and that when appropriate the costs of repairs, housing, and maintaining the collection be included". At the subsequent meeting of the Board (i.e., the first on 24 April), Dr. Spaulding agreed to amend his notice of motion by adding "when this Board considers it appropriate". The recommended financial committee was also formed at this meeting. It consisted of Dr. Hannah (still President), Dr. Neilson (Acting Managing Director), and a new Board member, Dr. John W. Scott. Dr. Neilson also reported that Mr. Hodgson was engaged in preparing new by-laws, which were being reviewed by Dr. Paterson and himself. It was also decided that honoraria for Board members would be discontinued when the Supplementary Letters Patent were granted.

The New Objectives of AMS

At the meeting of members on 24 April, the current objectives of the corporation were deleted and the following new ones were substituted by unanimous vote:

(a) To receive and maintain a fund or funds and to apply from time to time all or part thereof and the income therefrom for charitable purposes.
(b) Under the name of "The Jason A. Hannah Institute for Research into and Study of the History of Medical and Related Sciences" to establish, maintain and advance studies in the history of medical and related sciences by every available means;
(c) To encourage medical research and preventive medicine;
(d) To co-operate with organized medicine in the advancement of the standard of medical service;
(e) To acquire by purchase, donation or exchange and to retain any real or personal property conducive to the carrying out of its charitable purposes;
(f) For the further attainment of the above objects, to hold, manage, sell or convert any real or personal property from time to time owned by the Corporation; to invest and reinvest in such investments as the directors deem advisable without being limited to investments authorized by law for the investment of trust funds; to retain any real or personal property in the form in which it may be when received by the Corporation for such length of time as the directors may deem advisable; to acquire by purchase, lease, devise, gift and any other title and to hold any real property necessary for the carrying on of its undertaking and for the purpose of drawing a revenue therefrom; and to sell, lease, mortgage, dispose of and convey the same or any part thereof as may be considered advisable;
(g) To do all such other things as are incidental or conducive to the attainment of the above objects.

The motion want on to state that directors would serve without remuneration or profit, but could be paid reasonable expenses only when engaged in the business of AMS. Lastly, it was stated that:

Upon the dissolution of the Corporation and after the payment of all debts and liabilities, its remaining property shall be distributed or disposed of to promote medical education in the Province of Ontario.

Dr. Hannah Resigns as President

To the second Board meeting of the day, the President presented the 39th (his last) report for the annual meeting.[35] He expressed disapproval of the proposed new Letters Patent, and proposed that the university Hannah Chairs be financed by endowments. In the first meeting he had submitted his resignation as a director, effective at the close of the annual meeting for the fiscal year ending December 1975. The minutes record that his resignation was "primarily for reasons of health". Certainly, his outburst about endowments (to which he had previously always been opposed) seemed to owe much to the new Letters Patent and to his difficulty in facing resignation. The members received his report.

A closer reading of his report makes it clear that he then firmly believed that the concept of an institute for the history of medicine began in his mind in 1962, some nine years before the Board passed the necessary motion to set matters in motion. He wrote,

> The basic concept was to bring the five medical faculties into co-operation in order to raise the History of Medicine to the priority and standard essential for the better understanding of research, postgraduate study, and teaching.

An examination of the story told thus far will disclose that the idea of five chairs and an institute involving five medical faculties developed rather more gradually by a series of steps; that is, the whole idea was not conceived in 1962. The genesis of the idea can indeed be found in the records of that year, but development to the levels achieved by 1976 was tortuous and consisted of many peaks and valleys. It does seem very strange that the man who in conceiving the series of ideas had always maintained that the finances must remain with the corporation, should now be speaking of an alternative method of funding, namely, endowments.

He wrote:

> Despite the obvious success of A.M.S. and the ready approval for the concept of the Institute your President feels that the emphasis has been almost entirely on the monetary side of the problem. In his opinion there has been a lack of understanding of the more important concepts of the building of a new approach to research and advanced studies in the field of medical education necessary to bring medical history up to the priority it must have if we are to become a world centre for advanced teaching.
>
> A close study of the proposed Supplementary Letters Patent and the proposed revised By-law has reaffirmed these fears to your President.
>
> It is doubtful if there is a legitimate place for such an organization if it can only do what the universities are already doing, and for which they already have the organization and personnel. There is no doubt that the Institute will be almost overwhelmingly influenced by the universities in most of their activities. Therefore, in the opinion of your President unless we have more to offer than a duplication of the functions for which the universities are already equipped, the Institute could justly be considered as an expensive and unnecessary frill.

It is indeed unfortunate, most unfortunate, that in his last report – his swan-song as it were – Dr. Hannah should have professed to having lost his second great idea because of worries about possible happenings that time has shown did not take place. The universities have not been able, because of failing finances, to give history of medicine an honourable and active place without the considerable aid of an outside source of moneys. Nor have the universities "almost overwhelmingly influenced" the activities of the institute named for Dr. Hannah. Many nonuniversity activities also have been promoted. Few of the people working with or influenced by the Hannah Institute consider it a frill; many other jurisdictions envy Ontario Dr. Hannah's idea as it has developed.

When the second Board meeting of the day considered Dr. Hannah's wish to resign as a director, "There was general agreement among the Directors that this resignation should be accepted from which would follow that Dr. Hannah could not continue in the office of President."[36] He was elected to the position of Honorary President. The directors then elected as their new President (and Acting Managing Director) Dr. John B. Neilson.

Instead of being a very sad occasion, this day should have marked the successful transformation of AMS from the provision of prepaid medical care to the promotion of medical history, which change owed so very much to the dogged persistence of the retiring President, in the face of severe illnesses, decreased energy, and a distressing inability to understand or accept the ideas of the other persons with whom he needed to cooperate. In spite of these difficulties, the successful transformation owed more to Dr. Hannah than to anyone else.

He seldom visited the offices after his resignation. The Board did sponsor a fine reception for him in July 1976, which many old friends attended. His health continued to deteriorate, however, and he died 2 May 1977. Yet he did achieve his memorial. His name has gone down in history because of two great ideas. It may truly be said that he could have had "no better float through posterity".

A New President

The new President seized the opportunity to outline his views on the composition of AMS at the next meeting of the executive, 27 May 1976.[37] He believed there should be a President to administer AMS, an Executive Director to operate the Hannah Institute, and an Executive Committee to consist of the President and two designated Board members, which would meet three or four times a year or as required "to deal with policy matters and make recommendations to the Board". After much discussion, the general concept that the Hannah Institute should be perpetuated was approved.

The year 1976 proved to be the busiest year yet with respect to organization of the institute and reorganization of AMS. A total of ten Board and Executive meetings were held that year. Much credit is due the new President, his members of the Board (some of them new), National Trust, the auditors (Thorne Riddell), and the legal adviser to AMS (Mr. John Hodgson) for the speed with which they tackled the problems associated with the status of AMS and for the successes they achieved.

At the 27 May meeting of the Executive, Mr. Hodgson had to report that AMS was still under the scrutiny of the Department of Insurance (provincial) and would remain so until it should become a charitable foundation; but at the Board meeting of 21 June he was able to announce receipt of the Supplementary Letters Patent from the provincial government.[38] A few minor and insignificant changes only had been made. The new document had also been sent 7 June to the Department of National Revenue (federal) for approval. The solicitor was also able to present a further draft of new by-laws, which, among other things, made provision for the Hannah Institute, its composition and its duties.

A few changes only were necessary in June to make the by-laws ready for presentation to the next annual meeting. It was expected this status would be changed in 1977 by the government's new regulations. Under these AMS became a charitable organization, a new classification. However, until its status was confirmed by the government, the Board felt it should start a substantial level of expenditure as would be required of registered charities. A number of methods for doing this were suggested, but few were accepted, because the Paterson five-year plan was not to be presented to the Board until June. However, one expenditure made was a capital grant of $98,902 to the Academy of Medicine, Toronto, to construct a new rare book room with appropriate humidity and temperature controls. Libraries were discussed in May, for several collections were in the process of appraisal. A special committee of Board was struck "to investigate library holdings particularly regarding the printing of records into a computerized catalogue". Its work was the beginning of Medicat. A microfiche reader demonstration was given at that meeting of the new Executive Committee (Drs. Neilson, Spaulding, and Scott). It was also reported that the Osler Library had been acquired from California from Zeitlin-ver Brugge, and plans were under way to seek costs for reproducing it on fiche for the benefit of all five participating libraries.

At the 21 June meeting of the Board, the resignation of Mr. K.C. Hossick, longtime Board member and Chairman and Vice-President of AMS, was accepted. It was also declared that the office of Honorary President, to which Dr. Hannah had been elected on his retirement, was without responsibilities or duties. The position of Acting Managing Director was terminated, and the duties, responsibilities, and remuneration of the position were accepted by the new President. The chair grants were raised to $55,000, as recommended by the Executive Director, because of the higher rate of inflation. A draft budget for the institute was accepted. The Executive Director was instructed to visit Queen's University to discuss with the university authorities a submission for a capital grant to provide space for the Department of the History of Medicine.

A Five-Year Plan for the Institute and Chairs

The fundamental document of the Hannah Institute was ready for consideration by the Board on 21 June 1976. This was the report that the special committee had required of the Executive Director when I was appointed to that position 1 July 1975.[39] It extended to almost fifty pages, set forth thirty-four recommendations, and was intended to provide the guidelines for the period 1976-1981, during which time it was expected the five universities would appoint Hannah Professors and the Hannah Institute would become active in its role in the Hannah system.

Early in the report, I wrote:

> It was apparent early in the period under report that consultations would have to extend beyond the Deans to include many of their colleagues. The reasons for this are easily seen. Deans of Medicine are extremely busy men

and as a result must assign responsibilities to other personnel. Faculties of Medicine do not, in general, create a department for a new chair, no matter how prestigious the appointment, and therefore administrative arrangements terminating in the Dean's office are necessary. Financial implications to the Universities by reason of A.M.S.-University agreements are silhouetted sharply in days of stringent university financing by the province. Certain of the terms of the A.M.S.-University agreements require clarification and interpretation so that the universities will not feel they are committing without due consideration, funds and resources required for other programmes to which they assign higher priority than they do to History of Medicine. The Universities have felt, quite properly, they need reassurances concerning the availability of the resources necessary to carry out such a scheme properly.

Consequently, it was found essential to pay visits of several days to each of the five campuses (in one case, two such visits), to meet there with the Principals/Presidents, Vice-Presidents/Vice-Principals of Health Sciences, Deans and Associate Deans of Medicine, Professors and other resource and administrative personnel. It was felt necessary (and it was so expressed) to listen to what the universities were saying, to answer questions, to ask questions, all to develop cordial working relationships. In addition to availability of necessary resources, other major concerns of the universities have been identified as continuity of the funding possibility, academic freedom, review procedures, effects of inflation, the effects of academic isolation on the Hannah Professor and his/her activities, and the costs of search, appointment and removal.

Universities where appointments had already been made were visited first. At three universities where no appointment had yet been made, an essential element in the discussions, a Hannah Professor, was missing. Nevertheless, among the recommendations were those concerning: terminology used in the agreements; library policies; AMS special grants for library purchases (working collections, specialist collections, Canadiana material, one general rare book collection); costs generated in universities by AMS gifts; union catalogue – computerized cataloguing support system; Academy of Medicine, Toronto; problems associated with library purchases; archives; AMS publications policy (publications assistance, videocassettes); AMS research and graduate study support policies (grants-in-aid, fellowships, and studentships, major equipment grants; visiting scholar program, symposia, scheme of miscellaneous aid, payments of grants, publicity for research and graduate study support programs); awards programs (Hannah Medal, organization awards program); appropriate housing of Hannah Chairs; effects of inflation; Hannah Institute Advisory Council; a section on developments at each of the five universities; history of medicine in continuing education; relations with other medical and medico-historical associations (Ontario Medical Association, Canadian Medical Association, Canadian Society for the History of Medicine); a conclusion; and a summary of the thirty-four recommendations.

In my conclusion, I wrote:

> As is the case with all reports of this scope and length, there is not really an ideal time for its writing for all persons and matters concerned in its preparation. However, an honest effort has been made to listen to the universities, to answer their questions, to ask questions where needed, and to establish cordial working relationships. At all times too, the undersigned has tried to bear in mind §9 of the agreement.
>
> The spirit and intent of this agreement and time shall be of the essence of its fulfilment.
>
> It seems apparent that the five universities are prepared to work together and with us to bring into reality the dream of Dr. Hannah and Associated Medical Services, Inc. Perhaps the motto of the Hannah Institute should be, "Responsive to the Universities; Responsible to the Associated Medical Services, Inc."

Of special importance in this report, adopted with a few minor changes only when it was considered by the Board, was the recommendation that a Hannah Institute Advisory Council replace the dean serving ex-officio on the Board. The Council was to consist of the five deans of medicine or their nominees, together with two or three nominees of the Board of AMS. The AMS President would chair the Council, which would offer the advice of the five universities to the Executive Director.

The principal effect of this document, and of the Advisory Council that was established, was to create an atmosphere in which AMS and five universities could and would work together to bring into existence Dr. Hannah's second great idea. It is true that the Hannah system depended more on the universities and on individuals both within and outside the universities working toward a common cause than had been foreseen by Dr. Hannah when he worked out the agreements that had established its basis. As the system developed in this cooperative manner, some of the fears of early advisers to Dr. Hannah began to dissolve, and also the atmosphere of cooperation made it so much easier to approach individuals who should be concerned with the development of history of medicine and to ask for their help – in committee positions, as appraisers, as members of the AMS Board, and in so many other ways. It will be appreciated, then, that the Hannah Institute developed quite differently from existing institutes, such as Wellcome, Johns Hopkins, and the German institutes. It became an enabling body, both responding to ideas and initiating new plans.

Some of the recommendations after approval had to be fleshed out. Procedures had to be established for the new Advisory Council and for reviews of the chairs (not the Hannah Professors; that was the business of the universities) on a peer review system. Application forms, instructions, and procedures, as well as appropriate information, had to be designed so that each applicant would receive full information about and consideration of his/her request.

When the chairs were all filled by September 1977, it became apparent that periodic meetings of the Hannah Professors were a necessity. The first such was held in Toronto in October

1977, and there have been annual meetings ever since. More and more matters were sent to this group for decision or for advice. The Executive Director of the Hannah Institute chaired these meetings and served as a conduit for opinions of the professors to reach the Board of AMS. Each Hannah Professor, of course, had another route to the Board through his/her dean of medicine, and by that means to the Hannah Institute Advisory Council, which functioned as a committee of the Board as well as an advisory group to the institute.

In 1981, a second five-year plan was produced by the President of AMS and the Executive Director of the Hannah Institute after extensive interviews with many representatives of the five universities. Fortunately, on this occasion, all five Hannah Professors were able to take part, putting forward their observations and thoughts.

Reorganization of AMS Completed

One major problem remained to be resolved. This was the tax status of the corporation. At the 15 July meeting of the Board, Mr. Hodgson was able to report that the Department of National Revenue considered the draft application for registration as a charitable organization acceptable.[40] He said that when a signed copy in final form was lodged with the Department, it would "be put through". The President reported to the Board meeting of 12 October that he had received word from Mr. Hodgson: as of 15 July 1976, AMS was registered as a charitable organization under the Income Tax Act.[41]

Legal advice in connection with this procedure made it important that I maintain a diary of my activities from 1 July 1976 for a period of 18-24 months in order to prove, to anyone whose business it was, that my duties were academic, and that my administrative activities were necessary to the academic nature of the position. In this way was established the difference between AMS and certain other charitable foundations: AMS was directly involved in the working out of the projects in which it was concerned; the others were usually just sources of funding, having no deep concern in the results achieved by those funded.

Thus, by the summer of 1976 the change in nature of AMS's responsibilities to two levels of government – the charter derived from the provincial government, the tax-free status required from the federal government – had been achieved. Approximately a year later, all five Hannah Chairs were filled. The basic structures and procedures were in place to create and activate the Hannah system. It is true, there have been other developments. A new name for the institute – the Hannah Institute for the History of Medicine – was adopted in 1978. A new standing committee of Board was established in 1982, the Special Grants Committee, in order to examine requests for aid that did not fit the terms of reference of the Publications and Grants Committees. Special Grants aid was primarily if not inevitably in the field of history of medicine. Before the committee was set up, such requests used to come to the Executive (Investment and Finance) Committee. To have fair and full investigation, the new committee was required.

Most other developments, however, are more properly considered in the next chapter under the heading "Accomplishments". To record these for information of the public – after all, funds of charitable organizations are really a public trust – AMS has issued periodic reports of its financial status and of how and on whose projects it has spent its money.[42] It intends to go on doing so.

The files of the corporation and its institute tell the story of accomplishments in part. The activities of many people tell even more of the story.

CHAPTER VII

Accomplishments

Soon after he came to office in 1983 as President Neilson's successor, Dr. Donald R. Wilson decided that the corporation and the Hannah Institute should examine carefully what had or had not been accomplished in the first decade of the existence of the Hannah Chairs and the Hannah Institute. In 1985, he appointed a committee of the Board, chaired by Dr. William B. Spaulding, a former Vice-President and member of the Board, to examine the past decade and to make recommendations concerning future activities of AMS in history of medicine.

Appointment of this committee caused those involved in those first years of the Hannah system to examine memories and records of successes and failures. This chapter is based in part on the stimulus created by the committee's activities. An attempt is made here to illustrate the scope of work and the effects of the Hannah Chairs and the Hannah Institute provincially, nationally, and internationally.

Activities of the Hannah Chairs

It was always Dr. Hannah's intention that the universities themselves should search for possible appointees to Hannah Chairs and make appointments by their own methods. At no time did AMS or the Hannah Institute become involved in chair appointments, except to supply information to university officials that was being sought by applicants for chairs. AMS and the Institute always believed that each university and its officials had a different personality, which was reflected in its procedures for seeking applicants, for making appointments, for housing appointed Hannah Professors, for defining administrative routes, and so on. The differences also applied to the position of the subject in the curricula of the five faculties. Although it may be difficult for readers to appreciate, this attitude and the chair review procedure are believed to be responsible for the effective relationships between the five faculties and AMS and the Institute.[1] Institute policy was to allow as large a degree of autonomy as possible to the universities in advancing the history of medicine.

From early days, the role of the Institute in relation to the chairs was seen by AMS as similar to tightrope walking, judging when and when not to move as demanded by circumstances. Prominent among supportive measures has been the program of research awards for independent scholars, post-doctoral fellows, graduate students, and undergraduates from medicine and history. AMS sponsors meetings of Hannah Professors, and has funded and/or staged several Hannah symposia (and their publication) and many Hannah Lectures. Responsive reactions to ideas of Hannah Professors include publication in book form and on fiche of research aids and bibliographic tools. Space and shelving have been paid for to increase library facilities. Financial support to the national society has promoted the publication of research and provided places where scholarly contacts could be made. Individual projects of Hannah Professors have also met responses from the Hannah Institute. Initiatives have included purchase of subject libraries to match individual research interests, and distribution on rotating bases of medical historical exhibits.

Videotapes of prominent Canadian doctors began the setting up of a film bank (through purchases from CBC, BBC, ITV, and other sources), the primary purpose of which was to provide teaching aids for Hannah Professors. Archival collection and identification have provided stimulus for research at some of the Hannah Chairs.

Libraries

As has been noted previously, the first library purchased by Dr. Hannah, that of the Medical Society of London, stimulated the Board to become involved in history of medicine and also formed the nucleus of the Hannah Collection, ultimately established in the Fisher Rare Book Library of the University of Toronto, but regarded as a provincial resource. To that first purchase were added, before the Board decided against further large library acquisitions unless exceptional libraries were offered,[2] a second library from the Medical Society of London, two purchases from Dr. Thomas Lambo of Geneva, and the Rucker Library in obstetrics and gynaecology obtained from Henry Schuman-New York. AMS has made annual grants to add to the strengths of and fill gaps in the Hannah Collection. Decisions about such additions are made by the head of the Fisher Rare Book Library, Richard Landon, who has had grants of $15,000-$25,000 per annum for this purpose and for binding and repairs. The Hannah Collection now consists of approximately 5,000 volumes. Arrangements have been made so that Hannah Professors at universities other than Toronto may borrow from the collection by means of communication between the Fisher Library head and the chief librarian (or his/her representative) at the university seeking to borrow. This service, while not heavily used, has helped the research of several Hannah Professors.

Within the sum of the annual chair grants, all five universities are expected to acquire secondary library material in history of medicine.[3] For several years, a precise sum within that budget was designated to be used for such purchases. However, since in library matters each university acts individually, as it does in most other matters, the Board decided to give universities more responsibility for expenditure for non-salary items, while expressing general guidelines about the acquisition of secondary medical historical monographs and journals that it was considered the chairs would need for general use and scholarship.[4] In 1978, AMS engaged the services of Eric J. Freeman, chief librarian of the Wellcome Institute of the History of Medicine, to examine the cooperating university libraries and to make recommendations respecting library policy.[5] In the decade since an AMS library policy was first put forward, it is fair to say the five medical libraries have accumulated respectable working collections.

On several occasions, special purchases of secondary libraries and specialty libraries have been made, after which the books acquired have been installed at one or more sites appropriate to need for or content of the library acquired. One of the most important of such acquisitions was the working collection accumulated over many years by Henry and Ida Schuman of Henry Schuman, the distinguished publisher. When that firm finally closed in 1977, the library was bought by AMS, and a large part of it was sent to the University of Ottawa.[6] The remainder was added to other collections. A specialty collection of considerable interest was offered AMS by a West Coast dealer; it concerned history of military medicine. This was placed at Queen's for a number of reasons, among which was the presence in Kingston of the Royal Military College. In 1976, the Board had made policy that, when a special library was acquired and sent to one of the five universities where it caused the library to incur extra costs, the Board would consider seriously making a special grant to cover those additional costs.[7]

Sometimes the acquisition of a special library has started the Institute on a new activity. Such a case resulted from the purchase of an Osler collection from a California dealer. A library, of course, can be placed in its original form at one site only. The logical site for deposition in the Hannah system was McMaster University, since the only Ontario residence remaining at which Osler lived for a period of time is within a mile or two of McMaster. But Osler is a genuine (one of the few such) Canadian medical hero, and his writings should be available to all medical students in this country. A decision was taken to create ten copies on microfiche of the library purchased (and a few other works were added) so that each library in the system could make the Osleriana available to its students. This action provoked two other ventures that will be dealt with later: a much more extensive project on microfiche, and an Osler book for distribution to medical students. It should be noted here that two of the Hannah Professors played initiating and ongoing roles in these two projects, Professor Paul Potter at the University of Western Ontario and Dr. Charles Roland at McMaster University. The latter is the Hannah system's recognized Oslerian expert, and was one of the founders of the American Osler Society before his return to Canada.

All of the medical libraries have been asked to make a basic aim the acquiring of Canadiana so that medical and other students may appreciate developments in the field in their own country. In particular, those associated with chairs having a special interest in the history of Canadian medicine (Queen's and McMaster) as well as the Hannah Collection have responded to this request.

It will have been appreciated that the Academy of Medicine, Toronto, has over the years possessed two most influential libraries, the clinical one and the rare book library, both of interest to Dr. Hannah prior to and at the time he considered establishing his institute at the Academy. In the light of the outcome of those negotiations, it seems appropriate that later Boards should have decided to help the Academy in two ways. One was to make available to the Academy for a period of five years an annual sum for the addition to the library of secondary materials in history of medicine. The second form of help was much bigger in scope and expenditure. The Board agreed with the Academy's contention that their rare book collection was suffering from improper storage conditions. At the time of the Academy's reconstruction in 1976, the Board agreed to a grant of almost $100,000 to the Academy in order that it might install appropriate air conditioning and humidification within the basement area of the older building retained in the renewal project.[8] Subsequently, this facility was named in honour of Dr. Arthur D. Kelly, a member of the first Publications Committee of the Institute, who died in December 1976. This was a fine gesture on the part of the Academy, for Dr. Kelly had done much for many Canadian medical organizations, including the Academy. The reason given by the AMS Board for this major expenditure was a strong belief that the Academy's treasured books were essential to the success of the program in history of medicine.

It is difficult to know precisely how much has been spent by AMS for library resources for the Hannah system, primarily because many secondary and research materials are bought with funds from the annual chair grants. Excluding these purchases, but adding to direct purchases by the parent organization sums expended on making library resources available to users, it would appear the total, in all likelihood, exceeds $1,300,000 since the inception of the program.

Medicat

Within the decade of the AMS program in history of medicine, applications of modern technology to libraries and to use of their contents have increased exponentially. The Hannah Institute showed an early awareness of the value of such applications. Indeed, Dr. Hannah had early recognized the likelihood that AMS would have to involve itself in this field.

From the early 1970s, the Ontario government had supported an experiment in the cooperative library development of an automated on-line cataloguing support system in partnership with the Council of Ontario Universities and certain Ontario university and other libraries. During the course of the experiment, it was joined by a number of Quebec libraries, mostly in the universities. This, of course, was the project called Unicat.[9] It had proven, by the time the Hannah system began operations, most successful in providing access to machine-readable bibliographic sources previously unavailable on-line, access to a union file of records from all participants, the ability to produce catalogue cards or book catalogues mechanically, and the ability to produce associated products such as book cards and labels mechanically. These services had been made available to participants at a significant and provable cost reduction, while making possible elimination of duplication of cataloguing expertise and permitting better use of such expertise at each university. It had also been proven possible to create a union catalogue, which has provided increased capability for rationalizing library collections and cooperative university program development.

From 1975, AMS, through the Hannah Institute, had been interested in extending Unicat principles to medical sciences library holdings, including those in history of medicine, in order to achieve the benefits noted for this area of specialization and to obtain maximum value from its own expenditures. Moreover, the Board believed that Unicat principles would make possible a province-wide approach to location and use of library resources for such purposes as medical services planning, medical sciences research, personalized continuing education, and maintenance by individuals of their professional competence. It will be seen AMS still had a lively interest in other areas of medical education and practice, as permitted by its charter, and that its total thinking and resources were not devoted to history of medicine.

To examine the first aim of AMS with respect to the library materials for history of medicine, the Board in 1975 established a special library committee,[10] to be chaired by the Executive Director of the Hannah Institute, and to consist ultimately of two members of the Board (Dr. John W. Scott and Dr. John B. Neilson); Ralph E. Stierwalt, Director of the Office of Library Coordination, Council of Ontario Universities; and William Newman, Acting Chief Librarian of York University. It was Dr. John Deutsch who, during his short time on the Board of AMS, in conversation with the author on the subject of rationalization of AMS medical historical library expenditures, suggested a contact with Dr. J.B. Macdonald, former president of the University of British Columbia and in 1975 chairman of the Council of Ontario Universities. Dr. Macdonald assigned Mr. Stierwalt to work with AMS and the Hannah Institute to study the applicability of Unicat and its principles to monographs in medical historical libraries. Mr. Newman was asked to serve on the AMS committee because, as librarian of a university not having a medical school or a Hannah Chair, he would not be in conflict of interest. When Dr. Neilson became President of AMS, he continued his involvement with the special committee in an *ex-officio* capacity but appointed Dr. S.B. Upper, a returning Board member, to serve on the committee.

The committee quickly decided that the constituency of history of medicine was not sufficiently large to be treated by itself by means of Unicat principles. The AMS charter, of course, permitted activity in medical education generally, and broadening the concept to all medical science library resources could serve many other professional and public concerns. Thus the committee began to use the term Medicat to describe the application of Unicat to the medical sciences.[11] The committee also took the view that a conference of chief librarians of the universities having faculties of medicine would contribute to an assessment of the size that Medicat could assume.

The conference, termed a meeting between the Hannah Institute and the Office of Library Coordination, and attended by the chief librarians or their nominees, took place 19 February 1976.[12] From the meeting came agreement of cooperation in helping the Office of Library Coordination determine the extent of medical science library holdings in the five universities and five other medically oriented libraries in Ontario. The Office and the Institute then worked together in the AMS special committee to produce a medical proposal, which was ready by early April 1976.[13] As none of the libraries had a rate of new acquisitions in the medical sciences sufficient to justify the installation of terminal and printer, the proposal was enlarged to include existent holdings as well. Several months later, a proposal with respect to the ten libraries considered showed that during the next three years, nearly half a million titles of monographs could be taken into a Medicat file at an estimated cost of somewhat more than $2,000,000.[14]

Obviously, such a sum in addition to the costs associated with five Hannah Chairs and a proposed support system for research and publications was beyond the capability of AMS acting alone. There were many valid reasons for involving government in the Medicat plan, for it would yield many benefits to medical practice. These included continuing education that might in future be required of registrants (but not until library resources were available to all practitioners) and availability of up-to-date medical knowledge to isolated practitioners. A proposal concerning Medicat was prepared by AMS and the Hannah Institute in 1977 for discussion with government, foundations, and other organizations.[15] In late 1977, the President of AMS and the Executive Director of the Hannah Institute obtained separate appointments with two highly placed civil servants to make a reconnaisance concerning possible government support. An answer came back in a few weeks suggesting that AMS fund a pilot study that would yield more information about feasibility. This answer was said to reflect the proverbial shortage of funds in government coffers.

In 1977, a proposal for a pilot project came to the Board of AMS from McMaster University. In December 1977, the Board approved the project, which was designed "to demonstrate the feasibility of establishing a machine readable data base of library holdings in the medical sciences and including history of medicine at a cost of $99,000".[16] The proposal, put forward by Dr. Will Ready, McMaster's chief librarian, and by Mrs. Mariu Kraav, Associate Librarian – Technical Services, was designed to put approximately 36,000 titles on-line with the cooperation of the McMaster library staff (both Main Library and Health Sciences Library), the director and staff of the University of Toronto Library Automation System (UTLAS), the director and staff of the Office of Library Coordination of the Council of Ontario Universities, and staff members of AMS and the Hannah Institute. The project also required access to computer files of the National Library of Medicine (NLM) in Bethesda, files that would require adaptation for use at McMaster. The Board approved the project since it would complement NLM's Medline information system and reduce monograph cataloguing costs.

Much more adaptation of the NLM files than was anticipated proved necessary. However, an evaluation was prepared and presented to the Board in March 1980.[17] At a cost quite comparable to that for standard, pre-computer cataloguing, the library's essential (and fuller than ever before) bibliographic information had been placed on-line in a Medicat file maintained by UTLAS. Savings of considerable size would result for each successive user of the file – one of the original aims of the pilot project.

Recommendations of the writers of the final report (representative of McMaster, UTLAS, OLC, and AMS) included means of making the results and possible implications known to a wide variety of potentially interested organizations or at least persons and units who should be interested. The list included medical librarians, medical organizations, some practising physicians and surgeons, historians of medicine, government health agencies, the federal Minister of State for Science and Technology, other Ontario health-oriented foundations, and the previously contacted provincial government departments as sell as other Canadian, American, and international authoritative bodies.

A Conference on the Future of Medicat was held in Don Mills, 21 January 1981.[18] The participants included the chief librarians of all five participating libraries in the Hannah system, along with members of their staffs, and representatives from

McGill University, Dalhousie University, and Memorial University of Newfoundland (all were playing a role in Medicat) and from the Canadian Institute for Scientific and Technical Information (CISTI). By the time this conference took place, a number of factors had changed on the Ontario scene. The complexities included increasing costs of centralized computer functions and access; decided trends towards acquisition by universities of their own computers, which served both library and other needs (decentralization); ever more stringent budgets for library acquisitions and cataloguing; the need for libraries to prove economy of use as well as interests of library users in maintaining or extending computer applications; and the demise of the Office of Library Coordination of the Council of Ontario Universities. All these factors, along with changes in government personnel, delayed resuming talks with civil servants; such talks would have tried to make clear the widespread uses and economies possible in medical practice and education with a constantly enlarging Medicat file. The time was not ripe for a steady development of the Medicat file, and Medicat subsided into a holding pattern for several years. In spite of the reasons given for this state of affairs, the President of AMS and the Executive Director of the Hannah Institute, between them, did communicate individually with each chief librarian involved in the conference, in order to determine whether in their minds AMS had made a mistake in funding the pilot project. Although they felt sure that some day something would develop from this experimental project, there were times when it seemed this would not be so and the time had not come for proselytizing.

The situation has changed so that it is now possible to feel Medicat was an idea ahead of its time, one that is now reaching towards at least part of its potential. UTLAS contacted the Hannah Institute in October 1984 to give a report on the growth of Medicat, both principle and file.[19] It was learned that fourteen of the sixteen Canadian universities with medical libraries were not only accessing the machine-readable records made possible through Medicat but were also, on an ongoing basis, contributing new title information to the database. Moreover, the two remaining medical libraries were using the files for reference and inquiry. The UTLAS-NLM relationship was still in place, and the NLM file size had grown to approximately 200,000 records. The conclusions drawn by UTLAS personnel were that the medical content of the UTLAS database was significant, and that the Hannah Institute had every reason to be proud of its stimulus to the Medicat project. It is worth noting too that several foreign universities had picked up the idea.

Microfiche Projects

Earlier, the first microfiche project, that which enabled AMS and the Institute to distribute libraries of Osleriana to all five Ontario medical schools, was mentioned. The Osler fiche, and the publication of a book, *An Annotated Bibliography of Canadian Medical Periodicals, 1826-1975*, by two Hannah Professors, C.G. Roland and Paul Potter (subsidized by a grant and published by the Hannah Institute, 1975), led to the second fiche project, a much larger contribution to the literature and to research and researchers in the history of Canadian medicine.

This was the placing on fiche cards of the contents of every Canadian medical periodical issued between 1826 and 1910 (the year before the *Canadian Medical Association Journal* began publication) that could be borrowed – borrowed because nowhere did there exist a complete set of all these treasures. The libraries that lent journals for the project were those of the Academy of Medicine, Toronto, and the universities of Toronto, Western Ontario, Manitoba, British Columbia, and McMaster; the Osler Library at McGill University; and the National Library of Medicine at Bethesda, Maryland. Many individuals contributed advice to the promoters of the task.

Approximately thirty libraries and individuals subscribed to the project. The devotion of the staff of the Hannah Institute is measured by two factors: their promotion of the project and obtaining of subscriptions, and their surviving the bankruptcy of two microfiche-producing firms during the many months it took to complete it.

Medical Archives

Related to the microfiche project just described and producing more material for researchers in the history of Canadian medicine was a program initiated at a meeting, in 1978, of the Hannah Professors. This constituted an effort to catalogue known Ontario medical archives and to identify previously unknown ones. The Board accepted the recommendation of the Hannah Professors that a researcher be hired for a period of time to undertake these tasks and to produce *A Directory of Medical Archives in Ontario.*[20] Carrying out these aims was the task assigned Miss Margaret Dunn, appointed by AMS to the post of archives researcher in July 1978 for a period of two years.

During the course of her work, Miss Dunn identified known and, in a surprising number of cases, previously unknown medical archives – in the Public Archives of Canada; the Archives of Ontario; the archives of educational institutions, particularly those of the five Ontario universities in Ontario having medical schools; various county and municipal archives; the records of professional and other associations and councils; the organizational but not medical records of hospitals; and those of some religious communities and churches. In the course of her work, Miss Dunn proved to be a very fine ambassador for history of medicine and for AMS and the Institute.

In the preface to the *Directory*, the Institute's Executive Director expressed the book's aims in the following way:

> The book is intended to help hospitals and other institutions to appreciate the archival value of their records. It is intended also to help historians of medicine organize fund requests and plan research trips by informing them where relevant material may be held and where holdings do not exist. Of course, the principal aim behind this work is to make all more archives-minded, those who possess archives, those who preserve such, those who work with them in writing history.

Of course, the book could not possibly be complete. Therefore, the Board established policy that would make it possible for those who unearthed fresh archival material, or transferred it from one site to another, to report the facts to the Institute, which would edit accordingly the word processing disks containing the text of the *Directory*. A later addition to the usefulness of the contents of the book was a series of indexes, prepared during the summer of 1984 by Miss Colette Morin, as part of an undergraduate project, funded by a Hannah Studentship.[21]

The cause of medical archives has been stimulated in a variety of other ways, such as a one-day conference co-sponsored with the Ontario Hospital Association, speeches, and personal consultations.

Many individuals and organizations have helped in this crusade. Especially helpful has been the Public Archives of Canada, a member of whose staff helped select Miss Dunn for her job. Many archivists in that organization aided with on-the-job training, with availability when advice was needed, and with the production of a travelling exhibit (to be described below).

Publications

The origin and terms of reference of the Publications Committee have been dealt with in the previous chapter. The first book submitted for a subsidy to effect publication actually caused the formation of an *ad hoc* committee from which came the Publications Committee. That first book was *The Miracle of the Empty Beds: A History of Tuberculosis in Canada* (University of Toronto Press, 1977). It was written by Dr. G.J. Wherrett, for many years the executive secretary of the Canadian Tuberculosis Association. The subvention given, including editorial assistance provided to the author, totalled $10,100. For a second book, *A Century of Medicine At Western*, by Dr. Murray L. Barr (University of Western Ontario Press, 1977), the subvention was $10,000.

Publications assistance has been given by grant, loan, or both for manuscripts submitted by authors or their publishers and for works initiated by Hannah Professors or by the Hannah Institute. In some cases the Institute has also been the publisher. In certain instances, contributions have been made to the costs of publishing proceedings of conferences, including several Hannah Conferences.

Other forms of publication besides monographs have been subsidized also. These include special numbers of a bulletin or journal featuring some aspect of history of medicine, a Hippocratic Concordance, a reprint of a classic, and several series of seven or eight articles each by Dr. William E. Swinton that had been originally published in the *Canadian Medical Association Journal.*[22] A pamphlet of 56 pages published in 1977 has mildly embarrassed the Institute – not because of its contents (three excellent papers given by Drs. M.L. Barr, G.D. Hart, and R.B. Salter at a special symposium sponsored at the XXV International Congress of the History of Medicine) – but rather because it called itself Volume I, Number 1, and neither Number 2 nor Volume II has ever appeared. The idea of an Institute bulletin or regular publication was, to say the least, premature.

At one time, Canadian medical students used to receive copies of Sir William Osler's *Aequanimitas* from one of the major drug houses. Dr. Paul Potter, Hannah Professor at the University of Western Ontario, drew the fact that this practice had ceased to the attention of a meeting of the Hannah Professors, who recommended that the Board of AMS fill the void.

The Board agreed, and asked the Hannah Professors to devise a method (and to choose an editor, who proved to be Dr. C.G. Roland) for determining the contents of an appropriate publication. *Sir William Osler 1859-1919: A Selection for Medical Students* was issued in time for its initial distribution to a class of medical students at each of the five Ontario medical schools in September 1982.[23]

In 1985, a decision was taken by the Board to reprint the book and also to translate it into French so that it might be offered to all sixteen Canadian medical schools.[24] It has been bought by several American schools for their students as well.

The microfiche projects referred to constituted another form of publication, as has a series of films and videocassettes produced for the Hannah Institute under the title *Making Canadian Medical History*.

This series, as originally conceived, had two specific purposes within the overall objective of producing audiovisual teaching materials for universities and secondary schools. One purpose was to record Canadian medical history by means of filmed biographies of famous Canadian physicians (containing not only on-camera interviews but also archival materials); and the other was to promote role models for young medical, premedical, and would-be medical students.

The first seven productions were made for the Institute by the staff of Instructional Media Services of the Faculty of Medicine, University of Toronto, on the following subjects: Dr. William Boyd, distinguished pathologist and teacher; Dr. Jason A. Hannah, neuropathologist and innovative medical economist; Dr. Robert B. McClure, medical missionary extraordinary; Dr. Charles H. Best, superb medical researcher and one of the discoverers of insulin; Dr. Gustave Gingras, a dedicated leader in rehabilitation medicine; Dr. W.G. Bigelow, famed cardiovascular surgeon; and Dr. E. Harry Botterell, outstanding neuroscientist and medical educator. Two more recent films in the series, portraits of Dr. Charles G. Drake, famed neurosurgeon, and Dr. Murray L. Barr, discoverer of the Barr body and distinguished anatomy teacher and researcher, were produced by W.J. Brady of CFPL (London).

Other films, not commissioned by the Hannah Institute, have been acquired so that the film bank now totals between 35 and 40 films. Dr. W.C. Gibson's 1973 CBC series on medical explorers, dramatic presentations and series, and several tributes have been added to the film bank. The total cost of these audiovisual resources is in excess of $100,000. In addition, the Ontario Medical Association was given aid to produce a centennial film, *The Battle to Serve* (1980).

In total almost $500,000 has been spent by AMS on promoting publications in one form or another.

Exhibits and Conferences

AMS funded in 1977 and 1978 the research necessary for and the costs of production of a teaching exhibit for cardiovascular surgery residents at the Toronto General Hospital. This permanent exhibit, requested by Dr. W.G. Bigelow, is entitled

Valve Surgery: Two Main Valve Types (Biological and Prosthetic).[25]

Other exhibits produced have been less permanent; but they should, of course, never exist for a week's use only. Nor do they. Board policy has been that exhibits will be promoted for multiple usage. Most exhibits produced for or by the Hannah Institute have made their debuts at annual meetings of the Royal College of Physicians and Surgeons of Canada; indeed, each year since 1977 an exhibit has been displayed for education in history of medicine.

The first exhibit of this type ever sponsored by the Institute was created with the aid of the Academy of Medicine, Toronto, for display at the XXV International Congress of the History of Medicine at Quebec in August 1976. The three subjects that formed the whole of the exhibit were Canadian health stamps, Amerindian medicine (one of the Congress topics), and the autopsy of Nakht, the Egyptian mummy, that had been performed several years before in Toronto. All three exhibits were placed on display first at the Academy of Medicine after the Congress. Subsequently, in 1977, the latter two parts of the exhibit were shown at the Royal College meetings in Toronto.

In succeeding years, exhibits were prepared on East African medicine (from the personal collection of Dr. Edward Margetts) for Vancouver in 1978 and on pharmaceutical equipment (from the collection of Mr. William Lebow) for Montreal in 1979. In 1980 came a great step forward. The Institute was permitted by the Royal College to plan a symposium as well as an exhibit for the annual meetings in Ottawa. The choice of subject was Canadian medical archives. A very great deal of most valuable aid was given the Institute by the Public Archives of Canada and members of its staff. Miss Dunn (the Institute's archives-researcher), two Hannah Professors (Drs. Roland and Shortt), and I combined to select and display on appropriate exhibit panels material on three subjects – cholera, health care delivery, and the scope of medical archives. After the 1980 Royal College meeting, this exhibit was shown for some weeks to visitors to the Public Archives of Canada. Then it travelled across Canada for almost three years, stopping at some fifteen locations for display purposes. At a number of places, it provoked planned sessions concerning history of medicine. It is impossible to estimate how many people saw this exhibit and may possibly have been influenced by it. A most useful catalogue was produced by the Public Archives of Canada to aid viewers.[26]

For the 1981 Royal College meetings in Toronto, the Institute borrowed an exhibit, *Crucial Experiments in Medical Sciences*, created by Dr. Kenneth B. Roberts, John Clinch Professor of the History of Medicine and of Physiology at Memorial University of Newfoundland. Dr. Roberts had first shown his display at the meetings of the Federation of Biological Societies. For the 1982 Quebec meetings of the Royal College, Dr. Jacques Bernier, Assistant Professor of History, Laval University, and some of his colleagues in the Canadian Society for the History of Medicine created en exhibit entitled *The Medical Profession in Quebec in the 19th Century*. It travelled to London and Hamilton for additional viewings, as did Dr. Roberts' exhibit of the previous year.

In 1983, the Institute and Ortho Pharmaceuticals combined to produce an exhibit, *A History of Contraceptives*, based on the permanent museum of Ortho Pharmaceuticals. The exhibit was first shown at the Calgary meetings of the Royal College, and later both the Institute and Ortho made use of the exhibit at different sites. For the Institute, the display made the rounds of the Ontario universities having Hannah Chairs. The 1984 exhibit for Montreal celebrated the fiftieth anniversary of the founding of the Montreal Neurological Institute, and was designed and assembled by the staff of that Institute. For 1985 (Vancouver), the Hannah Institute prepared an exhibit, *Medicine and Exploration*, having received much help from the National Maritime Museum of Greenwich, England, McGill-Queen's University Press, and Dr. Roger Amy, pathologist at the University of Alberta. This exhibit has also made the rounds of the University of Calgary and Ontario universities.

One of the most interesting and unusual experiences with an exhibit caused a return to the first one prepared for Quebec in 1976. When the Egyptian Society for the History of Medicine was host to the XXIX International Congress of the History of Medicine in December 1984, the Canadian delegate was approached by the Egyptian congress president to see if his society might borrow the exhibit on Nakht, the Egyptian mummy. The Board of AMS decided to give the Egyptians a copy of the exhibit. It was received and displayed with a great deal of pleasure and interest. Thus it was that a portion of the first exhibit was reused almost a decade later, and the story of an Egyptian mummy's experience in Canada returned to the land of his birth, several millennia after his death.

The exhibit for the 1986 Royal College meetings (Toronto) is called *Medicine in Political Prints.*

Beginning with the 1980 meetings of the Royal College, at which a symposium on medical archives was presented, it has become customary for the Hannah Institute to plan a symposium for each annual meeting. In addition, a representative of the Institute sits on the Royal College's planning committee. The 1980 and 1985 experiences, where the symposia subjects matched the themes of the exhibits and drew greater audiences to the symposia, have produced the point of view that where feasible this linkage should be utilized for future exhibits and symposia.

In most years since 1975, AMS has also promoted, both financially and morally, programs in history of medicine within the annual meetings of the Canadian Medical Association. Generally, these programs have been related to the locales of the meetings.

Equally, if not more, important has been the aid given the Canadian Society for the History of Medicine/La Société Canadienne d'Histoire de la Médecine in two ways. These are the provision of funds for a Hannah Lecturer, since 1981, at the annual meetings with the Learned Societies, and a subsidy for two years (recently extended a further two years) to permit the beginning of the Society's *Canadian Bulletin of Medical History/Bulletin canadien d'histoire de la medecine,* first appearing in 1984.

It is a smaller step than one would think from support of a lecture to sponsorship of a conference, even a conference lasting up to three days. Among the groups and societies given grants towards costs of conferences and/or publication of the proceedings have been the XXV International Congress of the History of Medicine; the Canadian Science and Technology History Association (for three biennial conferences at Queen's University); the Institute for the History and Philosophy of Science and Technology of the University of Toronto; the Academy of Medicine, Toronto; the American Osler Society (for an annual meeting held at Hamilton); the Canadian Society for Eighteenth Century Studies; the Osler Library (McGill University) for a celebration of the fiftieth anniversary of the library and for publication of the proceedings; the Canadian Society for History and Philosophy of Science for the Third International Conference on History and Philosophy of Science (in Montreal); the Association of Canadian Medical Colleges; and various Ontario medical student societies.

In the Executive Director's report of 1976, it was suggested that Hannah Conferences be held biennially at campuses where a Hannah Professor would take major responsibility for organizing a conference on some aspect of the history of medicine.[27] The first such was held in Hamilton in May 1982, organized by McMaster's Hannah Professor, Dr. C.G. Roland. The proceedings of the three days' sessions have been published as *Health, Disease and Medicine: Essays in Canadian History*.[28] The second Hannah Conference, held in October 1984 at the University of Western Ontario, was organized largely by Dr. John Nicholas, Chairman of the Department of the History of Medicine and Science. The proceedings are being published as *Moral Priorities in Medical Research* by Wilfrid Laurier University Press.

Oral History

In 1977, Dr. R.S. Harris, University of Toronto Historian, requested from AMS financial aid for the medical portion of his task of interviewing influential academics with knowledge of the university over the past fifty to sixty years. Two interviews with medical faculty had already been conducted by Mrs. Valerie Schatzker at that time.

The funding given in 1977 and later extended has produced forty-six interviews, of which more than forty concern the history of the Faculty of Medicine, its departments, and its teaching hospitals. In addition to further funding, AMS, through the Hannah Institute, took over administration of this phase of the university project. An advisory committee was set up to select subjects for interview, consisting of Dr. John D. Hamilton, Dr. K.J.R. Wightman, Dr. Harris, President J.B. Neilson, Mrs. Schatzker, and myself. It was not a particularly effective committee and it met twice only. Nevertheless, the experience stimulated us to identify individuals of significant achievement. This knowledge might be of value to a medical historian in the future who takes on the task of writing a history of the Faculty of Medicine.

Other parts of the province claim that there is too much concentration on Toronto (a point with which the author agrees). One correction of this imbalance was an excellent oral history project done at Hamilton by Drs. W.B. Spaulding and C.G. Roland under the title *The Development and Evolution of the Faculty of Health Sciences, McMaster University*. To have the story from the participants themselves of the founding of one of Canada's youngest medical schools is a most valuable accomplishment. In addition, AMS has responded to grant requests involving oral history techniques from both individuals and such institutions as the Faculty of Nursing, University of Toronto, and the Canadian Anaesthetists' Society. In total, a sum in excess of $100,000 has been expended on this activity.

The Hannah Institute, treating the tapes and transcripts of the interviews as archival sources, has deposited the original tapes and a copy of each transcript in the Public Archives of Canada, after obtaining release forms from those interviewed. By agreement, the Public Archives of Canada has prepared cassette copies of the tapes for the Archives of Ontario, the University of Toronto Archives, the Hannah Institute, and each interviewee. The Institute provides an edited, bound transcript of the interview.

The Hannah Medal and the Neilson Award

In September 1975, the Institute's Executive Director recommended to the Board that AMS establish an awards program for achievements in history of medicine at those universities with Hannah Chairs.[29] In a lengthy report that examined awards made by other societies (e.g., American Association for the History of Medicine, the American Institute for the History of Pharmacy), he recommended establishment of an *ad hoc* committee to consider the whole subject of awards.[30] Shortly after, a special committee was established. It consisted of Dr. J.M.S. Careless, Professor of History, University of Toronto, as chairman; Dr. D.G. Bates, McGill's Professor of the History of Medicine; Dr. D.O.W. Waugh, as a representative of the Board; and the Executive Director acting as secretary. From this committee came a motion that a Hannah Medal be established, if possible through the Royal Society of Canada, to honour the author of a monograph in Canadian history of medicine. ("Canadian" referred to citizenship, residence, or content.) At the Board meeting of 21 June 1976, I was able to report that I had met with the Awards Committee of the Royal Society of Canada (chaired at that time by Dr. Antoine d'Iorio of the University of Ottawa) and that the committee was recommending to the Society's Council that the Hannah Medal be established for excellence of publications in Canadian history of medicine.[31] Frances Gage, the artist who had made the head of Dr. Hannah, was commissioned to design and cast the Hannah Medal using the head as a model for the portrait.

The Hannah Medal was first awarded in 1978 to Dr. Henri Ellenberger of the University of Montreal for his book *The Discovery of the Unconscious.*[32] Subsequently, it has been awarded to Dr. John Farley (1979) of Dalhousie University, for his book *The Spontaneous Generation Controversy from Descartes to Oparin;*[33] to Dr. Malcolm G. Taylor (1980) of York University, for *Health Insurance and Canadian Public Policy;*[34] to Dr. Michael Bliss (1983) of the University of Toronto, for *The Discovery of Insulin;*[35] to Dr. Harvey G. Simmons (1984) of York University, for *From Asylum to Welfare;*[36] to Dr. A. Margaret Evans and Dr. C.A.V. Barker (1985) of the University of Guelph, for *Century One;*[37] and to Dr. W.G. Bigelow (1986) of Toronto, for *Cold Hearts.*[38]

When Dr. John B. Neilson retired as President of AMS in April 1983, the Board desired to recognize his service by establishing the Neilson Award. It was further decided to give the award to a Canadian medical practitioner who, while making his/her career in some other branch of medicine, had nevertheless made important contributions to history of medicine in Canada. The Neilson Award was made for the first time in the autumn of 1984 to two joint winners, Dr. Sylvio LeBlond of Quebec and Dr.

Harold Segall of Montreal. In May 1985 it was given again, this time to Dr. Edward Bensley of Montreal. These presentations were made by Dr. Neilson in Montreal. The 1986 winner of the Neilson Award was Dr. Claude Dolman of Vancouver.

Support of Research and Researchers

From the earliest days of Dr. Hannah's planning for the institute and the chairs in history of medicine, there appeared frequently applicants for funds with which to pursue their research interests. Dr. Hannah and I both felt strongly that research in history of medicine would best serve to promote interest in the subject. Forms of research support were on the agenda of all meetings the Executive Director conducted with personnel at the five universities when gathering material and impressions for the 1976 Executive Director's report. It has been noted previously that an *ad hoc* grants committee, established to review early applications, was made a standing committee and given terms of reference it itself had largely determined.

The grant-in-aid for independent scholars has been looked on as the core form of research support. For grants-in-aid, the general definition for Canadian history of medicine has been utilized. The preference for post-doctoral fellowships was intended not only to favour the further development of young scholars but also to counteract academic isolation on the part of Hannah Chair occupants. Post-doctoral fellowships and scholarships have thus, in the first decade of the Hannah system, been restricted to the five Ontario universities having Hannah Chairs. Scholarships have always been intended to aid the early development of younger scholars.

In recent years (i.e., since 1981), a global support budget for research has been employed, so that all applicants, whether for grants-in-aid, fellowships, or scholarships, have been competing for their share of the total budget. At the same time, the Grants Committee has been enlarged and is now representative of Canada and the United States. In 1983, AMS initiated undergraduate studentships, usually held in the summer period, for undergraduates in medicine, history, or some other relevant field. A maximum of ten such awards has been made available for each academic year.

By the end of the 1985/86 year, nearly $1,500,000 had been spent on or committed to these forms of research aid. In several cases, the end-point of the research has been a manuscript that has gained publication assistance from AMS. In many other cases, the product has been a scholarly paper given to a learned society and published later in a scholarly journal. The distinct impressions of the Board of AMS confirm the original feeling that research support may well be the most important program offered by the Hannah Institute.

The Spaulding Committee Report

At the beginning of this chapter, it was recorded that "after ten years of activity supporting medical history A.M.S. decided to strike a committee to review the current status and make recommendations for the future". The committee consisted of Dr. William B. Spaulding as chairman (Dr. Spaulding is a former director and vice-president of AMS), with Miss Ray Godfrey and Dr. Robert A. Macbeth as additional members. Both of the latter two are current members of the Board. Their report was received by the Board on 13 January 1986.[39]

In its report, the committee stated its aims as:

> to assess the effectiveness of the A.M.S. contribution to the history of medicine in Ontario over the last ten years through the program now in place and to recommend ways in which the resources of A.M.S. and the Hannah Institute may be most effectively used to promote interest in and understanding of medical history in Canada.

The general conclusion of the committee was expressed as follows:

> A great deal has been accomplished by A.M.S. in the last decade. Important books have been published, visiting speakers and professors have been invited to our universities, many research projects have been supported, archives

> have been catalogued, a Canadian journal has been subsidized, films and other audio-visual programmes have been produced, meetings have been sponsored, and Hannah Chairs have been established. In consequence the visibility of medical history in Ontario and Canada has increased markedly. The Hannah Institute and its activities are now recognized internationally.

The Spaulding committee chose to concentrate its thinking on the chairs, particularly those that had proven most successful. The committee wrote, "Achievements by the Hannah Professors have been impressive, especially in the medical schools most supportive of medical history." In cases of less successful chairs, the committee seemed to think more effort and involvement on the part of those universities would produce better results. With respect to medical history in parts of Canada outside Ontario, the committee thought the Institute should adopt a more aggressive initiating role rather than a reactive one. Because of the perceived limitation of funds that would not permit doing both, the committee came down in favour of continuing to fund chairs rather than establishing one central physically distinct institute with a critical mass of scholars. The latter course would abolish what the committee saw as the chief role of AMS – that is, making history of medicine available to medical students, other students interested in becoming health sciences professionals, and medical practitioners. In addition, they were not convinced scholarly output would increase in such an institute.

> It is our judgment that a central, physically distinct Institute of Medical History would not achieve the purposes of the A.M.S. program more effectively than the Hannah Chair programs. There are a number of reasons for this opinion. Institutes are highly dependent on leadership to succeed and tend to wax and wane in their influence and productivity depending upon who is in charge. The risk is considerable that a leader of world stature would not be available and that a succession of such leaders could not be found in the future. To attract scholars from other coun-

> tries, as the Wellcome Institute is able to do, would require a world class library. Acquiring, housing and maintaining such a library at to-day's costs would be a great strain on the resources of A.M.S. Furthermore, existing Hannah Chair programs would be markedly diminished or might disappear with the appearance of a central Institute. Finally, there is no guarantee that scholarly productivity would equal or exceed that of the Hannah Chair programs.

The committee then made a series of recommendations regarding Hannah Chairs, other programs, support of the history of medicine outside Ontario, organizational changes, and the current model of the Hannah Institute. Interesting suggestions concerning the order of responsibilities of Hannah Professors were included in the recommendations in the following terms:

> Educational responsibilities of Hannah Chairs should be directed toward students interested in a career in the health professions (particularly medicine and nursing), medical and nursing graduates, other university students, high school students, primary school students, the public-at-large in that order of priority. In addition to orienting students to medical history over the ages and to topics specially selected by the Hannah Professors, Canadian Medical History, the development of medical care in the western world, and the history of ethical issues should be emphasized.
>
> Scholarly Activity. These educational responsibilities should be linked with rigorous academic research in medical history. Hannah Professors are expected to make presentations of original work at national and international meetings; they should publish their results in peer-reviewed journals.

To make all this possible, the committee recommended certain actions on the part of AMS and the individual universities to provide security for the incumbent, greater collegial interaction, and an increase in the number of post-doctoral fellowships.

Staggered appointments and defined teaching responsibilities for the fellows, it was thought, would "augment the educational impact of the Hannah Professors". The committee also expressed the view that improved selection and quality of training of graduate students would enrich the chairs.

A move away from too parochial a view, usually felt to be due to the fact that the AMS reserves had been realized in Ontario, was very evident. Initiatives recommended included

> an offer to support a series of lectures or workshops on selected history of medicine topics at medical schools where interest is manifest; to distribute selected books to medical libraries and students; to offer a professional consultation service on how to set up an effective program; to sponsor a one or two day annual workshop organized by one individual in each medical school and to offer some financial support for a faculty member who has taught history of medicine effectively and wishes to devote more time to this.

There would be a condition attached to such support. The faculty member would be designated a Hannah Lecturer.

It was thought that an AMS newsletter should be sent after each Board meeting to the Hannah Professors. At the same time, an annual meeting of the Hannah Professors with the Board and receipt by Board members of the Hannah Professors' newsletter would improve communications. The subject of mini-institutes was also discussed, but was of interest to the Hannah Professors only if they were the initiators of such developments, which were natural outgrowths of local successes and initiatives at their own schools.

Initial Board reactions to the report took place at the meeting at which Dr. Spaulding presented the report of his committee.[40] Further consideration was left for the next Board meeting of 9 April.

New Board Policies

Before the Board met again to discuss the Spaulding report in depth, it was referred to the Hannah Institute Advisory Council for consideration by the deans followed by discussion at a Council meeting 13 March. The minutes of this meeting indicated a lengthy discussion.[41] The reaction of Council members to the report was generally very favourable, although there were reservations with respect to certain of the recommendations.

One of the reservations expressed concerned the degree of the universities' share of financial support for the programs proposed. The deans believed in general that any immediate commitment by the universities could only result in severe budgetary problems. The deans also stressed the contributions of their faculties to the Hannah programs in the form of assumption of overhead costs. Nevertheless, there was agreement in principle that there should be some sort of shared responsibility financially.

The universities preferred not to use the words "security" and "tenure" but rather to speak of "commitment" to occupants of the Hannah Chairs. "There was agreement that there should be a commitment in measurable terms from both AMS and the Universities on a long-term basis." A consensus was found with respect to the review process: (a) an internal review of the incumbent after the first three years of the appointment, (b) an external review of the program after five years, and (c) a ten-year funding commitment by AMS where such reviews had evidenced a satisfactory standard of performance of the program and its incumbent.

The deans preferred collegial interaction to be strengthened by increased numbers of post-doctoral fellows rather than by second appointments. "The personality and attitude of the incumbent was seen as a major factor in enhancing the profile of history of medicine on campus, in capitalizing on an already existing interest in the subject, and in establishing links with other departments and broader interest groups."

There was agreement that, although provincial graduate scholarship is already a complex subject, there is a need to examine it from the points of view of inter-university study, supervision, and cross-appointments. It was agreed that scholarship stipends should be equivalent to those provided by other granting agencies.

There was some reluctance to consider AMS support of history of medicine programs outside Ontario. The deans appeared to believe that such interests were at least partially served by research and publication support. They were afraid that increasing the number of programs beyond the province might create problems for the well-established bases in Ontario.

Lastly, the Advisory Council considered the role of the Hannah Institute. It was seen by the Council to be different in relation to the chairs than to its other activities in the history of medicine. For the chairs, the role was seen as more of an executive nature.

When the Board met next on 9 April, it was in a position to correlate the thinking of its members with the report of the Hannah Institute Advisory Council.[42] Discussions centred initially on the responsibilities of AMS, the five universities, and the Hannah Professors. The President of AMS, Dr. Wilson, expressed the view, with which the Board agreed, that AMS should prepare a summary of its expectations of the universities, as well as of guidelines acceptable to them. The Board then proceeded to discuss policy, with the expectation that the President and the Executive Director of the Institute would draft the guidelines, which would come back to Board for approval or revision, after which they would be discussed in an autumn meeting of the Advisory Council.

Concerning finances, it was agreed that a draft letter to the deans should be precise with respect to AMS expectations of shared funding within the next five years. After much discussion, members of Board agreed that long-term funding would be acceptable to AMS after a three-year internal review and a five-year external review, with a supporting annual statement of performance from the dean. It was accepted that there should be a written statement to this effect that included an appropriate grandfather clause. It was also agreed that a definite percentage of the annual budget should be allotted to library purchases, after the expenditures of the past five years were examined by the Executive Director.

Both the Spaulding committee report and the Grants Committee report[43] proposed a broadening of the rules as to where Hannah post-doctoral fellowships could be held. The Board accepted this recommendation, provided the priority of award, all other factors being equal, should be Hannah Chairs, other Canadian sites, and then non-Canadian sites.[44] It was also determined that the Grants Committee should have the power to recommend initial two-year fellowships, if indicated.

In discussing expansion of support outside Ontario for other than the present support programs (research grants and publication assistance), it was agreed the concept should be accepted in principle, contingent on satisfactory ground rules being enunciated and each application being dealt with on an individual basis. The Board thought this kind of support could be very positive for AMS and for history of medicine in Canada.

Finally, before accepting the Spaulding report, the Board agreed that guidelines for ancillary programs need not be spelled out to the deans but should be dealt with separately, that administration and organization should be reviewed separately, and that communication between Board and the Hannah Professors should be strengthened. In closing the discussion, the President "noted the three facets of the report requiring addressing in guidelines" as chairs, supplementary programs, and administration.

It will be seen, then, that acceptance of the Spaulding report will lead to continuation and expansion of AMS activities in history of medicine, and that a number of the activities will serve to remove certain parochial aspects of the first decade of the corporation's involvement in the discipline on which it has chosen to concentrate much of its expertise and resources. It will also be apparent that AMS believes it has spent its funds devoted to history of medicine in a worthwhile manner.

Summary

Has Jason Hannah's second great idea proved to be a success? The answer of the Spaulding committee is a definite *yes*. The story set forth in these pages would seem to warrant the committee's conclusion.

Will the Hannah program in history of medicine continue to be a successful addition to the world's institutes and chairs devoted to promoting the subject? It is the view of the Board that, because the program has been built on a quite solid base with the aid and goodwill of many interested persons, it will go on to further successes.

Has Jason Hannah gone down in history as he so dearly wished to do? It is the belief of the writer that the answer must be a resounding *yes*: he has gone down in history, perhaps in a more impressive way than even he himself imagined or hoped would be the case. Perhaps, on the other hand, what has been achieved is of the order of what he hoped for as his memorial.

CHAPTER VIII

Looking Back and Looking Ahead

In the previous seven chapters, I have attempted to tell the story of Dr. Hannah's second accomplishment, AMS involvement in history of medicine. Before attempting to look into the future, I think it wise to summarize what has thus far happened.

Dr. Hannah made a success of his first entrepreneurial role, both in the provision of what a section of the public needed and could afford, and in a business sense. He displayed ability, an ability shared with a number of other persons and with government officials, to foresee the future of prepaid medical care (as he preferred to call it) or comprehensive health insurance, as government named it.

His unusual personality was first evident, in all likelihood, at an early age. In the period under consideration in this book, it first became apparent in the extra clauses inserted in the charter, those clauses that made it possible for AMS to consider alternative actions when it had played out its first role. At no time did he ever consider the available option of winding-up and turning the corporation's assets over to general government revenues. His unusually determined character showed itself again in his resolute pursuit of a memorial by which he would be known to succeeding generations. It is difficult to estimate how much time he spent during the 1960s and early 1970s in his search for immortality.

It is even more difficult to estimate how much time – and patience – of others he used up, in his quest for lasting fame. He was never, at any time after 1937, comfortable with any activity other than prepaid medical care and its ramifications. Diversification, in retrospect, seems to have been an illogical series of exercises whose only purpose was to unearth the memorial he so ardently desired. His memorial had several requirements in his thinking. The AMS accumulation of funds in the operation of the prepaid medical care program had to remain under his/AMS control. Others – individuals and institutions – had to pay part of the cost of his memorial. If the identity of the memorial were established and if it did not fit his criteria of control, then the memorial would have to change to fit his thinking.

After his meeting Dr. Gibson, who was himself an entrepreneur, but on behalf of medical history rather than medical economics, it was only a matter of time until an action and/or opportunity within that discipline, history of medicine, would initiate the specific designation of a memorial he regarded as suitable and as his due. That situation arose in 1971 when, seemingly without Board approval, he purchased a portion of the library of the Medical Society of London – with AMS funds, it must be emphasized, and without his having planned ahead with respect to where it should or could, under his terms, be placed. Uneasy relationships and contentious exchanges with the Academy of Medicine, Toronto, and Massey College occurred when he sought space for the library. The coupling of an institute for the history of medicine and five academic chairs with his library seems also to have emerged from chance happenings arising from relations established with individuals who really cared about the discipline. They were, however, happenings upon which he seized because of his anxiety to build his memorial during the remainder of what seemed to himself and others to be a rapidly shortening life.

If his institute could not be established at the Academy or within a part of the university, the two sites he recognized as most desirable in Toronto, then he would have to set up his own institute, which would then, of necessity, have to assume a different form. True, he had come to realize he needed some sort of link with academia. He proceeded then to obtain agreements with the five universities in Ontario that had faculties of medicine. Obtaining these agreements was arguably his greatest achievement. To do it while suffering severe ill health was nothing short of a magnificent accomplishment. However, what to do to implement the agreements in a manner acceptable to the universities was beyond his failing physical abilities, his rigid distrust of government and universities, and his determination to retain full control of AMS resources. Others had to put flesh on the bones of the agreements he had obtained. The dedicated work of many persons – new officers and Board members of AMS, the staff of the Hannah Institute, academics and practitioners, non-medical personnel, Hannah Professors, willing committee members from Canada, the United States, and the United Kingdom – was necessary to create a viable Hannah system. It may be possible that never have so many contributed so willingly to establish a useful organization about whose origins they knew so little.

It has been stated previously that Jason Hannah has his memorial; his name has gone down in history, but rather in analogy to that of the bibliographer who has become better known that those whose works are annotated or listed in the bibliography. Hannah Professors, Hannah research grantees, postdoctoral fellows, scholars, those granted special funds for original ideas, books, and numerous other projects have carried the name Hannah around the world.

But having adopted history of medicine as the field that would provide his memorial, Dr. Hannah stated as one of his objectives that medical students should be influenced in their future careers by means of their understanding on whose shoulders they stood. Has this happened? It is certainly not apparent yet that it has. Perhaps it is too early to see an effect such as he wished. At one time, he suggested it would take at least a generation to see any effect. That much time has not yet elapsed. Shall we ever see such a result? If we or our successors do not, will the venture have been in vain? I think not, for I believe that the most valuable feature of the story of the second great idea of Jason Hannah has been the way it has served to unite people from so many different areas of interest and study in common cause. Some of the activities of the Hannah Institute have contributed to this belief; some have not. The report of the Spaulding committee seems to suggest a positive balance, as I hoped in my preface.

The Future?

A changing world – and most of us prefer to live in a changing world – demands adaptation to change. AMS will have to adopt new policies as time goes by. If the foundation is firm enough, change, modification, revision can all be accommodated. Among things changing – it has happened before – may well be attitudes of students to a subject such as history of medicine, methods of interesting students and practitioners in the subject, what is important to those with interest in or nostalgia about history of medicine. During the decade and a half since Dr. Hannah bought the first library, we in AMS and the Hannah Institute have seen a remarkable increase of interest in history of medicine among non-medical persons. True, some of the increased interest may be because of the availability of research funds, but I doubt that that is a major factor in explaining the increased activity. One has only to examine public attitudes to recognize greater desire to know more about current medicine and its methods. Similarly, it seems logical that general, social, and other historians and academics in other fields, as well as members of the general population, should show much more interest in medicine's past than has previously been the case. The desire to know more about medicine or history of medicine even though one is not medically trained is not to be criticized; rather is it to be welcomed.

There are then two constituencies that must be considered in the future, as they should have been in the past: those medically trained, and those not. How will they be informed on whose shoulders physicians stand? Is it at all important that they should be so informed? I believe it is. One of the negative factors in a rapidly changing world is the tendency to lose one's roots, to fail to appreciate progress made in our lifetimes, in the lifetimes of our predecessors. To know these things is to acquire a greater understanding of where we and events are going. What is the best way to have history of medicine play a part in mapping the future? By becoming more popular? By becoming rigorous in study, research, and communication? By using modern technology to communicate fascinating information rather than the trash so common on television? All of these thoughts and questions are raised as a consequence of reading some of the Hannah ramblings.

The Spaulding committee's report, and the Board of Directors in adopting the report, have come down in favour of retaining the system of Hannah Chairs as the principal means of disseminating knowledge of the history of medicine – this rather than the establishment of a centralized institute. The members of the committee have given sound reasons for not attempting the latter, which could probably be done only at the expense of the chairs, which have shown a considerable measure of productivity. To improve the current level of productivity of all the chairs, recommendations have been made that would increase their impact by providing for larger concentrations of scholars at each of the five sites. Help is also promised those other Canadian schools that demonstrate initiatives. These two measures, in the opinion of the author, should increase not only the visibility but also the productivity in teaching and in research of the Hannah Chairs.

One serious question does arise, however, as a result of these actions. What will be the future of the individuals trained in history of medicine as a result of this increased scholarship? While it is true that half of Canada's sixteen medical schools do not have chairs in the subject, and while it is true that the Hannah system is becoming widely known internationally, it is also true there are unlikely to be sufficient medical academic opportunities available to all those trained in an expanded program. When this happens in other fields, other types of opportunities must be found for those trained. One or two current trainees have attempted to couple training in other related fields with advanced qualification in history of medicine. These other fields include primary activity in some other branch of medicine, some other branch of history, archival work, or government policy. It would seem realistic to study such alternatives.

I have already mentioned that many history departments of universities not having medical faculties have witnessed the adoption of history of medicine as research majors by some of their scholars and staff members. This may lead to professorships in the subject in history departments, particularly in the field of social history. One must never forget either that training in history of medicine may well lead to other opportunities not yet explored – politics, civil service, service aspects of research in history of medicine, and related fields.

Whether these possibilities are explored or accomplished depends to a very great extent on continued commitment and funding from AMS, as well as on a continuing funding of research by the Social Sciences and Humanities Research Council and the Medical Research Council. It would seem, in the opinion of members of the Spaulding committee, that an extended involvement on the part of the participating universities will also be needed. One cannot of course predict the future interest and activity of all these organizations. Board action on the Spaulding report, and the past record of AMS, do strongly suggest the desire to maintain history of medicine as a major activity on the part of the corporation.

Because its entry into the field of history of medicine a decade and a half ago has provoked a large number of positive developments, it seems reasonable to assume that the Board's continuing interest and adaptation to changing times and circumstances will lead the way to further progress in this fascinating branch of history. It is certainly to be hoped this will be the case.

APPENDIX I

The Hannah Institute for the History of Medicine in the Academy of Medicine, Toronto

J.W. Scott, B.A., M.A., M.D.

At the present time in the University of Toronto, there is not a chair in the History of Medicine, nor is there a medical historical museum. The cataloguing of the University Library does not facilitate the study of the history of medicine. There is a collection of rare and ancient books, but the medical books are not separated from other disciplines. The Academy of Medicine holds the only significant medical museum in Canada, and has in addition a significant collection of ancient and rare medical texts. This is supported by a section in the library dealing with medical biography and history.

Within the School of Graduate Studies at the University of Toronto, there is an Institute for the History and Philosophy of Science and Technology, which is well established in the fields of the physical sciences, technology and mathematics, but is relatively weak in the biological field. There is no one whose main interest is the History of Medicine. This institute is authorized to train students for the degree doctor of philosophy.

For an Institute in the Academy to be successful, it must be headed by an outstanding medical historian, who has adequate support staff, both academic and technical, with access to the university to train graduate students. Funds should be available to attend meetings, learned societies and temporary studies at other centres where books and manuscripts are available.

Facilities should also be provided for graduate students and post doctoral fellows.

Such an Institute established within the Academy could be

associated with the School of Graduate Studies of the University of Toronto. There is precedent for this in the Pontifical Institute for Mediaeval Studies, which is not part of the University of Toronto, yet several members of its staff hold honorary appointments within the University, and have academic status in the School of Graduate Studies. Consequently they can present their students to the University for degrees.

The Director of the Institute should be a senior internationally known medical historian. He would be charged with the organization and operation of the programme of the Institute. He would assist in supervision of the museum, presumably there would be a curator of the museum, he would assist in supervision of the rare book collection, and be responsible for adding to this collection.

There should be an assistant who could be either the curator of the museum, or a post doctoral fellow. The museum will need a full time curatorial assistant and conservationist. If the museum continues to grow additional staff may be required.

A librarian to care for the rare books and historical collection should be provided; for the rare books should be readily available, must be adequately supervised and receive appropriate tender loving care.

Secretarial assistants must be available and until the size of the staff is known, the amount of secretarial help cannot be predicted, at least one, perhaps two to begin with.

As a start the staff should probably consist of a Director, a curatorial assistant, a librarian and appropriate secretarial help.

Before long a second historian with sufficient seniority to obtain academic status should be appointed and consideration given to post doctoral fellows and graduate students. At the present time limitations of space will be serious until a new building is available. Space should be rented in either the Medical Arts Building or in a nearby house on Huron Street.

Dr. Swinton could serve as an Acting Director until a permanent Director is chosen, he could then continue as the Director of the museum.

APPENDIX II

The Agreement signed by Associated Medical Services, Incorporated and each of the five universities. (Draft No. 4, 2 October 1973).

AN AGREEMENT MADE BETWEEN ASSOCIATED MEDICAL SERVICES, INCORPORATED AND QUEEN'S UNIVERSITY, OTTAWA UNIVERSITY, McMASTER UNIVERSITY, UNIVERSITY OF WESTERN ONTARIO, AND THE UNIVERSITY OF TORONTO FOR THE PURPOSE OF ESTABLISHING "THE JASON A. HANNAH CHAIR IN THE HISTORY OF MEDICAL AND RELATED SCIENCES".

---

1. WHEREAS Associated Medical Services, Incorporated (hereinafter referred to as A.M.S.) desires to promote the study and dissemination of the knowledge of the History of Medical and Related Sciences; and

2. WHEREAS A.M.S. is prepared to make a grant of fifty thousand dollars ($50,000) for a period of not less than five (5) years for the cost of maintenance of a Chair to be known as "The Jason A. Hannah Chair for the History of Medical and Related Sciences"; and

3. WHEREAS each of the universities; Queen's University, University of Toronto, University of Western Ontario, McMaster University and Ottawa University have each separately and collectively indicated by signing similar agreements, their desire and willingness to co-operate with A.M.S. and each with the other, in this respect; and

4. WHEREAS A.M.S. is prepared to make a grant of fifty thousand dollars ($50,000) to each of said universities for a period of five years, the funding for the program to begin on the date of appointment and actual commencement of duties of the Professor to direct it. The grant may be renewed or extended under conditions satisfactory to A.M.S. The individual appointed as Professor and Director shall devote his full time to the objectives of "The Jason A. Hannah Chair for the History of Medical and Related Sciences". Such appointee shall, however, co-operate in the establishment of an overall Institute for research into the History of Medicine and Related Sciences; and

5. WHEREAS the universities herein indicated have agreed to participate in the development of an Institute to be known as "The Jason A. Hannah Institute for Research Into and Study of the History of Medical and Related Sciences", which shall be for the purposes of the Jason A. Hannah Chairs beyond the confines of the universities, which Institute shall also be financed by grants from A.M.S. to the extent of fifty thousand dollars ($50,000) each year for a period of five (5) years, renewable under conditions and circumstances satisfactory to A.M.S., such grant to commence at a date satisfactory to A.M.S.

6. The purposes and objects of The Jason A. Hannah Chair (and Institute when established) shall be: –

(a) Generally to assist and advise A.M.S. in making grants for the study of; research into; and dissemination of knowledge in respect of the History of Medical and Related Sciences.

(b) For which purpose each university shall provide from within the funds made available through the Annual grant suitable housing and administrative support. However, at no time and in no event shall more than ten percent (10%) of the Annual grant be utilized for the provision of suitable housing and administrative support, and under no circumstances shall any part of the grant be used for capital construction.

(c) To enable the universities to provide and maintain a suitable center through which acceptable persons may advance their personal and the general knowledge of the History of Medical and Related Sciences through study and research.

NOW, THEREFORE, each of the universities named in paragraph 3 above agrees with A.M.S. and each with the other as follows: –

EACH UNIVERSITY AGREES THAT IT SHALL:

(a) Within a period of time agreed upon by each university individually and A.M.S., make available a program in the History of Medical and Related Sciences for Students of the University as a whole. While not limited to medical students, they shall be given preference if for any reason such an excess of applicants for the program the numbers admitted has to be restricted.

(b) That no portion of the grant made by A.M.S. for The Chair and/or Institute for the Study of the History of Medical and Related Sciences shall be utilized for any purpose [other] than set forth in this agreement; except with the express written consent of A.M.S.

(c) That the University shall design a five-year program, and shall submit to A.M.S. annually a full report on the activities, progress and budget of the program during the previous year and proposals and a budget for the succeeding year. There shall be an overall review at the end of three years to determine whether or not the A.M.S. grant shall be continued.

(d) Each and every one of the universities agrees to assist and co-operate fully with A.M.S. in fulfilling the terms of this agreement in spirit as well as in letter.

(e) The university and A.M.S. accepts that this agreement may only be terminated or amended with not less than two years notice, if in the opinion of A.M.S., the terms hereof have been abrogated or the university or its agents or servants fails to fulfill them.

8. A.M.S. AGREES:

(a) TO make grants as indicated in 4. above in twelve (12) equal monthly grants to a total of fifty thousand dollars ($50,000) each year for a period of five (5) years, which shall be renewable under circumstances and conditions satisfactory to A.M.S.

(b) TO assist the university to accomplish the objects herein set forth.

9. The spirit and intent of this agreement and time shall be of the essence in its fulfillment.

10. SIGNED, SEALED AND DELIVERED at __________
this ________ day of ________________, 1973,

____

____

____

ASSOCIATED MEDICAL SERVICES, INCORPORATED

APPENDIX III

Biographical Sketches of Hannah Professors

POTTER, Paul Melvin Joseph, University of Western Ontario; born in Hamilton, Ontario. Education – B.Sc. in Chemistry/Mathematics, McGill 1966; M.D.C.M., McGill 1968; M.A. in Greek, McMaster 1970; D. Phil. in Greek/Latin and History of Medicine, Kiel University 1973. Appointed Assistant Professor in the Hannah Chair, September 1974. Currently Associate Professor. Research interest – Hippocratic and Roman Medicine. Books – *Hippokrates: Über die Krankheiten*, III, Akademie Verlag, Berlin; *Hipprocrates* (Loeb Classical Library), Volume 5, Harvard University Press.

HODGKINSON, Ruth G., Queen's University; born in England. Education – B.Sc. (Hons.) in Economic History, London School of Economics and Political Science, University of London, 1946; Ph.D. in Modern Social History, University of London 1950. Appointed to the Hannah Chair as Professor, January 1975. Resigned September 1978. Research interests – social history of medicine, national health service, Thomas Hodgkin. Book – *The Origins of the National Health Service.*

MAZUMDAR, Pauline M.H., University of Toronto; born in England. Education – M.B., B.S., University of London 1958; M.Tech. in Immunology, Brunel University 1972; Ph.D. in History of Medicine, Johns Hopkins 1976. Appointed Associate Professor in the Hannah Chair, December 1976. Research interests – history of physiology and immunology, history of eugenics in Britain.

ROLAND, Charles Gordon, McMaster University; born in Winnipeg. Education – premedicine, University of Toronto 1952-1954;

M.D., B.Sc. (Med.)., University of Manitoba 1958. Appointed Hannah Professor, July 1977. Previously was in private practice in Ontario, then senior editor, *Journal of the American Medical Association*; then Associate Professor and Professor, Mayo Medical School, Rochester, Minn. Research interests – bibliographic research, history of military medicine, prisoners of war. Publications – numerous publications on Osler; *Secondary References in the History of Canadian Medicine*; co-editor with P.M.J. Potter of *An Annotated Bibliography of Canadian Medical Periodicals 1826-1975.*

GELFAND, Toby, University of Ottawa; born in Philadelphia. Education – B.Sc. (Biology), Ursinus College 1963; Ph.D in History of Medicine, Johns Hopkins 1973. Appointed Associate Professor in the Hannah Chair, September 1977. Was previously Assistant Professor at Princeton University and at the University of Minnesota. Research interests – French social history of medicine in the 18th century, medical professionalization. Book – *Professionalizing Modern Medicine and Institutions in the 18th century.*

SHORTT, Samuel Edward Dole, Queen's University; born in London, Ontario. Education – B.A. (Hons.) in Political Science and History, McGill 1968; M.A. in Canadian Studies, Carleton 1969; Ph.D. in History, Queen's 1973; M.D., University of Western Ontario 1977. Appointed as Associate Professor in the Hannah Chair, July 1979. Resigned June 1984. Research interests – history of Canadian psychiatry, professionalization in 19th century medicine. Books – *The Search for an Ideal: Six Canadian Intellectuals and Their Convictions in an Age of Transition; Medicine in Canadian Socitey, Historical Perspectives* (editor); *Psychiatric Illness in Physicians.*

APPENDIX IV

Dr. Hannah's Plan for the Hannah System, 1974

GRAPHIC STRUCTURE

ASSOCIATED MEDICAL SERVICES, INCORPORATED, 1937

JASON A. HANNAH INSTITUTE

ADMINISTRATION – FINANCING – PROVIDING ITINERANT LECTURERS – ESTABLISHING PRIZES, GRANTS COOPERATION WITH CMA, OMA, & LOCAL SOCIETIES, ETC.

OTTAWA	McMASTER	QUEEN'S	TORONTO	WESTERN

UNDERGRADUATE & GRADUATE STUDIES & RESEARCH COOPERATION WITH LOCAL SOCIETIES IN PROMOTING & DISSEMINATING MEDICAL & RELATED SCIENCES HISTORY & OTHER INTERESTS

COOPERATION WITH EACH OTHER THROUGH THE INSTITUTE ESTABLISHING RELATIONS & MAINTAINING CONTACT WITH THE INSTITUTE AND WORLD-WIDE MEDICAL AND RELATED SCIENCES THROUGH UNIVERSITIES, LIBRARIES, SOCIETIES, ETC.

OTHERS	U.S.A.	GERMANY	BRITISH ISLES	GREEK & ROMAN	ARABIC & ANCIENT	CANADIAN ENGLISH FRENCH

IT IS HOPED AND EXPECTED THAT EACH UNIVERSITY WILL SPECIALIZE IN ONE AREA, AS WELL AS KNOW THE GENERAL FIELD. IT IS ESSENTIAL THAT THE PROFESSION AND PUBLIC IN GENERAL ALSO BE MADE AWARE OF OUR HISTORICAL BACKGROUND.

REFERENCES

Chapter I: Diversification

[1] Letters Patent to Associated Medical Services, Incorporated, 9 April 1937.
[2] J.A. Hannah, Diary, 25 September 1961; AMS, Board of Directors, Minutes, 11 December 1960.
[3] Ibid., 12 February 1961.
[4] Diary; letter to R.L. Bradbury, 24 September 1961.
[5] AMS, Board of Directors, Minutes, 11 June 1961.
[6] AMS, Managing Director's Report to Board of Directors, 2 June 1961.
[7] AMS, Board of Directors, Minutes, 6 May 1962.
[8] Ibid., 1 June 1962.
[9] Ibid., 2 September 1962.
[10] Ibid., 1 September 1963.
[11] S. Boyd Upper, personal communication, June 1986.
[12] V. Schatzker, oral history of Dr. J.B. Neilson, 29 March 1982, p. 200.
[13] AMS, Board of Directors, Minutes, 21 October 1962 and 10 February 1963.
[14] Ibid., 1 September 1963.
[15] Ibid., 22 December 1963.
[16] Ibid., 3 May 1964.
[17] Ibid., 6 September 1964.
[18] Ibid. and AMS, Annual Meeting, 9 May 1965.
[19] S. Boyd Upper, personal communication, June 1986.
[20] E.H. Botterell, personal communication, 16 October 1985.
[21] AMS, Board of Directors, Minutes, 29 August 1965.
[22] S. Boyd Upper, personal communication, June 1986.
[23] AMS, Board of Directors, Minutes, 6 February 1966.
[24] AMS, Board of Directors, Minutes, and Annual Meeting, 15 May 1966.

[25] S. Boyd Upper, personal communication, June 1986.
[26] AMS, Board of Directors, Minutes, 4 September 1966.
[27] D.B. Strudley, letter to Dr. J.A. Hannah, 9 September 1966.
[28] AMS, Board of Directors, Minutes, 18 December 1966.
[29] Ibid., 3 September 1967.
[30] Ibid., 17 December 1967.
[31] AMS, President and Managing Director's Report, 21 August 1968.
[32] AMS, Board of Directors, Minutes, 8 September 1968.
[33] S. Boyd Upper, personal communication, June 1986.
[34] AMS, President and Managing Director's Report, 4 December 1968.
[35] AMS, Board of Directors, Minutes, 15 December 1968.
[36] AMS, President and Managing Director's Report, 28 August 1969; AMS, Board of Directors, Minutes, 7 September 1969.
[37] Ibid., 18-19 October 1969.
[38] Ibid., 14 December 1969.
[39] J.A. Hannah, An Evaluation of AMS, Its Personnel, and Future as of 31 December, 1969, dated 7 April 1970.
[40] AMS, Board of Directors, Minutes, 12 April 1970.
[41] S. Boyd Upper, personal communication, June 1986.
[42] AMS, Board of Directors, Minutes, 7-8 August 1970.
[43] AMS, Report of the Managing Director, 1 December 1970.
[44] AMS, Board of Directors, Minutes, 13 December 1970.

Chapter II: Libraries

[1] J.A. Hannah, letter to Dr. Malcolm D.W. Low, 19 April 1968.
[2] J.A. Hannah, letter to Dr. W.C. Gibson, 19 April 1968.
[3] J.A. Hannah, letter to Dr. J.A. Corry, 22 April 1968.
[4] J.A. Hannah, letter to All Members of the AMS Board of Directors, 24 April 1968.
[5] J.A. Hannah, letter to Dr. Malcolm D.W. Low, 26 April 1968.
[6] J.A. Hannah, letter to Dr. W.C. Gibson, 3 May 1968.
[7] J.A. Hannah, letter to Dr. W.C. Gibson, 6 May 1968.
[8] AMS, Board of Directors, Minutes, 5 May 1968.

[9] AMS, President and Managing Director's Report, 21 August 1968.
[10] J.A. Hannah, memorandum to file, telephone conversation with Dr. W.C. Gibson, 16 November 1968.
[11] J.A. Hannah, letter to Dr. W.C. Gibson, 21 November 1968.
[12] J.A. Hannah, letter to All Members of the AMS Board of Directors, 31 January 1969.
[13] J.A. Hannah, Proposal Regarding the Establishment of a Province-Wide Medical Library System, Draft No. 1, 27 January 1969.
[14] AMS, Managing Director's Report, 7 September 1969.
[15] AMS, Board of Directors, Minutes, 14 December 1969.
[16] Ibid., 12 April 1970.

Chapter III: Academy of Medicine, Toronto

[1] A. Primrose, "The Faculty of Medicine," in W.J. Alexander, general editor, *The University of Toronto, 1827-1906* (Toronto: The University Library, 1906, pp. 168-179).
[2] H.B. Anderson, *Bull. Acad. Med., Toronto*, 5, 34-39 (1932).
[3] E.S. Ryerson, *Bull. Acad. Med., Toronto*, 5, 26-31 (1932).
[4] J.W. Scott, letter to Dr. J.A. Hannah, 17 February 1972.
[5] AMS, Board of Directors, Minutes, 18 October 1969.
[6] J.A. Hannah, letter to Dr. Mary C. McEwan, 5 December 1969.
[7] J.W. Scott, Outline of Course in History of Medicine for students in Art Applied to Medicine, Faculty of Medicine, University of Toronto, 1971-1972; in letter to Dr. G.A. Pengelly, 15 July 1971.
[8] Medical Society of London, Minutes, 8 March 1971.
[9] Ibid., 26 April 1971.
[10] *Bull. Hist. Med.*, 58, 565 (1984).
[11] J.A. Hannah, Memorandum to Members of the Board of Directors, AMS, 10 May 1971.
[12] W.E. Swinton, personal communication, 25 February 1985.
[13] Mary C. McEwan, letter to Dr. W.E. Swinton, 2 June 1969.
[14] W.C. Gibson, letter to Dr. J.A. Hannah, 21 May 1969.

[15] J.A. Hannah, Memorandum to Members of the Board of Directors, AMS, 18 May 1971.
[16] J.A. Hannah, The Origin of Sources of Finances, 19 May 1971.
[17] AMS, Board of Directors, Minutes, 15 May 1966.
[18] J.A. Hannah, The Jason A. Hannah Canadian Institute for Medical History, Guidelines, 25 June 1971.
[19] J.A. Hannah, letter to Dr. G.A. Pengelly, 25 June 1971.
[20] J.A. Hannah, Memorandum to all members of the Board of Directors of Associated Medical Services, Incorporated, 21 July 1971.
[21] J.W. Scott, Memorandum for discussion; Proposed Institute for the History of Medicine in the Academy Medicine, Toronto, 15 July 1971.
[22] J.A. Hannah, file, The London Medical Society Library, 13 August 1971.
[23] G.R. Paterson and M. Wildridge, personal recollection.
[24] J.A. Hannah, letter to Dr. G.A. Pengelly, 12 August 1971.
[25] J.A. Hannah, letter to Dr. G.A. Pengelly, 16 August 1971.
[26] J.W. Scott, personal communication, 29 August 1985.
[27] Minutes, Meeting between the Executive of the Toronto Academy of Medicine and AMS, 17 August 1971 (T.E. Alderwick, recorder).
[28] Minutes, Meeting between the Executive of the Toronto Academy of Medicine and AMS, 15 November 1971 (S. Boyd Upper, recorder).
[29] J.A. Hannah, memorandum to file, The Toronto Academy of Medicine, 9 November 1971.
[30] J.A. Hannah, private and confidential letter to Dr. G.A. Pengelly, President, Academy of Medicine, Toronto, 15 December 1971.
[31] Mrs. B. Edwards, To All Members of the Board of Directors of A.M.S., 26 November 1971.
[32] Report of the Managing Director to the Board of Directors of Associated Medical Services, Incorporated for the Meeting of 12 December, 1971, dated 2 December 1971.
[33] J.W. Scott, personal communication, 29 August 1985.
[34] AMS, Board of Directors, Minutes, 12 December 1971.
[35] J.A. Hannah, letter to the Executive Committee, Academy of Medicine, Toronto, 19 January 1972.

[36] J.W. Scott, letter to Dr. J.A. Hannah, 20 January 1972.
[37] G.A. Pengelly, letter to Dr. J.A. Hannah, 21 January 1972.

Chapter IV: Massey College

[1] Massey College in the University of Toronto, n.d., p.2.
[2] J.A. Hannah, letter to Dr. Robertson Davies, 15 December 1971.
[3] AMS, Board of Directors, Minutes, 12 December 1971.
[4] W.E. Swinton, personal communication, 25 February 1985.
[5] W.C. Gibson, personal communication, 19 April 1985.
[6] J.A. Hannah, Bursaries, Prizes, Fellowships, etc. for the Jason A. Hannah Institute in Medical History at Massey College, and Rules re Fellowships at the Jason Hannah Institute of Medical History, Draft No. 1, 4 January 1972.
[7] J.A. Hannah, Memorandum of Agreement, Draft No. 2, 21 December 1971.
[8] Report of the President and Managing Director to the Board of Directors for Board Meeting at Massey College, 22 January, 1972, dated 13 January 1972.
[9] S. Boyd Upper, personal communication, 6 August 1985.
[10] C.E. Friesen, letter to Dr. Jason A. Hannah, 20 January 1972.
[11] J.W. Scott, Seminars on the History of Medicine to be given at the Academy of Medicine, Toronto, 288 Bloor Street W. Dates – 19 January to 19 April 1972.
[12] J.A. Hannah, letter to Dr. Robertson Davies, 14 February 1972.
[13] Robertson Davies, letter to Dr. Jason A. Hannah, 22 March 1972.
[14] AMS, Board of Directors, Minutes, 30 April 1972.

Chapter V: An Institute and Five Chairs

[1] Report to the Board of Directors of AMS by the President and Managing Director for meeting of 16 April 1972, dated 4 April 1972.

[2] AMS, Board of Directors, Minutes, 30 April 1972.
[3] Report of the President and Managing Director to the Board of Directors of Associated Medical Services, Inc., 15 July 1972.
[4] AMS, Board of Directors, Minutes, 10 September 1972.
[5] J.J. Lussier, identical letters to Dr. F.L. Holmes, Dr. J.W. Scott, Dr. A.A. Travill, Dr. C.B. Mueller, 13 October 1972.
[6] J.A. Hannah, Memorandum of Agreement re the *Jason A. Hannah Institute for the History of Medical and Related Sciences*, 18 October 1972.
[7] J.W. Scott, letter to Dean J.J. Lussier, 24 October 1972.
[8] C.B. Mueller, *Guidelines*, Notes made at meeting of Committee of COFM, 20 October 1972.
[9] J.A. Hannah, letter to Dean J.J. Lussier, 23 October 1972.
[10] W.C. Gibson, personal communication, 19 April 1985.
[11] Report of the Special Committee appointed by the Board of Directors of Associated Medical Services (A.M.S.), 7 December 1972.
[12] J.A. Hannah, Presentation to the Premier of Ontario, The Honourable William Davis, regarding the proposed *Jason A. Hannah Institute for the Study of the History of Medicine and Related Sciences*, 5 October 1972.
[13] F.N.L. Poynter, letter to Dr. J.A. Hannah, 17 October 1972; Hannah, letter to Poynter, 19 October 1972; Poynter, Letter to Hannah, 26 October 1972; Hannah, letter to Poynter, 30 October 1972.
[14] J.A. Hannah, file, Luncheon, 20 October 1972.
[15] J.A. Hannah, letter to the Hon. William Davis, Premier of Ontario (n.d., but other evidence seems to suggest 2 November 1972).
[16] J.A. Hannah, letter to Drs. J.J. Lussier, J.W. Scott, F.L. Holmes, A.A. Travill, C.S. [*sic*] Mueller, 7 November 1972.
[17] F.L. Holmes, personal communication, 14 May 1985.
[18] J.A. Hannah, letter to Dr. F.L. Holmes, 16 November 1972.
[19] J.A. Hannah, letter to the Deans of the Medical Faculties in All Universities of Ontario, 27 November 1972.
[20] J.A. Hannah, letter to Dr. Robertson Davies, 11 February 1972.
[21] J.R. Evans, letter to Dr. J.A. Hannah, 30 November 1972.
[22] D. Bocking, letter to Dr. J.A. Hannah, 2 January 1973.

[23] J.A. Hannah, memorandum of a meeting held at 3.00 p.m. at the Toronto General Hospital on March 1, 1973.
[24] J.A. Hannah, Proposed Agreement with Each of the Five Universities in Ontario which include Medical Faculties, namely Queen's, Toronto, McMaster, Western and Ontario, Draft No. 1, 24 April 1973.
[25] J.A. Hannah, letter to Dr. John R. Evans, Dr. Roger Guindon, Dr. D. Carlton Williams, Dr. A.N. Bourns, Dr. John Deutsch, 13 July 1973.
[26] J.A. Hannah, letter to Dr. D. Bocking, 7 August 1973.
[27] J.A. Hannah, letter to the Heads of all the Universities in Ontario with Medical Faculties, 17 August 1973.
[28] AMS, Board of Directors, Minutes, 15 August 1973.
[29] J.D. Hamilton, letter and Proposed Draft No. 3 to Dr. J.A. Hannah, 13 September 1973.
[30] An Agreement made between Associated Medical Services, Incorporated and Queen's University, Ottawa University, McMaster University, University of Western Ontario, and the University of Toronto for the purpose of establishing "The Jason A. Hannah Chair in the History of Medical and Related Sciences", Draft No. 4, 2 October 1973.
[31] J.A. Hannah, letter to Ms. Sydney Dymond, 3 May 1973; Hannah, letter to M.C. Wills, 3 May 1973.
[32] P.M.J. Potter, letter to Dr. J.A. Hannah, n.d., received 27 March 1973.
[33] J.A. Hannah, letter to David Esplin, 2 February 1973.
[34] J.A. Hannah, file, Conversation with Mr. Esplin in regard to the London Medical Society Library, 12 February 1973.
[35] G.E. Barr, Memorandum of a Meeting in the afternoon of 31 January 1973 at the home of Dr. J.A. Hannah, 5 February 1973.
[36] G.E. Barr, Memorandum of Agreement between Associated Medical Services, Incorporated and the Board of Governors of the University of Toronto, Draft No. 1 (27 April 1973); Draft No. 2 (7 May 1973); Draft No. 3 (10 May 1973).
[37] G.E. Barr, Memorandum to Dr. J.A. Hannah re Meeting with Mr. D.G. Esplin, 27 April 1973.
[38] T.C. Hunt, letter to Dr. J.A. Hannah, 3 April 1973.

[39] Memorandum of Agreement between Associated Medical Services, Incorporated and the Governing Council of the University of Toronto, 6 and 12 June 1973.
[40] AMS, Board of Directors, Minutes, 30 May 1973.
[41] J.D. Hilton, letter to Dr. J.A. Hannah, 4 December 1972; S.B. Upper, letter to Mr. Robin Scott, 10 January 1973.
[42] R. Scott, letter to Dr. B. Upper, 25 January 1973.
[43] J.A. Hannah, file, Discussion with Dr. Urquhart, Friday, 9 February 1973, dated 12 February 1973.
[44] J.A. Hannah, letter to Dr. Douglas Wright, 14 September 1973.
[45] J.A. Hannah, letter to Dr. L.G. Stevenson, 7 June 1973.
[46] L.G. Stevenson, letter to Dr. J.A. Hannah, 13 June 1973.
[47] L.G. Stevenson, letter to Dr. J.A. Hannah, 28 June 1973.
[48] J.A. Hannah, letter to Dr. L.G. Stevenson, 5 July 1973.
[49] J.A. Hannah, letter to Dr. W.C. Gibson, 10 August 1973.

Chapter VI: Organization of the Hannah System

[1] J.A. Hannah, letters to Dr. W.C. Gibson, 21 September and 17 October 1972.
[2] J.A. Hannah, letter to Dr. H.G. Kelly, 16 January 1974.
[3] J.A. Hannah, letter to Dr. W.C. Gibson, 14 July 1974.
[4] W.E. Swinton, personal communication, 26 August 1985.
[5] Interim Report Number (2) Two of the Managing Director to Directors of Associated Medical Services, n.d. (stamped, received 19 November 1973).
[6] Robertson Davies, letter to Dr. J.A. Hannah, 1 November 1973.
[7] J.A. Hannah, letter to Dr. Robertson Davies, 9 November 1973.
[8] Robertson Davies, letter to Dr. J.A. Hannah, 12 November 1973.
[9] Robertson Davies, letter to Dr. J.A. Hannah, 26 November 1973.
[10] Draft Memorandum of Agreement between Associated Medical Services, Incorporated, and Massey College, University of Toronto, 19 November 1973.

[11] AMS, Board of Directors, Minutes, 13 December 1973.
[12] Report of the President and Managing Director for the meeting of the Board of Directors, AMS, 13 December 1973.
[13] G.R. Paterson, personal recollections of interview by Dr. J.A. Hannah on 23 April 1974.
[14] W.E. Swinton, personal conversation, 26 August 1985.
[15] AMS, Board of Directors, Minutes, 18 September 1974.
[16] J.A. Hannah, letter to Mr. Colin Friesen, 25 July 1974.
[17] AMS, Board of Directors, Minutes, 9 January 1975.
[18] J.A. Hannah, Notice of Motion for 38th Annual General Meeting for the year ending December 31, 1974, n.d.
[19] J.A. Hannah, (?) An Agreement Made between Associated Medical Services, Incorporated, and Queen's University, Ottawa University, McMaster University, University of Toronto and University of Western Ontario for the purpose of establishing the "Jason A. Hannah Chair in the History of Medical Related Sciences", Draft No. 4, 2 October 1973.
[20] J.J. Deutsch, Walter Little, and J.B. Neilson, Report to the Board of Directors, AMS, 17 July 1975.
[21] AMS, Board of Directors, Minutes, 17 July 1975.
[22] Ibid., 6 February 1975.
[23] G.R. Paterson, Report on Libraries, September 1975.
[24] AMS, Board of Directors, Minutes, 22 September 1975.
[25] G.R. Paterson, Report on the History Videotape Project, September 1975.
[26] G.R. Paterson, Report on the Sculpture of Dr. Hannah and a Proposal with Respect to It, 18 September 1975.
[27] Royal Society of Canada, *Calendar*, 1977-1978.
[28] R. Brewerton, letter to Dr. J.A. Hannah, 24 October 1975.
[29] AMS, Board of Directors, Minutes, 9 December 1975.
[30] Ibid., 10 March 1976.
[31] J.B. Neilson, Report of a Committee Appointed to Consider the Status of A.M.S. as a Tax Exempt Organization, n.d.
[32] AMS, Board of Directors, Minutes, 25 March 1976.
[33] Ibid., 24 April 1976.
[34] Minutes, Members of AMS, 24 April 1976.
[35] Report of the President to the Annual Meeting for 1975 (39th.) of the Members of the Associated Medical Services, Incorporated, 24 April 1976.

[36] AMS, Board of Directors, Minutes, second meeting, 24 April 1976.
[37] AMS, Executive Committee, Minutes, 27 May 1976.
[38] AMS, Board of Directors, Minutes, 21 June 1976.
[39] G.R. Paterson, Report of the Executive Director, Hannah Institute for the History of Medical and Related Sciences, 30 April 1976.
[40] AMS, Board of Directors, Minutes, 15 July 1976.
[41] Ibid., 12 October 1976.
[42] J.B. Neilson and G.R. Paterson, Report, Associated Medical Services, Incorporated; Hannah Institute for the History of Medicine, 1972-1978; ibid., 1978-1980; ibid., 1980-1982.

Chapter VII: Accomplishments

[1] G.R. Paterson, Procedure for a Five-Year Review of a Hannah Chair for the History of Medical and Related Sciences, 7 February 1977.
[2] See Chapter III.
[3] AMS, Board of Directors, Minutes, 8 December 1976.
[4] G.R. Paterson, Report on Libraries, September 1975; J.B. Neilson, letters to Deans T.J. Boag, R.B. Holmes, M. Hollenberg, G.D. Hurteau, J.F. Mustard, 4 April 1979.
[5] E.J. Freeman, Library Provision for the History of Medicine, 14 July 1978; J.B. Neilson, letter to Members of the Hannah Institute Advisory Council, 4 April 1979.
[6] G.R. Paterson, Schuman Reference Library as Working Library at the University of Ottawa, February 1977; AMS, Board of Directors, Minutes, 9 March 1977; G.R. Paterson, Schuman Reference Library, May 1977.
[7] G.R. Paterson, Report of the Executive Director, Hannah Institute for the History of Medical and Related Sciences, April 1976.
[8] AMS, Board of Directors, Minutes, 15 June 1977.
[9] Ibid., 24 April 1976.
[10] AMS, Executive Committee, Minutes, 24 April 1976; Board of Directors, Minutes, 27 May 1976.

[11] Office of Library Coordination, Council of Ontario Universities, Unicat/Telecat, October 1975; G.R. Paterson, Accessibility to Library Resources, in Report, Associated Medical Services, Inc. and Hannah Institute for the History of Medicine, 1972-1978, pp. 13-14.

[12] Minutes of the Meeting between the Hannah Institute and the Office of Library Coordination, Council of Ontario Universities, 19 February 1976.

[13] Office of Library Coordination, *Medicat*, a Proposal for the Establishment of a Data Base of Records for Medical Research Resources, 2 April 1976.

[14] R.E. Stierwalt, *Medicat, a Three Year Project*, 1976.

[15] G.R. Paterson, *Medicat*, a Proposal by Associated Medical Services, Inc. and the Hannah Institute for the History of Medical and Related Sciences, June 1977.

[16] W. Ready and M. Kraav, *Proposal for a Pilot Project to Demonstrate the Feasibility of Establishing a Data Base of Records for Medical Research Resources*, December 1977.

[17] M. Kraav, E.E. Minett, R.E. Stierwalt, and G.R. Paterson, Evaluation Report on *Medicat*, March 1980.

[18] G.R. Paterson, ed., *Conference on the Future of Medicat*, 21 January 1981; includes four papers: (i) G.R. Paterson, "Associated Medical Services, Inc., the Hannah Institute and Medicat". (ii) G.R. Hill, "Medicat: Looking Forward, Looking Back". (iii) B.H. Robinow, "The Pilot Project Medicat at the Health Sciences Library, McMaster University". (iv) M. Kraav, "Machine Readable Files – Toys or Tools?"

[19] H. Velazquez, letter to Dr. G.R. Paterson, 23 October 1984.

[20] M. Dunn with M. Baldwin, ed., *A Directory of Medical Archives in Ontario* (Toronto: Hannah Institute, 1983).

[21] C. Morin, Indexes to *A Directory of Medical Archives in Ontario* (Toronto: Hannah Institute, 1984).

[22] W.E. Swinton, Physicians in Literature, eight articles published in *Can. Med. Assoc. J.* between 8 November 1975 and 20 March 1976; Physician Contributions to Non-Medical Sciences, eight articles published in *Can. Med. Assoc. J.* between 18 September 1976 and 8 January 1977; Physicians as Explorers, eight articles published in *Can. Med. Assoc. J.* between 3 September

and 17 December 1977; and seven miscellaneous articles published in *Can. Med. Assoc. J.* between 8 November 1980 and 1 December 1981.

[23] C.G. Roland, ed., *Sir William Osler 1849-1919: A Selection for Medical Students* (Toronto: Hannah Institute, 1982).

[24] French translation available early 1987.

[25] J.B. Neilson and G.R. Paterson, Report, Associated Medical Services, Inc. and Hannah Institute for the History of Medicine, 1972-1978, pp. 21, 23.

[26] Canadian Medical Archives, A selection of archival material relating to the history of medicine in Canada/Archives médicales du Canada, L'histoire de la médecine au Canada à travers les documents d'archives, Ottawa, June 1980.

[27] See note 7 above.

[28] C.G. Roland, ed., *Health, Disease and Medicine: Essays in Canadian History* (Toronto: Hannah Institute, 1984).

[29] AMS, Board of Directors, Minutes, 22 September 1975.

[30] G.R. Paterson, Report on the Sculpture of Dr. Hannah and a Proposal with Respect to It, 18 September 1975.

[31] AMS, Board of Directors, Minutes, 21 June 1976.

[32] H. Ellenberger, *The Discovery of the Unconscious: The History and Evolution of Dynamic Psychiatry* (New York: Basic Books, 1970).

[33] Baltimore: Johns Hopkins Press, 1974.

[34] Montreal: McGill-Queen's University Press, 1978.

[35] Toronto: McClelland and Stewart, 1982.

[36] Downsview, Ont.: National Institute on Mental Retardation, 1982.

[37] Guelph: The Authors, 1976.

[38] Toronto: McClelland and Stewart, 1984.

[39] W.B. Spaulding, Report of the AMS Review Committee, December, 1985.

[40] AMS, Board of Directors, Minutes, 7 January 1986.

[41] Hannah Institute, Advisory Council, Minutes, 13 March 1986.

[42] AMS, Board of Directors, Minutes, 9 April 1986.

[43] AMS, Report of the Grants Committee, 13-14 February 1986.

[44] AMS, Board of Directors, Minutes, June 1986.

INDEX